Volume 3

Exam Oriented

Anatomy
Questions and Answers

Second Edition

❑ **Head**   ❑ **Neck**   ❑ **Face**

Shoukat N Kazi MS (Anatomy), DTCD, BSc, LLB

Principal, Dr Tasgaonkar Medical College and
Research Centre, Karjat, Maharashtra
Ex-Principal, Prasad Institute of Medical Sciences
Banthara, Lucknow (UP)
Ex-Professor
Rajshree Medical Research Institute, Bareilly
SRM Medical College Hospital and Research Centre, Potheri, Chennai
Chennai Medical College Hospital and Research Centre, Trichy
Dr DY Patil Medical College, Pimpri, Maharashtra
Dr DY Patil Vidyapeeth (Deemed to be University), Pimpri, Pune

CBS

CBS Publishers & Distributors Pvt Ltd

New Delhi • Bengaluru • Chennai • Kochi • Kolkata • Mumbai
Hyderabad • Jharkhand • Nagpur • Patna • Pune • Uttarakhand

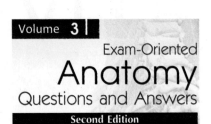

Volume **3**

Exam-Oriented

Anatomy

Questions and Answers

Second Edition

ISBN: 978-93-90046-12-6

Copyright © Author and Publisher

Second Edition: 2021

First Edition: 2005

Published by Satish Kumar Jain and produced by Varun Jain for

CBS Publishers & Distributors Pvt Ltd

4819/XI Prahlad Street, 24 Ansari Road, Daryaganj, New Delhi 110 002, India.

Ph: 011-23289259, 23266861, 23266867 Fax: 011-23243014   Website: www.cbspd.com
e-mail: delhi@cbspd.com; cbspubs@airtelmail.in

Corporate Office: 204 FIE, Industrial Area, Patparganj, Delhi 110 092

Ph: 011-4934 4934   Fax: 011-4934 4935   e-mail: publishing@cbspd.com;publicity@cbspd.com

Branches

• **Bengaluru:** Seema House 2975, 17th Cross, K.R. Road, Banasankari 2nd Stage, Bengaluru 560 070, Karnataka

Ph: +91-80-26771678/79   Fax: +91-80-26771680   e-mail: bangalore@cbspd.com

• **Chennai:** 7, Subbaraya Street, Shenoy Nagar, Chennai 600 030, Tamil Nadu

Ph: +91-44-26260666, 26208620   Fax: +91-44-42032115   e-mail: chennai@cbspd.com

• **Kochi:** 42/1325, 1326, Power House Road, Opp. KSEB, Power House, Ernakulam 682018, Kochi, Kerala

Ph: +91-484-4059061-65   Fax: +91-484-4059065   e-mail: kochi@cbspd.com

• **Kolkata:** No. 6/B, Ground Floor, Rameswar Shaw Road, Kolkata 700014 (West Bengal), India

Ph: +91-33-2289-1126, 2289-1127, 2289-1128   e-mail: kolkata@cbspd.com

• **Mumbai:** PWD Shed, Gala No. 25/26, Ramchandra Bhatt Marg, Next to JJ Hospital, Gate No. 2 Opp. Union Bank of India, Noorbaug, Mumbai 400009, Maharashtra, India

Ph: +91-22-24902340/41/42   Fax: +91-22-24902342   e-mail: mumbai@cbspd.com

Representives

• **Hyderabad**	0-9885175004	• **Jharkhand**	0-9811541605	• **Nagpur**	0-9421945513
• **Patna**	0-9334159340	• **Pune**	0-9623451994	• **Uttarakhand**	0-9716462459

Printed at Nutech Print Services, Faridabad, India

To
_____

My parents
Late Haji Nizamsaheb K Kazi
Late Hajjan Mrs Jainnabbi N Kazi

My wife Kamartaj

For tolerating my preoccupation

And my daughter Sadiya

For understanding me
And

Students

For appreciating my way of teaching and
providing me a continuous stimulus to write the book

Foreword to the Second Edition

Prof SN Kazi's *Exam-Oriented Anatomy,* 2nd edition, is going to compete with all other books on the subject available in the market. It is not only simple, digestible and very attractive but also exceptionally informative and rich into the extent that even heavy textbooks do not carry so much information. I have great respect for him, for his dedication and lust for writing book. I wish him all the best.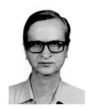

Dr Nafis Ahmad Faruqi
Professor
Department of Anatomy
Jawaharlal Nehru Medical College
Aligarh Muslim University, Aligarh, UP
India

Foreword to the First Edition

Prof SN Kazi's book is intended to help medical students rapidly master complex intricacies of human anatomy that is essential to clinical care.

This book was written to fulfill the need for a brief, but readable, summary of the relevant anatomy, with succinct notes on applied anatomy wherever indicated. It addresses the diverse and mounting need of medical students preparing for professional examinations. The text will not only enhance the knowledge to an extent sufficient to satisfy the examiners but will also equip the readers with the necessary understanding of applied anatomy for future practice. A recurring problem in medical education is the common inability of the students to relate the large body of factual knowledge to practical application in their future clinical training. A commendable endeavour has been made by Prof Kazi to bridge the gap between rote anatomy and clinical relevance. The mnemonics and humour in this book do not intend any disrespect for anyone, rather they are employed as an educational device, as it is well known that the best memory techniques involve the use of ridiculous association. Stephen Goldberg in his unique book titled "Clinical Neuroanatomy Made Ridiculous Simple" has already demonstrated their efficacy superbly.

Books	LAQs	SAQs	SNs	Keywords	Line diagrams	Tables
Above diaphragm	93	20	156	91	254	47
Below diaphragm	47	38	125	49	254	47

This book is not designed to replace standard reference textbooks, but rather is to be read as a companion text before appearing in an examination. This will enable the student to gain an overall perspective of essential anatomy.

My best wishes for the success of this endeavour which merits appreciation.

Prof (Dr) Mahdi Hasan
MBBS, MS (Hons.), FICS, FAMS, PhD,DSc, FNA
Professor Emeritus
INSA Senior Scientist, Department of Anatomy
Chhatrapati Shahuji Maharaj Medical
University (King George's Medical University)
Lucknow, UP (India)

Formerly
Professor and Chairman, Department of Anatomy and
Founder Director
Interdisciplinary Brain Research Center
Dean, Principal and Chief Medical Superintendent Jawaharlal Nehru Medical College, Aligarh
Muslim University, Aligarh, UP (India)

Foreword to the First Edition

All the medical colleges in the state of Maharashtra were affiliated to eight different conventional universities in the state up to 1997. After the establishment of Maharashtra University of Health Sciences in the state in 1998, all of them were affiliated to this single state level university. Previously syllabi and pattern of examination were different but the new pattern (1 + 1½ + 2 years) of curriculum recommended by the Medical Council of India while the conventional universities were following the old (1½ + 1½ + 1½ years) pattern. First time in the examination, LAQ, SAQ and MCQ patterns were introduced by MUHS. On the background of the reduced duration for both students (for learning) and teachers (for teaching) of I MBBS, there was a need for examination-oriented revision book.

It is really a great pleasure for me to introduce this book on human anatomy written by one of my ex-colleagues, Dr SN Kazi. I have gone through the manuscript of this book which adequately covers the subject. Usually students have to purchase separate books for anatomy, histology, embryology, general anatomy, genetics, etc. Dr. Kazi has tried to cover all these branches in simple language with the help of computerized line diagrams. It is designed to meet the need of the undergraduate exam going students. Most of the information are given in tabular forms, easy to compare and remember and clinical applications of the subject have been touched adequately.

The book speaks the long experience of the author in the subject and will minimize the stress and strain of a medical student during pre-examination period. I congratulate the author for this venture and wish the book great success.

Shingare PHMS
Professor and Head
Department of Anatomy
Grant Medical College and
Sir J J Group of Hospitals
Byculla, Mumbai
Director of Medical Education and Research,
Maharashtra
Ex-Dean, Faculty of Medicine, North Maharashtra University
Ex-Controller of Exam, MUHS, Nashik
Ex-Chairman, BoS Preclinical, MUHS, Nashik
Member of BoS Preclinical Faculty of
Medicine and Faculty of Dentistry, MUHS
Ex-Vice Dean UG, Grant Medical College, Mumbai
Ex-Vice Dean PG, Grant Medical College, Mumbai

Preface to the Second Edition

I am very much excited to present the 2nd edition. Initially I thought it will not take much time, but as I started preparing for the 2nd edition, new ideas start clouding in my mind and the ideas went on increasing.

In the last 15 years, I received many feedbacks about inadequate answers, too much simplicity of the text, too many mnemonics. I reviewed various books on memory techniques and came with various ideas. I am happy to share the experiences of teaching in different parts of country. In north and central part of India, the main barrier is writing skills. The students are either from Hindi medium or language of regional medium. The immediate challenges after joining medical course is communication and managing vast syllabus.

I have made an attempt to write in very simple language. In the first reading only, the student should be able to understand the contents. I have used the symbols for most of the words. It is rightly said "A picture is equal to thousands of sentences. A cartoon is worth of thousands of pictures". **Visual memory** works better for the pictures than the texts. **Colours** have deep impact than black and white. Kinesthetics have far more effect as compared to auditory and visual. Combined effects of auditory, visual and kinesthetic have profound effect on memory.

A sincere attempt is made not only to give the contents of the subject, but also to make the student remember the subject by using various techniques. The author has attended the lectures of the many anatomists, studied the delivery of lectures. He has picked up the concepts and presented in the form of book. The book is collections of techniques used by well-known anatomists of India.

Memory Technique

1. Association memory
    A. Day-to-day examples: City bus for ascending and descending tracts.
    B. Association of letters
        a. After "C" to recollect the nuclei of cerebellum.
        b. ABCD for the normal constrictions of oesophagus
        c. Ruffini for red and Krause for cold receptor. This was contributed by **Dr Nandedkar madam**, a senior anatomist from AFMC.
    C. Association of digit 10 for 4 important information of oesophagus.
        a. Length of oesophagus
        b. Constrictions of oesophagus
        c. Opening in diaphragm at 10th thoracic vertebra
        d. First mark on the paediatric Ryles tube.
2. Use of one's hand for representation of various structures and relations
    A. Branches of splenic artery
    B. Intermuscular spaces
    C. Use of 3 fingers for transpyloric plane at lower 1st lumbar
    D. Branches of basilar artery
    E. Tributaries of coronary sinus
3. Framing the rules for registration of information
    A. Rule of alternate framed by honorable late Padmashree Dr Mahdi Hasan to
        a. Recollect the

        I. Paired and unpaired branches of abdominal aorta

        II. Peritoneal and retroperitoneal structures.

    b. Dropping the alternate letters to recollect the names of extrapyramidal tracts.

  B. Use of jiggle "Carotico parotico Tonsilii Tympani" to complete the distribution of glossopharyngeal nerve. This is contributed by famous anatomist and surgeon Dr Kadasne, author of many textbooks.

  C. Use of fingers to differentiate to walls of artery and vein. This is contributed by Dr Krishna Garg madam, editor of world famous textbook *BD Chaurasia's Human Anatomy*.

4. Link technique

5. Meaning of words

  A. Dura—hard, durable   B. Dia—in between

6. Peg technique Mnemonic—Laila Loves Majnu for the branches of lateral cord of brachial plexus.

7. Simile: Course of hepatic artery represented by badly driven nail. Referred from Surgical Synopsis.

8. Picture mnemonic to represent Cri du chat syndrome.

9. Stories

  A. A girl from South and boy from Chandigarh had friendship in Jaipur. They got married in Jaipur but marriage could not survive because of different culture and food habit. They got divorced. Boy went back to Chandigarh and got married in own community. This story is appealing for origin, course and distribution of accessory nerve. The story was fabricated by Dr Aruna Mukherjee, a well-known anatomist.

  B. A story of water pipe for the course of internal pudendal artery.

10. Text in simple English.

11. Things added with religious sentiments: Dr Mysorekaraneminent, Professor of AFMC, used to teach functions of thalamus by giving simile of thalamus to God Nandi and cerebrum with Lord Mahadev.

12. The concept of mind mapping, introduced by Tony Buzan, is used to depict the branches of brachial plexus.

13. Use of celebrities

  A. Mary Kom—action of serratus anterior

  B. Ajay Devgn for overriding of horse to make understand the features of Fallot's tetralogy.

14. Use of key **advertisements** as the keywords—PRO V for features of Fallot's tetralogy.

15. Use of airplane and navies for reminding suprascapular artery and nerve, above and below the suprascapular ligament.

16. Use of pictures of anatomy students whose passion is body building. A photo of Wasim Khan is used to display the actions of sternal and clavicular head of pectoralis major.

17. Fruit of pine tree to show pineal body.

18. Use of symbols and pictures of muscles to boost the memory.

It was a feedback from the passed-out students that there is mismatch between what is taught in applied anatomy in the first year and what is expected in clinical posting. To fill up the gap, the author has reviewed the applied anatomy from physician, general surgeon, ENT surgeon, ophthalmologist, orthopaedic surgeon, and geneticist. The author has reviewed various regions from senior anatomists.

All the feedback has been meticulously rectified.

Separate boxes are introduced for the understanding of the subject and for memorization.

Shoukat N Kazi

Acknowledgements to the Second Edition

I recollect the days, when I determined to write for the second edition. I thought of getting all the books of anatomy that are freely available and accessible. I collected books from all the old book bazar in Delhi, Mumbai, Pune, Pimpri, Lucknow, Ahmedabad, Rajkot. I am very much thankful to Dr TC Singel, Professor, Department of Anatomy, Zydus Medical College, who took me to various old bookstores in Ahmedabad and made them available. He also lent me the library books. It was a great help. I could get the books which are not available in any of the college library. I am very much grateful to him.

I cannot afford to forget the continuous encouragement given by Mr Bhagwan Yadav, Chairman, Managing Director, Prasad Institute of Medical Sciences, Lucknow.

Scanning of the book was done by our office staff, namely Prajakta, Rhutuja. I am thankful to them. I need to mention the name of Mr Rehan Ansari, (HR, Prasad Institute of Medical Sciences, Lucknow) who got the books scanned in a very short time.

There were vital technical issues, because of which I was handicapped. The problems were resolved by my nephew, Mr Wahab Kabir Kazi. I am very much thankful to him.

The basic suggestions of diagrams were made by a corel artist Mr Sanjay, CBS Publishers & Distributors. I am thankful to him.

I am really lucky to have the contributions from many professors.

To start with, Mrs Jasmine Naik drew some of the diagrams in corel draw but because of her child's health she could not continue. The work was continued by Mrs Zeenat Shaikh. She really put her heart in diagrams. She learnt all the intricacies of anatomy subject and gave her 100% to make the diagrams right. She is very much concerned for the success of the book.

The repeated editing of the text and layout of diagrams, sequencing of questions, was done untiringly by Miss Parveen Shaikh and Mrs Jyoti Dhage. In addition to editing, Miss Parveen Shaikh has kept an eye on all the activities and coordinated in a very efficient way. They are the backbones of the book, without their help, the quality of the book was not possible. I am really blessed to have the staff, namely Miss Parveen Shaikh, Mrs. Jyoti Dhage and Mrs Zeenat Shaikh. Mrs Maya Bhujbal, and Mr Uday Jadiye, who have helped in minute layout of the book.

I am indebted for the help my brother Mr Kabir Kazi has extended to me. He has helped me in organizing guest lectures, workshops and made me tension free to write the book. It was a continuous support to me.

The continuous inspiration and motivation was given by my brothers Mr Shikandar, Allabaksh and Najir Kazi.

The technical support was given by Mr YN Arjuna Senior Vice-President—Publishing, Editorial and Publicity, and his team. He has understood me and helped without any hesitation.

The real financial help was extended by Mr Satish Kumar Jain, CMD, CBS Publishers & Distributors. His help was stress bursting to me. The quality of the book has reached only because of his timely help, and the patience he has shown to me. We have very good bonding for so many years.

I am really thankful from the bottom of my heart to Mr Varun Jain, Director, who is dynamic in implementing various technology in the books. The animation of neuroanatomy and upper limb and abdomen is being introduced, only because of his initiation. I owe him a lot.

The real tolerance and patience were given by my better half Mrs Kamartaj and my daughter Miss Sadiya. I did not give any time and attention to family activities. I appreciate their understanding.

Special Thanks

I am extending my sincere and special thanks to the following persons, without whom the book would not have been completed.

- **Dr PH Shingare,** Professor and Head, Department of Anatomy, Grant Medical College, Mumbai, has meticulously corrected the text and has given solutions to diagrams. He has tolerated my disturbance at odd hours in his busy schedule.
- **Dr (Mrs) Kanaklata Iyer,** Professor of Anatomy at Somaiya Medical College, Sion, Mumbai, has really given a breakthrough to the problems of diagrams. She has helped out rightly by sparing her valuable time through her busy schedule by taking keen interest. She has contributed diagrams of gross anatomy of abdomen, inferior extremity and general embryology.
- **Dr Savgaonkar,** Professor of Anatomy at BJ Medical College, Pune, has drawn histology diagrams of abdomen section. He being my close friend, understood the difficulties and offered his help by completing the diagrams in very short time.
- **Dr Anjali Dhamangaonkar,** Associate Professor, in Anatomy at GS Medical College, Mumbai, has contributed to the general embryology diagrams. It was very difficult for her to give some time. But her desire to help me has solved the problems.
- **Dr Manvikar Purushottam Rao,** Lecturer in Anatomy at Dr DY Patil Medical College, Pimpri, has drawn some of the diagrams of general histology. He is the main push for animation work.
- **Dr Kadasne DK,** the author of *Kadasne's Textbook of Anatomy (Clinically-oriented),* has allowed me to use some of the diagrams from his book.
- **Dr Umarji,** Professor and Head, Department of Anatomy, Krishna Institute of Medical Sciences, Karad, has drawn a few diagrams of general anatomy.

Shoukat N Kazi

Contributors

Arudyuti Chowdhury MS, DGO

Associate Professor, SRM Medical College, He was my roommate at SRM Medical College, Chennai. Dr Arudyuti Chowdhury is constant motivators. He has helped me in all the activities. His word of suggestion is important for me.

Ashok Kumar Rawat MS (Ortho)

Assistant Professor, Department of Orthopedics, Associate Professor, Prasad Institute of Medical Sciences, Lucknow.

He has helped in giving fine touch of applied aspects of joint.

Gangane

Professor and Head, Department of Anatomy, Medical College, Navi Mumbai. Thank you very much for finding time for approving the contents.

Jyoti Kulkarni

Professor in Anatomy in Nepal
She has gone meticulously in all the texts and diagrams of books and given valuable suggestions. The quality of the book is definitely improved because of her suggestions. I am very much obliged and thankful for her help.

Manvikar

Professor and Head, Department of Anatomy, Padmashree, Dr DY Patil Medical College, Pimpri, Pune. Thanks very much for giving genetic inputs.

MC Srivastav

Medical Superintendent and Associate Professor of Medicine, Prasad Institute of Medical Sciences, Lucknow. He is kind enough to add EKG changes in blockage of coronary arteries.

Murugan Kutty Gopalan

BSc, MBBS, DMA (USA)

Head, Departments of Medical Illustrations, Digital Health, Clinical Skills Simulation Center and Telemedicine, Amrita Institute of Medical Sciences and Research Center, Kerala, India. He is involved in the **Simulation-Based Medical Education** in giving training in various clinical skills. He is intensely working on introducing new generation **Medical Haptics**, **Robotic Surgery**, **Cardiac-Neuro-Ortho interventional Simulaids** for the super-specialty branches in Medicine and Surgery. He has won several regional, national and international awards for his innovative illustrative works.

All histology diagrams of 2nd edition are fabricated by Dr Gopalan. Apart from contributions to the book, he is my very close friend, whose door I can knock for any help any moment. I am heavenly blessed to have a friend like Dr Gopalan.

He is courageously fighting his health issue like a warrior. I know him since last 15 years. He is very much energetic. The energy and enthusiasm have increased many folds after he met his health issue. I think adverse situations boost his energy. I do not know from where he gets energy to do such activities. I pray God to give him long healthy life.

Nayana Karodpati

Professor (ENT, DYPMC), Pimpri, Pune
She edited the text and added the topics which are of clinical importance. Hearty thanks for the help.

P Vatsalaswamy MD

Director of DYPMC, Pimpri, Pune
In spite of her busy administrative activities and family commitments, she could spare time and could help me. I am very much obliged.
She has reviewed superior extremity. She has gone in details of each word of text and given the feedback.

Salamat Khan

Professor of Surgery, Prasad Institute of Medical Sciences, Lucknow. Dr Salamat Khan has voluntarily helped me in reviewing applied anatomy of limbs, abdomen, head, neck, face, thorax, and brain. He has gone word to word and gave the suggestions. I salute him for his help.

Sunita Nayak

Assistant Professor
All India Institute of Medical Sciences, Patna

Ubaidur Rehman

Medical Superintendent, Prasad Institute of Medical Sciences, Lucknow. He has helped in updating ophthalmology chapters. I was lucky to be associate with him.

Vaishali Bharambe MD, PhD

Ex-professor, DY Patil Medical College, Pimpri, Pune
Presently she is working as a Professor and Head, Symbiosis Medical College, Pune. She was very much busy in preparation of PhD. In spite of her hectic schedule, she could review the diagrams of lower limb. I owe her.

Vinod Kathju

Former additional Principal, Dr SN Medical College, Jodhpur
I am very much thankful for his kind guidance and contribution

Contents

Head, Neck and Face

Head, Neck and Face

Attention Please

All the text in boxes are not to be written in the examination.

All the shapes of muscles are required not to be drawn in the examination.

The shape of the muscles is drawn only to memorize the words. It may
• Signify the meaning of the word.
• Match the shape of the muscles in the body.

All the cartoons are drawn to make the subject to be memorized. They may not have any role in the subject. They are not supposed to be drawn while writing the answers of the question.

Introduction and Osteology

SN-1   Bones of the skull

The skull consists of cranium with mandible. The bones of the skull are classified as

1. Paired, and

2. Unpaired.

1. *Paired:* These are one on each side.

Paired bones of skull

Box 1.1

They can be recollected by a sentence. 🔑

<u>N</u>ow <u>Z</u>ee <u>T</u>V <u>P</u>rogramme <u>M</u>akes <u>I</u>ndian <u>P</u>eople <u>L</u>augh

<u>N</u>asal,

<u>Z</u>ygomatic,

<u>T</u>emporal,

<u>P</u>arietal,

<u>M</u>axilla,

<u>I</u>nferior nasal concha,

<u>P</u>alatine, and

<u>L</u>acrimal.

---

2. *Unpaired:* They are situated in the midline.

Unpaired bones of skull

Box 1.2

- To recollect the bones, imagine interior of the base of the skull.
- Visualise, that you are sliding your finger from anterior to posterior in the midline.
- It slides on frontal, ethmoid, sphenoid and occipital bone.
- Now slide the finger on the exterior of base of the skull.
- The finger slides on occipital, sphenoid, vomer and mandible.
- Vomer is situated between the two choanae.

All unpaired bones are summarized as
- Frontal,
- Ethmoid,
- Sphenoid,
- Occipital,
- Vomer, and
- Mandible.

SN-2   Pterion

Pterion (Gr. *Pteryx*—wing)
1. It is **H**-shaped suture presents on the lateral side of the skull.
2. **Formation:** It is formed by four bones.
   A. Frontal,
   B. Parietal,
   C. Sphenoid, and
   D. Temporal.

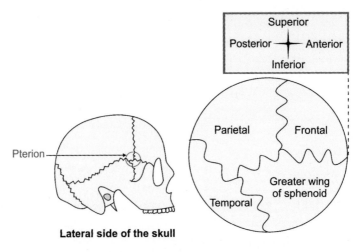

Lateral side of the skull

Fig. 1.1: Norma lateralis showing pterion

3. **Situation:** It is situated 4 cm above the midpoint of zygomatic arch and 2.5 cm behind the frontozygomatic suture.
4. **Relations:** Structures deep to pterion.
   A. Middle meningeal vessels.
   B. Stem of lateral sulcus of cerebral hemisphere (Sylvian point).

5. **Applied anatomy**
   ➤ Fracture of the pterion can be life-threatening because it overlies the anterior branches of the middle meningeal vessels. The vessels lie in the groove on the internal aspect of the lateral wall of the skull.
   ➤ The extradural haematoma exerts a local pressure on the corresponding cerebral cortex. The motor area lies deep to the haematoma.
   ➤ The centre of the pterion is an important landmark for a neurosurgeon to make Burr holes.
   ➤ An untreated middle meningeal artery haemorrhage may cause death.

| **SN-3** | **Suprameatal triangle (MacEwen's triangle)** |

It is a ▲ lar depression, present above and behind the external acoustic meatus.
1. **Boundaries** (Fig. 1.2): Margins of suprameatal triangle are: ◆━ SET
   A. Above by supramastoid crest.
   B. Anteriorly by posterosuperior margin of external acoustic meatus.
   C. Behind by tangential line drawn from posterior margin of external acoustic meatus.

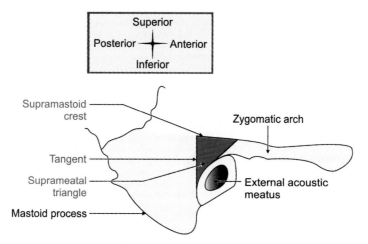

Fig. 1.2: Boundaries of right suprameatal triangle

2. **Applied anatomy**
   ➤ The suprameatal triangle corresponds with cymba concha of the auricle and the mastoid antrum.
   ➤ At birth, mastoid antrum is situated 1 mm deep to the suprameatal triangle. It increases by 1 mm/year till puberty. In an adult, it is situated 12 mm deep to the suprameatal triangle.

SN-4   Mastoid process

(*Masts*—breast, *oid*—like)

It is a large projection from the lower part of mastoid part of temporal bone. It forms the lateral wall of the mastoid notch.

1. **Situation:** Posteroinferior part of external acoustic meatus.
2. **Types of mastoid process:** Depending upon the distribution of air cells, it is of following types:
   A. **Pneumatic:** It shows many air cells.
   B. **Sclerotic:** It has few or no air cells.
   C. **Mixed:** It contains air cells and bone marrow in equal proportion.
3. **Development**
   A. It develops in 2nd year of life and is usually better developed in males ♂ than in females ♀.
   B. It is an example of traction epiphysis.
4. **Attachments:** Following muscles are attached from superficial to deep.

    SSC LC.

   <u>S</u>ternocleidomastoid (spinal root of accessory nerve),
   <u>S</u>plenius <u>c</u>apitis (**C1** to **C6** nerves), and
   <u>L</u>ongissimus <u>c</u>apitis (dorsal rami of cervical nerve).

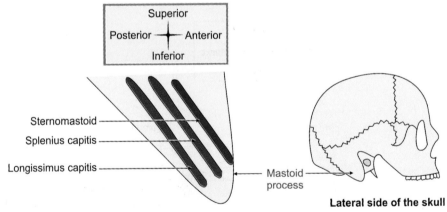

Fig. 1.3: Muscles attached to the right mastoid process

5. **Relations**
   A. It is grooved on the deep aspect by digastric notch for the origin of posterior belly of digastric. Medial to the notch is a groove for the occipital artery, facial nerve, and stylomastoid branch of posterior auricular artery.
   B. Stylomastoid foramen is present between mastoid process and styloid process. It transmits
      a. Facial nerve, and
      b. Stylomastoid branch of posterior auricular artery.

6. Applied anatomy

➤ The facial nerve is likely to get damaged in application of forceps during assisted delivery.

➤ At birth, the stylomastoid foramen is more superficial because of following reasons.

• Mastoid process is not developed at birth, and

• The external acoustic canal is short.

SN-5   Styloid process

Styloid {stylo—stake (wooden or metal post-pointed at one end), oid—resemblance}

It is a long, slender and pointed bony process. It measures about 2.5 cm, it arises from inferior surface of temporal bone. It is directed downwards and forwards.

1. **Site:** It is present on the inferior surface of petrous part of temporal bone.

2. **Parts of styloid process**

    A. **Tympanohyal** {Hyal—hyoid **U** (shaped like a Greek letter upsilon (u)}: It is covered by tympanic plate.

    B. **Stylohyal:** It is the lower part of styloid process.

3. **Relations**

    A. **Medially:** From anterior to posterior

        a. Internal carotid artery,

        b. **IX, X** and **XI** cranial nerves, and

        c. Internal jugular vein.

    B. **Laterally:**

        a. At base: Facial nerve,

        b. At apex: External carotid artery,

        c. Overlapped by parotid gland.

4. **Attachments (Fig. 1.4)**

Table 1.1: Structures attached to styloid process and their nerve supply

Parts of styloid process	Structure	Nerve supply
• At the tip and anterior surface	• Styloglossus muscle	• Hypoglossal (XII)
• Medial surface	• Stylopharyngeus muscle	• Glossopharyngeal (IX)
• Posterior surface	• Stylohyoid muscle	• Facial nerve VII
• Tip of styloid process and anterior surface	• Stylomandibular ligament	———
• Tip of styloid process	• Stylohyoid ligament	

A. Styloid process + structures attached to styloid process = styloid apparatus.

Head, Neck and Face

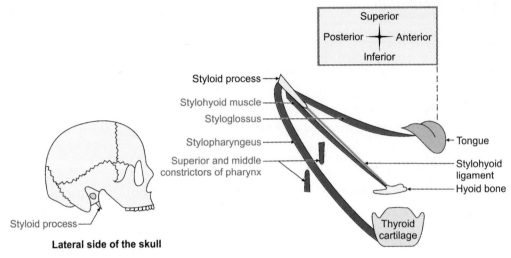

Fig. 1.4: Attachments to right styloid process

5. **Development:** It is developed from the cartilage of 2nd pharyngeal arch.
   A. Its tympanohyal part ossifies before birth.
   B. The stylohyal part ossifies after birth.

SN-6   Foetal skull

1. **Features**
   A. Disproportion between cranial vault and facial skeleton. The vault is very large in proportion to face.
   B. The vertical diameter of the orbit equals the sum of vertical height of maxilla and mandible.
   C. The bones of the skull and of the face are loose. They are readily disarticulated in the macerated skull.
   D. The bones of the vault do not interdigitate in sutures but are separated by linear attachments of fibrous tissue.
   E. Anterior fontanelle lies between two parietal bones and two halves of frontal bones (Fig. 1.5).

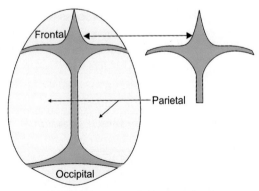

Fig. 1.5: Shape of anterior fontanelle

F. Posterior fontanelle lies between apex of occipital bone and posterior borders of parietal bone.

G. Stylomastoid foramen is near the lateral surface of the skull.

H. External acoustic meatus is wholly cartilaginous.

2. **Ossification of bones**

A. **Frontal bone:** It consists of two halves separated by a median metopic suture.

B. **Temporal bone:** It consists of four parts

   a. Petromastoid part,

   b. Squamous part,

   c. Styloid process, and

   d. Tympanic plate.

C. **Mandible is in two halves**.

D. **Occipital bone is in four parts**

   a. Squamous—1

   b. Basilar—1

   c. Condylar—2

E. **Sphenoid is in three pieces**

   a. Central part formed by body and lesser wing,

   b. Lateral part formed by greater wing, and

   c. Pterygoid process.

3. **Following structures are absent in foetal skull.**

A. Glabella, superciliary arch and mastoid process.

B. Bony part of external acoustic meatus.

C. There is no diploe in bones of cranial vault.

D. Tympanic part is present as C shaped ring.

E. Maxillary air sinus is narrow slit.

4. **Following structures are of adult size in foetal skull**

A. Tympanic membrane

B. The bones of the middle ear (malleus, incus and stapes).

C. Middle ear, internal ear and mastoid antrum. These are enclosed in petromastoid part of the temporal bone.

5. Applied anatomy : As the stylomastoid foramen is near the lateral surface of the skull, the facial nerve is unprotected and vulnerable.

SN-7   Fontanelle (fonticuli)

Introduction: They are membranous gaps present at the 4 angles of parietal bone.

1. **Features:** They are paired and unpaired.

2. **Unpaired**

A. Anterior fontanelle, and

B. Posterior fontanelle.

Head, Neck and Face

Head, Neck and Face

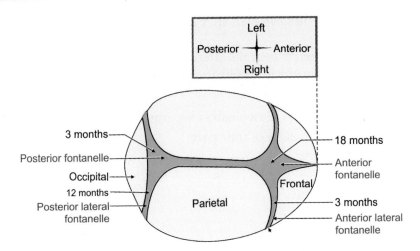

Fig. 1.6: Norma verticalis of foetal skull to show various fontanelles

3. **Paired**
    A. Anterolateral fontanelle, and
    B. Posterolateral fontanelle.

Table 1.2: Features of different fontanelles

Features	Anterior	Posterior	Sphenoid	Mastoid
• Number	• Unpaired	• Unpaired	• Paired	• Paired
• Situation	• At the bregma, junction of frontal and parietal bones	• At lambda, the junction of sagittal and lambdoid suture	• At pterion	• At asterion
• Shape	• Diamond	• lar	• Irregular	• Irregular
• Size	• Largest	• Large	• Small	• Small
• Obliteration	• 18 months	• 2–3 months	• 2–3 months	• 12 months

4. **Applied anatomy**

> It helps to determine the age of the child. If it persists after 2 years, it indicates
  • Disturbance in calcium metabolism or/and
  • Deficiency of vitamin D.
> Abnormal bulging indicates increased intracranial tension.
> Abnormal depressed fontanelle indicates dehydration.
> Superior sagittal sinus can be punctured at the anterior fontanelle to
  • Collect the venous blood for investigation (Fig. 1.7).
  • Start the infusion of fluid.
  • Transfuse blood.
> Nowadays, puncture of superior sagittal sinus is not used for above purposes. Central venous catheterization is used for above puposes.
> Cerebrospinal fluid can be obtained by introducing a needle from its lateral angle in a downward and lateral direction.

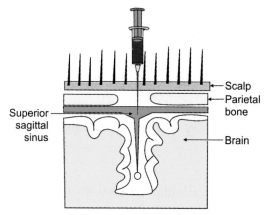

Fig. 1.7: Puncture of superior sagittal sinus to get venous blood

➤ It allows malleability of the foetal head (moulding of skull bones) during its passage through the birth canal at the time of delivery.
➤ It helps in diagnosis of the presentation, position and attitude of the foetal head.

| SN-8 | **Emissary veins** |

Emissary veins (*emissary*—drain, to send, messenger, ambassador)

Introduction: These veins connect the intracranial venous sinuses to extracranial veins (Table 1.3).

1. **Peculiarities:** They lack
   A. Valves,
   B. Smooth muscles, and
   C. Compressibility.
2. **Function:** They maintain intracranial pressure.

Table 1.3: Emissary veins connecting extracranial veins to the intracranial venous sinus

No.	Emissary vein	Foramen through which they pass	Connects	
			Veins outside skull	And venous sinus inside the skull
1	• Parietal e.v.	• Parietal foramen	• Veins of scalp	• Superior sagittal sinus
2	• Mastoid e.v.	• Mastoid foramen	• Veins of scalp	• Transverse sinus
3	• Emissary vein	• Foramen caecum	• Veins of root of nose	• Superior sagittal sinus
4	• Emissary vein	• Foramen ovale	• Pterygoid venous plexus	• Cavernous sinus
5	• Emissary veins	• Foramen lacerum	• Pharyngeal venous plexus	• Cavernous sinus
6	• Emissary vein	• Hypoglossal canal	• Internal jugular vein	• Sigmoid sinus
7	• Condylar e.v.	• Posterior condylar foramen	• Suboccipital venous plexus	• Sigmoid sinus

Head, Neck and Face

3. **Applied anatomy** : Infection outside the cranium spreads to the venous sinuses through the emissary vein.

OLA-1   Enumerate structures within parotid salivary gland.

They are grouped as

1. **Arteries:** External carotid artery and its two terminal branches
    a. Maxillary artery, and
    b. Superficial temporal artery.
2. **Veins:** Formation of retromandibular vein and its tributaries
    a. Veins forming retromandibular vein
        I. Maxillary vein, and
        II. Superficial temporal vein
    b. Tributaries of retromandibular vein
        I. Anterior division of retromandibular vein
        II. Posterior division of retromandibular vein
3. **Nerves**
    a. Terminal branches of facial nerve
        I. Temporal
        II. Zygomatic
        III. Buccal which subdivides into
            i. Upper buccal, and
            ii. Lower buccal
        IV. Mandibular
        V. Cervical
    b. Auriculotemporal nerve branch of posterior division of mandibular nerve.
4. **Parotid duct**

SN-9   Foramina of middle cranial fossa

1. **Optic canal**
    A. Optic nerve (kind cranial nerve) with meninges,
    B. Ophthalmic artery with sympathetic plexus, and
    C. Central artery of retina.

> Kind cranial nerve—Tip

Box 1.3

Optic nerve is called kind cranial nerve.

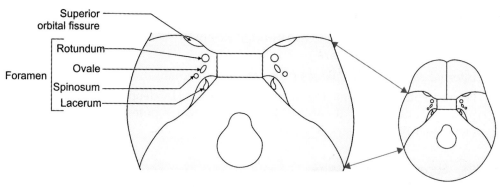

Fig. 1.8: Foramina of middle cranial fossa

2. **Superior orbital fissure**
   A. Outside tendinous ring (from above downwards)
      a. Vessels

      Meningeal branch of lacrimal artery M L A

      Anastomosing branch of middle meningeal artery AMMA
         I. Superior ophthalmic vein

      b. Nerves LFT

      Lacrimal branch of ophthalmic division of trigeminal nerve (**V1**)

      Frontal branch of ophthalmic division of trigeminal nerve (**V1**)

      Trochlear nerve (**IV**)

   B. In the tendinous ring
      a. Upper division of oculomotor nerve (**III**)
      b. Nasociliary branch of ophthalmic division of trigeminal nerve (**V1**)
      c. Lower division of oculomotor nerve (**III**)
      d. Abducent nerve (**VI**)

   C. Below the tendinous ring
      a. Inferior ophthalmic vein

      Foramen ovale ♂ MALE

      Trunk of Mandibular nerve, 3rd division of trigeminal nerve,
      Accessory meningeal artery (branch of maxillary artery),
      Lesser petrosal nerve (branch of tympanic plexus), and
      Emissary vein. It communicates cavernous sinus with
      b. Pterygoid venous plexus, and
      c. Anterior division of middle meningeal sinus.

3. **Foramen spinosum** 3M

   Middle meningeal artery (branch of maxillary artery)
   Middle meningeal vein
   Meningeal branch of mandibular nerve

4. **Foramen lacerum**

A. No structures pass through and through except ⬩━▪ MAP Meningeal branch of Ascending Pharyngeal artery.

B. Internal carotid artery passes from lateral to medial.

C. Nerve to pterygoid canal (Vidian nerve) is formed by deep petrosal (sympathetic plexus around internal carotid artery) and greater petrosal nerves (branch of facial nerve).

SN-10   Superior orbital fissure

1. **Location:** It is present in the superior wall of orbit.

2. **Shape:** Retort 〰 shaped.

3. **Features**

A. It is the gap present between greater and lesser wings of sphenoid bone.

B. It is completed laterally by the frontal bone uniting the two wings.

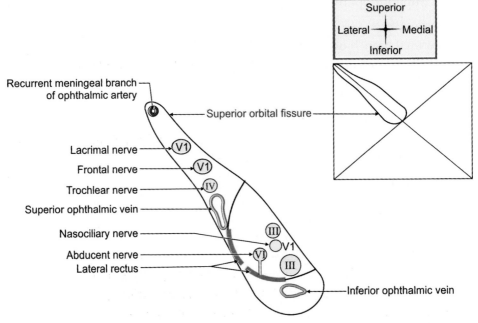

Fig. 1.9: Superior orbital fissure and its contents on right side

Note: The dimensions of various nerves

A. Optic nerve: Thickest sensory cranial nerve. It contains 1 million neurons.

B. Lower division of oculomotor nerve is thicker as compared to upper division. It has more branches.

C. Trochlear and abducent nerves are less thick than oculomotor nerve.

D. Nasociliary is thin nerve.

4. Contents

Table 1.4: Contents of superior orbital fissure

• Upper lateral part above the ring	• Orbital branch of middle meningeal artery (branch of 1st part of maxillary artery) • Meningeal branch of Lacrimal Artery M LA • Lacrimal nerve **V1** (ophthalmic nerve) • Frontal nerve **V1** (ophthalmic nerve) LFT • Trochlear nerve (**IV**) • Superior ophthalmic vein
• Middle part through the ring	• Upper division of oculomotor nerve • Nasociliary nerve • Lower division of oculomotor nerve • Abducent nerve
• Lower medial part below the ring	• Inferior ophthalmic vein

5. **Applied anatomy** : Fracture causing craniofacial disjunction may damage the 3rd, 4th and 6th cranial nerves in the superior orbital fissure.

SN-11   Inferior orbital fissure

1. **Location:** It is located between the upper margin of posterior wall of maxilla and the greater wing of sphenoid bone.
2. **Communication:** It communicates with
   A. Orbit superiorly,
   B. Infratemporal fossa laterally, and
   C. Pterygopalatine fossa medially.
3. **Contents** (Fig. 1.10)
   A. Maxillary nerve which continues as infraorbital nerve once it enters the orbit.
   B. Zygomatic nerve, a branch of maxillary nerve.

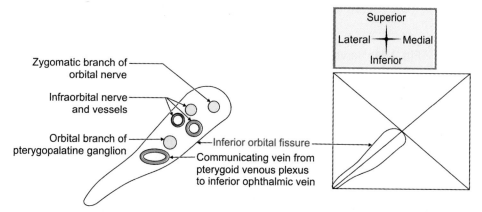

Fig. 1.10: Inferior orbital fissure and its contents on right side

C. Infratemporal artery, a branch of maxillary artery.

D. Infratemporal vein, a tributary of maxillary vein.

E. Connecting channels between inferior ophthalmic vein and the pterygoid plexus of veins.

4. **Applied anatomy**

➤ The infraorbital nerve is invariably damaged in depressed fractures of the zygomatic bone or in fracture of orbital floor.

➤ Malignant tumours of the maxillary sinus may cause pressure effects on the nerve. There may be pain or numbness of the cheek, lower eyelid, incisor teeth and adjacent gums.

SN-12   Arteries and nerves related to ramus of mandible

Following are the nerves and vessels related to mandible (Figs 1.11 and 1.12).

1. Masseteric nerves and vessels pass through the mandibular notch.

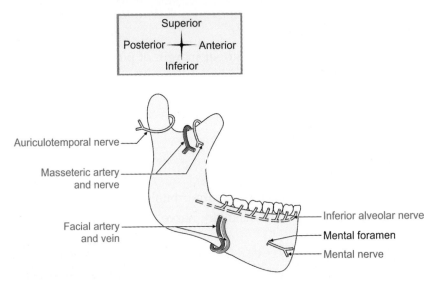

Fig. 1.11: Nerves and arteries related to lateral surface of mandible

2. Inferior alveolar nerves and vessels enter the mandibular canal through the mandibular foramen.

3. Mylohyoid nerves and vessels run forward in the mylohyoid groove.

4. Mental nerves and vessels emerge through the mental foramen.

5. Facial artery is closely related to the mandible.

6. Maxillary artery and some of its branches are related between lower border of lateral pterygoid and medial pterygoid.

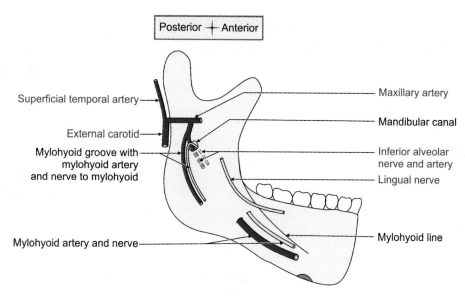

Fig. 1.12: Nerves and vessels related to medial surface of mandible

SN-13	Name the muscles attached to mandible

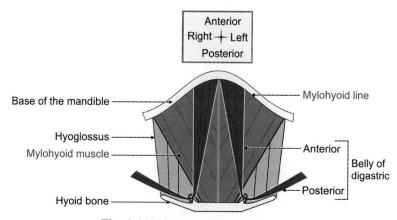

Fig. 1.13: Mylohyoid line and muscle

Table 1.5: Muscles attached to mandible and their nerve supply

Part of mandible	Muscles	Nerve supply
• **External surface of body** • Incisive fossa • Oblique line	• Mentalis • Orbicularis oculi • Depressor labii inferioris • Depressor anguli oris • Buccinator	• Facial nerve— 7th cranial nerve

• Internal surface of body
• Mylohyoid line
	• Mylohyoid	• Mandibular nerve—
		  3rd division of
		  5th cranial nerve

Contd.

Table 1.5: Muscles attached to mandible and their nerve supply (Contd.)

Part of mandible	Muscles	Nerve supply
• Behind mylohyoid line	• Superior constrictor of pharynx	• Pharyngeal plexus
• Genial tubercle	• Genioglossus	• Hypoglossal nerve
	• Geniohyoid	• C1 nerve
• Digastric fossa	• Anterior belly of digastric	• Mandibular nerve
• Near outer surface	• Platysma	• Facial nerve
• **Ramus of mandible**		
• Lateral surface	• Masseter	
• Medial surface	• Medial pterygoid	• Mandibular nerve
• Anterior border of coronoid process	• Temporalis	
• Medial surface of coronoid process		
• Pterygoid fovea of neck of mandible	• Lateral pterygoid	

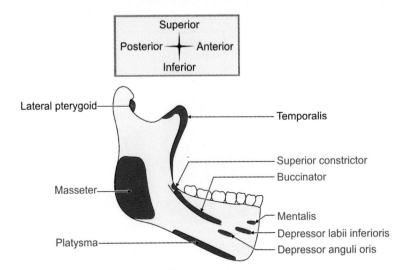

Fig. 1.14: Muscles attached to lateral surface of right side of body of mandible

SN-14   Spine of sphenoid

Introduction: It is an irregular downward projection arising from the inferior surface of **greater wing of sphenoid bone.**

1. **Attachment:** It gives attachment to sphenomandibular ligament.
2. **Relations**
   A. **Medially:** Chorda tympani nerve, a branch of facial nerve—7th cranial nerve.
   B. **Laterally:** Auriculotemporal nerve, a branch of posterior division of mandibular nerve.

3. **Applied anatomy**: The damage to the spine of sphenoid stops the secretion of all major salivary glands. This is because of its close association with chorda tympani and auriculotemporal nerve.

SN-15 Lateral pterygoid plate

Introduction: It is quadrilateral, thin plate arising from body of sphenoid bone.

1. **Surfaces:** It has medial and lateral surfaces.
2. **Features**
   A. Lateral surface forms the medial boundary of the infratemporal fossa.
   B. Medial surface forms the lateral wall of pterygoid fossa.
   C. Anterior border of lateral pterygoid plate forms the posterior boundary of pterygoid fissure.
3. **Attachments**
   A. Lateral surface—lower head of lateral pterygoid muscle.
   B. Medial surface—origin to medial pterygoid muscle.
   C. Posterior border—pterygospinous ligament.
4. **Ossification:** The pterygoid plate develops in membrane.

SN-16 Jugular foramen

(*Jugular*—pertaining to neck)

1. **Location:** It is situated between jugular process of occipital bone and petrous part of temporal bone.
2. **Features**
   A. The anterior wall is hollowed and forms the jugular fossa. It lodges the superior bulb of internal jugular vein.
   B. **It presents three canaliculi**
      a. Mastoid canaliculus transmits auricular branch of vagus nerve.
      b. Cochlear canaliculus transmits aqueduct of cochlea.
   C. Tympanic canaliculus transmits tympanic branch of glossopharyngeal nerve.

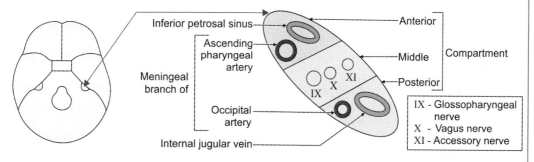

Fig. 1.15: Jugular foramen

Head, Neck and Face

3. **Contents:** It is divided into three parts. The contents are
   - A. Vessels in front
     - a. Inferior petrosal sinus.
     - b. Meningeal artery, branch of ascending pharyngeal artery.
   - B. Vessels behind
     - a. Internal jugular vein, a direct continuation of sigmoid sinus
     - b. Meningeal artery, branch of occipital artery
   - C. Three nerves in between
     - a. Glossopharyngeal nerve (**IX**),
     - b. Vagus nerve (**X**), and
     - c. Accessory nerve (**XI**).

SN-17 Anterior longitudinal ligament

1. **Attachment:** It is attached to upper and lower borders of anterior surfaces of bodies of all vertebrae.

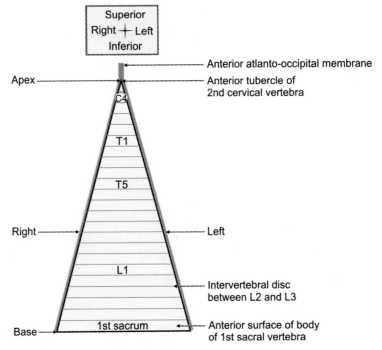

Fig. 1.16: Coronal section of vertebral column to show the attachments of anterior longitudinal ligament

2. **Extent:** It extends from anterior surface of upper sacral vertebra to anterior tubercle of axis (second cervical vertebra). **3A** Anterior ligament to anterior tubercle of axis.
3. **Variation in thickness:** It is ▲lar in shape. Base is at the upper sacral vertebra and apex at axis.
4. **Termination:** It continues as anterior atlanto-occipital membrane.

SN-18   Posterior longitudinal ligament

1. It is attached to the upper and lower borders of the posterior surface of bodies of all vertebrae (Fig. 1.17).

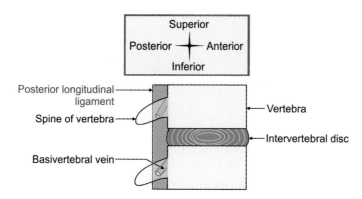

Fig. 1.17: Sagittal section of vertebrae showing attachments of posterior longitudinal ligament

2. **Extent:** It extends from the body of 1st sacral to the lower border of body of second cervical vertebra.

3. **Termination:** It continues as membrana tectoria (*tectum*—roof) above second cervical vertebra.

4. **Relations**

    A. **Anterior:** Basivertebral venous plexus,

    B. **Posterior:** Spinal cord with meninges.

5. **Variation in thickness:** Upper part is broad and has uniform width, lower part is narrow.

6. **Types of fibres**

    A. **Superficial fibres:** They join 3 to 4 vertebrae.

    B. **Deep fibres:** They merge with annulus fibrosus.

7. Applied anatomy: The posterior longitudinal ligament will be torn in excessive flexion of neck leading to prolapse of intervertebral disc.

SN-19   Dens (odontoid process)

Introduction: It is a strong tooth-like process projecting upwards from the body of axis (2nd cervical) vertebra.

1. **Evolution:** It represents the body of the 1st cervical vertebra.

2. **Articulations**

    A. Anteriorly with anterior arch of atlas.

    B. Posteriorly with transverse ligament of atlas

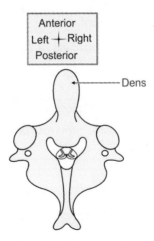

Fig. 1.18: Axis vertebra

3. **Attachments** (Fig. 1.18 and Table 1.6)

Table 1.6: Structures attached to parts of dens

Sr.	Location	Attachment
1	• Apex	• Apical ligament
2	• Side	• Alar ligament
3	• Anterior surface	• Longus colli • Anterior longitudinal ligament
4	• Posterior surface	• Posterior longitudinal ligament • Membrana tectoria.

SN-20   Foramen lacerum

(*lacerum*—irregular)

1. **Site:** Middle cranial fossa.
2. **Boundaries** (Fig. 1.19)
   A. Medially—body of sphenoid.
   B. Laterally—greater wing of sphenoid.
   C. Posteriorly—apex of petrous part of temporal bone
3. **Communications**
   A. Anteriorly, with pterygopalatine fossa.
   B. Posteriorly, with the carotid canal.
4. **Contents** (Fig. 1.19)
   A. No structures pass through and through except (Meningeal branch of Ascending Pharyngeal artery). **MAP**
   B. The structure crossing from lateral to medial is internal carotid artery.
   C. The structure formed is nerve of pterygoid canal (Vidian's nerve).

SN-21   Foramen magnum

(*Magnum*—great)

Introduction: It is the largest foramen of skull.

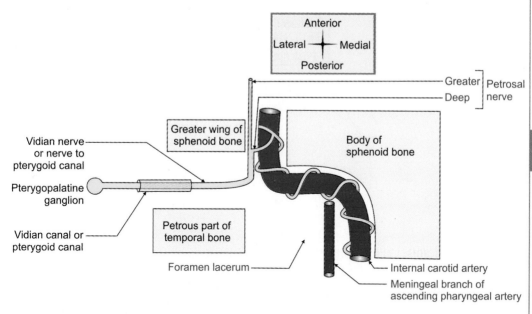

Fig. 1.19: Base of skull showing boundaries and contents of foramen lacerum on right side

1. **Site:** Posterior cranial fossa in occipital bone.
2. **Communication:** It connects posterior cranial fossa to vertebral canal.
3. **Shape:** Oval ⬤, it is wider in the posterior half.
4. **Structures passing (depending upon importance)** (Figs 1.20A and B)
   A. Most important structures: The lowest part of medulla oblongata with meninges.
   B. Important structures passing through subarachnoid space.
      a. Two vertebral arteries (branches of 1st part of subclavian artery) with sympathetic plexus

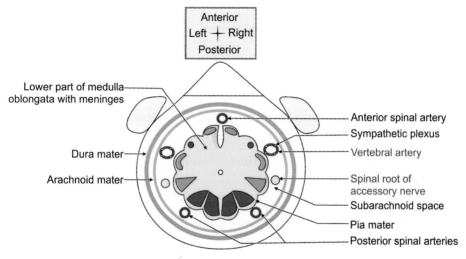

Fig. 1.20A: Important structures passing through foramen magnum

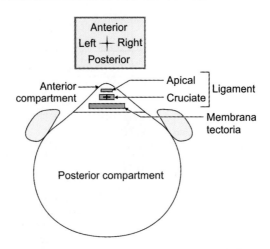

Fig. 1.20B: Less important structures passing through foramen magnum

b. One anterior spinal artery (branch of vertebral artery).

c. Two posterior spinal arteries (branch of vertebral artery).

d. Spinal roots of accessory nerves (**XIth cranial nerve**).

C. Less important

  a. Apical ligament of dens

  b. Vertical band of cruciate ligament

  c. Membrana tectoria

  d. Ligamentum denticulatum.

SN-22   Maxilla

It is a paired bone of the face forming upper jaw.

1. **Classification:** It is a pneumatic bone.

2. **Development:** It is developed in membrane.

3. **Side determination**

  A. It has frontal process pointing medially and upwards.

  B. Alveolar process is thick, arched and projects downwards (Fig. 1.21).

4. **Features:** It has body which is a hollow pyramid and has following surfaces.

  A. **Anterior surface:** It presents

    a. *Incisive fossa:* A fossa above the incisor teeth. It gives attachment to following muscles.

      I. Depressor septi from the fossa.

      II. Orbicularis oris below the fossa.

      III. Nasalis lateral to fossa.

    b. *Canine fossa:* It is lateral to incisive fossa. It gives origin to levator anguli oris

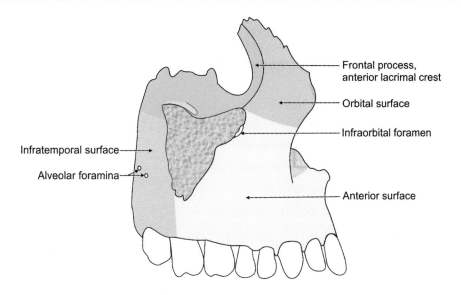

Frontal process, anterior lacrimal crest

Orbital surface

Infraorbital foramen

Infratemporal surface

Alveolar foramina

Anterior surface

Fig. 1.21: Lateral surface of right maxilla

    c. *Infraorbital foramen:* It lies above the canine fossa. It transmits
        I. Infraorbital artery, a branch of maxillary artery.
        II. Infraorbital nerve, a branch of maxillary nerve.
    d. Origin of levator labii superioris.
B. **Posterior (infratemporal) surface:** It has foramina for posterior superior alveolar vessels and nerves.
    It presents maxillary tuberosity: It has articular and non-articular surfaces.
    a. Articular surface articulates with pyramidal processes of palatine bone.
    b. Non-articular surface gives attachment to superficial head of medial pterygoid. It forms anterior boundary of pterygopalatine fossa.
C. **Superior (orbital) surface:** It forms the floor of the orbit. It is ▲ lar. It has
    a. Anterior, posterior and medial borders.
    b. It presents lacrimal notch which is converted into nasolacrimal canal.
    c. The surface presents infraorbital groove and canal for the infraorbital vessels and nerve.
    d. Inferior oblique muscle of eyeball arises from the surface.
    e. Its posterior border forms the inferior border of inferior orbital fissure. It transmits
        I. Infraorbital vessels,
        II. Maxillary nerve,
        III. Zygomatic nerve,
        IV. Sympathetic plexus, and
        V. Veins connecting ophthalmic vein to pterygoid plexus.
D. **Medial surface**
    a. It forms lateral wall of nose. It presents
        I. Maxillary hiatus: It leads to maxillary air sinus.
        II. Nasolacrimal groove,

III. Concha crest,

IV. Inferior meatus of nasal cavity, and

V. Atrium of middle meatus.

b. Processes

I. Frontal process: It has

i. Two surfaces: Lateral and medial

- Lateral surface presents
  - Anterior lacrimal crest that gives attachment to
  - Lacrimal fascia, and
  - Medial palpebral ligament.
  - Anterior smooth area that gives attachment to orbicularis oculi and levator labii superioris alaeque nasi.
- Medial surface forms a lateral wall of nasal cavity.

ii. Two borders: Anterior and posterior

iii. One end

II. Zygomatic process: A short process projecting laterally articulating with zygomatic process of temporal bone.

III. Alveolar process: It presents

i. Sockets for the teeth.

ii. Origin of buccinator muscle.

IV. Palatine process: It is strong, thick and plate-like. It articulates with its fellow of opposite side and forms the hard palate.

E. **Inferior surface**

a. It has

I. Pits for palatine glands.

II. Groove for greater palatine vessels and nerves.

III. Incisive canal which transmits terminal branches of greater palatine vessels and nasopalatine nerve.

IV. Anterior and posterior incisive foramina.

V. Nasal crest present on the medial border.

VI. Incisor crest is the anterior part of nasal crest.

VII. Anterior nasal spine is the anterior end of incisor crest.

b. **Processes:** It has four processes.

I. A process above—frontal process:

II. A process below and medially—palatine

III. A process laterally and above—zygomatic

IV. A process below and anteriorly—alveolar.

F. **Ossification:** It ossifies in membrane from a single centre which appears on the 6th week of intrauterine life. The centre appears in the canine fossa. Two more centres appear in the 7th week of intrauterine life.

5. **Applied anatomy**

➤ Pus in the maxillary sinus is not drained naturally because the antrum of Highmore is at higher level. In chronic maxillary sinusitis, the pus is drained by antral puncture or *antrostomy*. A trocar and cannula are passed through the nasal cavity in an upward and backward direction. It passes below the inferior nasal concha. A hole is produced in the lateral wall of nasal cavity.

   • **Note:** Nowadays, it has been taken over by endoscopic method of drainage.

➤ *Caldwell-Luc operation:* For adequate drainage in chronic sinusitis, a part of medial wall of the sinus below the inferior nasal concha is removed to avoid injury to infraorbital nerve.

➤ *Maxillary tumours* can produce a bulging in following adjacent structures.

   • Superiorly in the floor of the orbit,

   • Inferiorly in the roof of oral cavity,

   • Anteriorly in the face,

   • Posteriorly in the infratemporal fossa, and

   • Medially in the lateral wall of nose.

➤ There may be unilateral or bilateral fracture of maxilla.

   • Unilateral fracture involves alveolar process.

   • Bilateral fractures are subclassified depending upon involvement of zygomatic bone, orbit, and cranium. They are classified as

      – LeFort I,

      – LeFort II, and

      – LeFort III.

SN-23   Hyoid bone

(U shaped)

Introduction: It is unpaired midline bone of the neck. It is suspended by muscles and hence very much mobile.

1. **Classification:** It is irregular bone.

2. **Development**

   A. Smaller cornu and Superior part of body develop from second pharyngeal arch.

   B. Lower part of body and greater cornu develop from third pharyngeal arch.

3. **Features:** It has body, greater and lesser cornua.

   A. **Body:** It has two borders, and two surfaces.

      a. *Surfaces*

         I. Anterior surface: A median ridge divides into lateral halves. (The content of the brackets indicates the nerve supplying the muscles.)

            i. Geniohyoid (**C1**), mylohyoid (**V3**) and hyoglossus (**XII**) are attached to anterior surface.

            ii. Investing layer of deep cervical fascia is attached deep to mylohyoid.

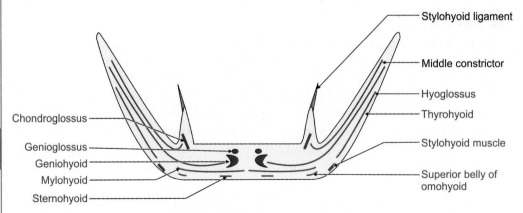

Fig. 1.22: Hyoid bone and its attachments

Labels (left, top to bottom): Chondroglossus, Genioglossus, Geniohyoid, Mylohyoid, Sternohyoid

Labels (right, top to bottom): Stylohyoid ligament, Middle constrictor, Hyoglossus, Thyrohyoid, Stylohyoid muscle, Superior belly of omohyoid

II. Posterior surface: It is related to
- Bursa,
- Thyrohyoid membrane, and
- Epiglottis

b. *Borders*

I. Upper border: It provides attachment to following structures from anterior to posterior
  i. Genioglossus muscle (XII)
  ii. Hyoepiglottic ligament.
  iii. Thyrohyoid membrane.

II. Lower border: Sternohyoid (ansa cervicalis) and omohyoid (ansa cervicalis) are attached to lower border.

B. **Greater cornu:** It has two borders and two surfaces.

a. *Surfaces:* Following muscles are attached to the anterior surface (from medial to lateral)
  I. Middle constrictor (pharyngeal plexus)
  II. Hyoglossus (XII)
  III. Stylohyoid (VII)
  IV. Intermediate loop of digastric.

b. *Borders:* They give attachments to following structures.
  I. Medial—thyrohyoid membrane
  II. Lateral—thyrohyoid muscle.

C. **Lesser cornu:** It has following attachments.
  a. Stylohyoid ligament
  b. Middle constrictor of pharynx.

4. **Joints:** Synovial joint is formed between lesser and greater cornua of hyoid bone and get obliterated in the later part of life.

5. **Movements**

   A. The suprahyoid muscle (mylohyoid, stylohyoid and geniohyoid)—elevators.

   B. The infrahyoid muscles (sternohyoid and omohyoid)—depressor.

6. **Ossification:** It ossifies from 6 centres. They are as follows

   A. Greater cornu (before birth)—2

   B. Body (after birth)—2, and

   C. Lesser cornu (at puberty).

7. **Applied anatomy**

   ➤ A postmortem finding of the fracture of the greater cornu is indicative of homicidal throttling.of the hyoid bone. This is true in case of

   • Sudden and

   • Unnatural death with other signs of suffocation.

   ➤ The hyoid bone moves with deglutination.

Head, Neck and Face

Scalp, Temple and Face

OLA-2   Why the infections of superficial fascia of scalp causes more pain?

Superficial fascia has abundant fibrous tissue and has rich nerve supply. Hence, infection of the superficial fascia irritates the nerve and one gets severe pain.

OLA-3   Why are sebaceous cysts and seborrhoea more frequently associated with the scalp?

Scalp has plenty of hair and sebaceous glands. The ducts of sebaceous glands are prone to infection and get damaged by combing. For this reason, scalp is a common site for sebaceous cysts. Hence, sebaceous cysts and seborrhoea are more common.

OLA-4   What is the "dangerous area of scalp" and why is it called so?

Third layer of scalp is loose areolar tissue. It is dangerous area of scalp. Any accumulation of blood in this area will not spread in following directions.
1. It cannot descend in neck because of firm attachment of epicranial aponeurosis to superior nuchal line.
2. It cannot descend laterally because of its attachment to superior temporal line.
   Only way it can spread is anteriorly. Hence, it accumulates deep to eyelid and results into black eye. This results in damage to eye hence it is called dangerous area.

OLA-5   What is "safety valve haematoma"? How the haemorrhage from the blood vessels of scalp is arrested?

1. Safety valve haematoma occurs due to the following reasons:
   A. Fracture of the bone of the scalp, and
   B. Intracranial bleeding (usually due to birth trauma in the newborn).
      The symptoms of intracranial bleeding are delayed due to leakage of blood. It spreads to the subaponeurotic layer from the fracture site. It expands to accommodate large quantity of blood. Since this haematoma delays the onset of symptoms of a serious condition, it is called safety valve haematoma.

2. By compressing at the site of injury, bleeding is arrested since underneath the scalp is cranium which is hard structure.

OLA-6 Why the wounds of face bleed profusely?

Scalp has *profuse* blood supply. It is supplied by *5 paired* arteries. These arteries pass through the dense connective tissue. Ruptured arteries of any part of the body are constricted by the contraction of smooth muscles present in walls of the vessel.

The vessels in the scalp pass through the dense connective tissue. The arteries of the scalp cannot overcome the resistance of the tough dens deep fascia. Hence, they are kept open and they bleed profusely.

OLA-7 What are the modifications of palpebral fascia?

The palpebral fascia of the two eyelids forms the orbital septum.

1. In upper eyelid becomes thick and forms tarsal plates or tarsi. Tarsi are thin plates of condensed fibrous tissue located near the lid margins. They give stiffness to the lids. The upper tarsus receives two tendinous slips from the levator palpebrae superioris.

   A. One from voluntary part, and

   B. Another from involuntary part.

2. At the angles, it forms palpebral ligaments.

OLA-8 What is stye (hordeolum)?

1. **Definition:** It is a suppurative inflammation of one of the glands of Zeis. It is large sebaceous gland.

2. **Clinical features**

   A. The gland is swollen, hard and painful.

   B. Lid is oedematous.

   C. Pus points near the base of one of the roots (follicle) of an eyelash.

OLA-9 What is chalazion?

Definition: It is inflammation of a tarsal gland, causing a localized swelling pointing inward.

SN-24 Modiolus

1. **Modiolus (nave, pillar):** It is a compact, mobile fibromuscular structure. It is present at about 1.25 cm lateral to the angle of the mouth opposite the upper 2nd premolar tooth.

2. The five muscles interlacing to form the modiolus are:

   A. Buccinator,

   B. Zygomaticus major,

Head, Neck and Face

C. Levator anguli oris,

D. Depressor anguli oris

E. Risorius.

3. **Shape:** Like a hub of a cart-wheel ⚙. The muscles radiate from it lie in different planes.

4. **Palpation:** It can be palpated between the opposed thumb compressing the skin at the angle of mouth and index finger simultaneously compressing the oral mucosa at the same point.

5. Applied anatomy : The complex integrated movements of modiolar muscles help in biting, chewing, drinking, sucking, swallowing and speaking apart from the facial expressions.

LAQ-1	Describe scalp under the following headings:
	1. Layers,
	2. Blood supply,
	3. Nerve supply, and
	4. Applied anatomy

1. **Layers** (Fig. 2.1): 🔑 SCALP

   A. <u>S</u>kin: *Skin is hairy and exceptionally thick.* It contains plenty of sebaceous glands. It is adherent to the underlying epicranial aponeurosis through the dense superficial fascia.

   B. <u>C</u>onnective tissue (superficial fascia): It is very dense and contains plenty of blood vessels and nerves. *It has the richest cutaneous blood supply in the body.*

   C. <u>A</u>poneurosis (galea aponeurotica or epicranial aponeurosis): This contains occipitofrontalis muscle. It has

   a. Occipital, and

   b. Frontal belly.

   a. Occipital belly arises from

      I. External occipital protuberance, and

      II. Highest nuchal lines and becomes continuous with epicranial aponeurosis.

   b. Frontal belly arises from epicranial aponeurosis and merges with the procerus, corrugator supercilii and orbicularis oculi. The direction of the fibres is antero-posterior. Thus, the occipital belly is attached to the bone and the frontal belly is attached to the dermis of skin.

   D. <u>L</u>oose areolar tissue extends

   a. Posteriorly from highest and superior nuchal lines,

   b. Laterally from superior temporal lines, and

   c. Anteriorly into the eyelids.

   E. <u>P</u>ericranium: It is loosely attached to the surface of the bone except near sutures. Hence, the fluid collected in this layer takes the shape of underlying bone.

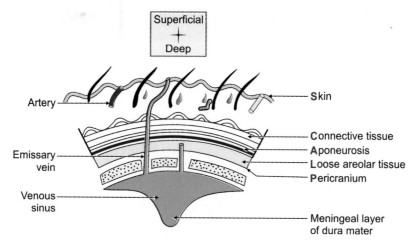

Fig. 2.1: Layers of the scalp

2. **Blood supply:** Scalp has rich blood supply.

A. Arterial supply (Fig. 2.2)

    a. In front of the auricle,

        I. Supraorbital artery (branch of ophthalmic artery), and

        II. Supratrochlear artery (branch of ophthalmic artery).

        III. Superficial temporal artery (branch of external carotid artery).

    b. Behind the auricle, it is supplied by

        I. Posterior auricular artery (branch of external carotid artery), and

        II. Occipital artery (branch of external carotid artery).

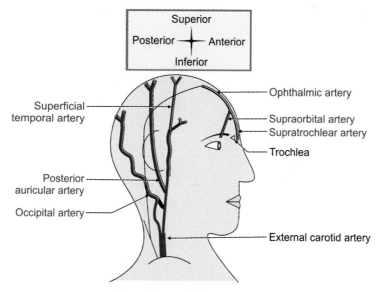

Fig. 2.2: Arterial supply of scalp

Head, Neck and Face

Sites of anastomosis of external and internal carotid arteries—Tip

Box 2.1

Note: Scalp is a site of anastomosis between branches of external and internal carotid arteries.

B. **Venous drainage** : It is described in Figs 2.3, 2.4 and Flowcharts 2.1 and 2.2.

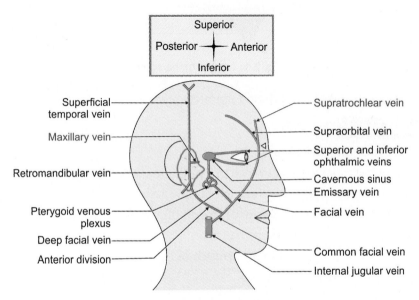

Fig. 2.3: Veins of the scalp draining into internal jugular vein

Flowchart 2.1: Veins of the scalp draining into internal jugular vein

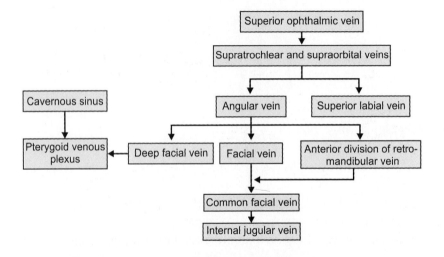

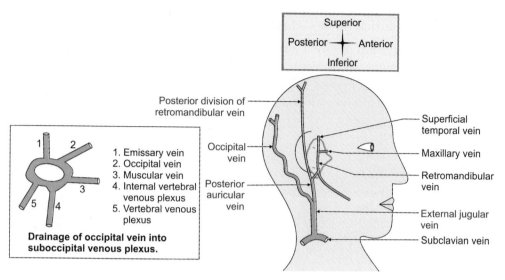

Fig. 2.4: Veins of the scalp draining into external jugular vein

Flowchart 2.2: Veins of the scalp draining into internal and external jugular veins

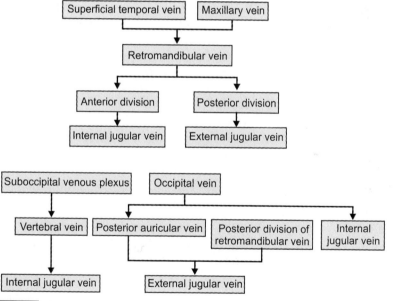

3. **Nerve supply**

A. **Sensory** (Fig. 2.5A)

   a. In front of auricle:

   I. Supraorbital and supratrochlear, branches of ophthalmic division of trigeminal nerve.

   II. Zygomaticotemporal a branch of zygomatic nerve which is a branch of maxillary division of trigeminal nerve.

   III. Auriculotemporal nerve—mandibular division of trigeminal.

b. Behind the auricle ⬤━ GaLeO - Go To

Posterior division of **G**reat **a**uricular nerve (ventral rami of **C2–C3**)
Lesser **O**ccipital nerve. Ventral rami of (**C2**)
Greater **O**ccipital nerve—dorsal ramus of **C2** spinal nerve.
Third **O**ccipital nerve—dorsal ramus of **C3** spinal nerve.

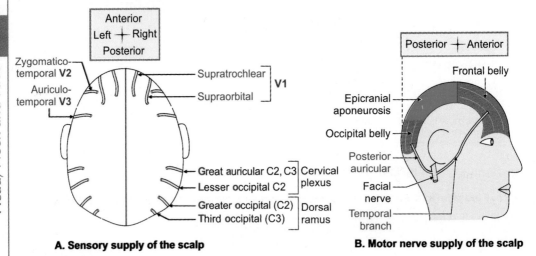

A. Sensory supply of the scalp   **B. Motor nerve supply of the scalp**

Fig. 2.5: Nerve supply of scalp

B. **Motor** (Fig. 2.5B)
   a. In front of the auricle: Temporal branch of facial nerve supplies frontal belly of occipitofrontalis.
   b. Behind the auricle: Posterior auricular branch of facial nerve supplies occipital belly of occipitofrontalis.

4. **Applied anatomy**

➤ **First layer**
   • Skin is thick and hairy. It is the common site of sebaceous cyst.
   • The infection of the scalp behind the ear may cause transverse venous sinus infection. It can be dangerous or fatal.

➤ **Second layer**
   • The bleeding in second layer is profuse. This is because of two reasons:
     – The scalp has rich blood supply (five arteries on each side),
     – The torn vessels are prevented from constriction because the walls of the blood vessels are adherent to the dense connective tissue. This prevents constriction of vessels.
     – The bleeding can be immediately arrested by compressing against hard bone, i.e. cranium.
     – As all the blood vessels of the scalp run from periphery to centre, bleeding from the scalp can easily be arrested by applying a tourniquet around the head.

➢ **Third layer:** The direction of injury to the scalp decides the rate of healing of the wound. There is rapid healing of the wound in injury parallel to direction of muscle fibres. There is delayed healing of wounds, in injury perpendicular to the muscle fibres.

➢ **Fourth layer**
  • This is the dangerous area of scalp. The infection from this layer spreads to the brain through emissary vein.
  • Accumulation of blood in this layer results in black eye.

➢ **Fifth layer**
  • Bleeding in 5th layer takes the shape of underlying bone. The condition is called **cephalohaematoma**.
  • **Caput succedaneum:** It is oedema occurring in and around scalp of newborn during labour.

OLA-10	Why do the wrinkles of face tend to gap?

As the person ages, the skin loses its elasticity (resilience) which results into wrinkles on the skin. If the skin incision is not parallel to these cleavage or wrinkle lines (Langer lines), it has tendency to gap.

OLA-11	In supranuclear lesion of facial nerve, only the lower part of the face is paralysed. Why the upper part of face is spared?

The supranuclear lesions are also called upper motor neuron lesions. It affects muscles of the lower ½ of the face only. The muscles of the upper ½ of the face are spared because muscles of the upper ½ of the face (muscles of forehead and eyebrows) are supplied by both cerebral hemispheres. This is called bilateral cortical innervation.

LAQ-2	Describe muscles of face under the following headings:
	1. Action,
	2. Nerve supply, and
	3. Applied anatomy

1. **Action:** The muscles of facial expression can be grouped as (mimetic muscles)
   A. **Muscles acting on the orifice of the orbit:** These are subgrouped as constrictor (sphincters) and dilators.
     a. **Frontal belly of occipitofrontalis** is responsible for elevation of eyebrows as in an expression of surprise and it also contracts in looking upwards. The action is antagonistic to the orbital part of orbicularis oculi.
     b. **Corrugator supercilii** drags the eyebrow medially and downward and protects the eye from bright sunlight. It produces vertical wrinkles of the forehead.
     c. **Orbicularis oculi** has three parts.
        I. Palpebral part closes the eye gently as in sleep and blinking.
        II. Orbital part closes the eye firmly as in dust storm.
        III. Lacrimal part dilates the lacrimal sac.

Head, Neck and Face

B. **Muscles acting on the orifice of the nose**

    a. **Procerus** (extended, tall). It is extended part of frontalis. It produces transverse wrinkles across bridge of nose as in frowning.

    b. **Nasalis** has two parts.

        I. Transverse part called *compressor naris*. It compresses the nasal aperture.

        II. Alar part called *dilator naris*. It dilates the anterior nasal aperture in deep inspiration.

    c. **Depressor septi** dilates anterior nasal aperture in anger.

Table 2.1: Muscles acting on openings of the face

Openings	Closing (sphincter)	Opening (dilator)
• Ocular (eyelids)	• Orbicularis oculi • Corrugator supercilii (frowning)	• Levator palpebrae superioris • Frontal belly of occipitofrontalis
• Lacrimal sac		• Lacrimal part of orbicularis oculi
• Anterior nasal aperture	• Compressor nasi	• Alar part of nasalis • Depressor septi (anger) • Levator labii superioris alaeque nasi (sadness)
• Oral opening	• Orbicularis oris (closing the mouth)	• Levator labii superioris • Levator labii superioris alaeque nasi (sadness) • Zygomaticus minor (contempt) • Levato ranguli oris (sadness)
• Angle of mouth		• Zygomaticus major (smiling and laughing) • Depressor anguli oris (grief)

C. **Muscles acting on the orifice of the mouth** (Fig. 2.6)

    a. **Closure:** Orbicularis oris closes the mouth.

    b. **Dilators**

        I. Subcutaneous layer: Risorius (*risus*—to laugh).

        II. Superficial layer:

            i. Zygomaticus major draws the angle of mouth upward and laterally as in laughing.

            ii. Zygomaticus minor elevates and everts upper lip.

            iii. Levator labii superioris alaeque nasi elevates and everts the upper lip and dilates the nostril.

        III. Middle layer

            i. Depressor anguli oris draws the angle of mouth downward.

            ii. Levator anguli oris

            iii. Depressor labii inferioris draws angle of mouth downward and somewhat laterally as in expression of irony.

            iv. Levator labii superioris elevates the lip.

IV. Deeper layer

   i. Mentalis protrudes the lower lip.

   ii. Buccinator flattens the cheek and forcibly expels the air between the lips (whistling).

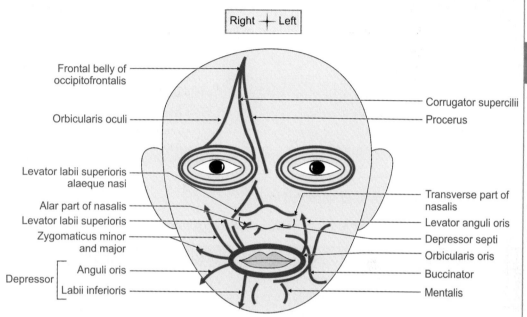

Fig. 2.6: Muscles of the face

2. Nerve supply : The muscles of the face are developed from 2nd pharyngeal arch and the nerve of the 2nd pharyngeal arch is facial nerve. Hence, all the muscles are supplied by facial nerve.

3. Applied anatomy

Table 2.2: Differences between upper motor neuron and lower motor neuron lesions

Particulars	Upper motor neuron lesion	Lower motor neuron lesion
• Synonym	• Supranuclear facial palsy.	• Infranuclear facial palsy, e.g. Bell's palsy
• Site of lesion	• Above the facial nerve nucleus, i.e. damage of corticonuclear fibres in the internal capsule.	• At and below the facial nerve nucleus, i.e. facial nerve
• Muscles paralysed	• Muscles of lower half of the face of the opposite side are paralysed.	• Muscles of the whole face of the same side.
• Clinical features	• Asymmetry of the face	• Asymmetry of the face

Head, Neck and Face

Contd.

Head, Neck and Face

Table 2.2: Differences between upper motor neuron and lower motor neuron lesions (Contd.)

Particulars	Upper motor neuron lesion	Lower motor neuron lesion
	• Inability of angle of mouth to move upwards. • Loss of nasolabial fold • Accumulation of food in the vestibule of the mouth • Dribbling of saliva • Inability to inflate the cheek laterally. • Able to close the eye • **Able to wrinkle the forehead**	• Inability of angle of mouth to move upwards. • Loss of nasolabial fold. • Accumulation of food in the vestibule of the mouth. • Dribbling of saliva • Inability to inflate the cheek laterally. • Inability to close the eye. • **Inability to wrinkle the forehead**

SN-25   Sensory nerve supply of the face

Table 2.3: Sensory nerve supply of the face (Fig. 2.7)

Source	Cutaneous nerve	Area of distribution
• Ophthalmic division of trigeminal nerve	• Supratrochlear nerve • Supraorbital nerve • Lacrimal nerve • Infratrochlear nerve • External nasal nerve	• Scalp up to vertex • Forehead • Upper eyelid • Conjunctiva • Root, dorsum and tip of nose.
• Maxillary division of trigeminal nerve	• Infraorbital nerve • Zygomaticofacial nerve • Zygomaticotemporal nerve	• Upper lip • Side and ala of nose • Lower eyelid, • Upper part of cheek • Anterior part of temple.
• Mandibular division of trigeminal nerve	• Auriculotemporal nerve • Buccal nerve • Mental nerve	• Lower lip, chin, lower part of cheek, • Lower jaw except over the angle, and • Lower margin, upper 2/3rd of lateral surface of auricle and side of head.
• Cervical plexus	• Anterior division of great auricular nerve (C2, C3). • Upper division of transverse (anterior) cutaneous nerve of neck (C2, C3).	• Skin over the angle of the jaw and over the parotid gland. • Lower margin of the lower jaw.

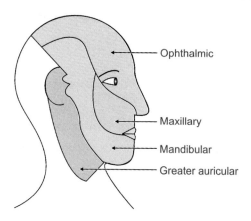

Fig. 2.7: Sensory nerve supply of the face

LAQ-3 **Describe facial vein under the following headings:**
1. Formation; 2. Relations; 3. Tributaries; 4. Termination; 5. Applied anatomy

1. **Formation:** The angular vein receives superior labial vein and continues as facial vein.

2. **Relations**
   A. It lies deep to
      a. Zygomaticus major,
      b. Risorius, and
      c. Platysma.
   B. From above downwards, it lies superficial to
      a. Buccinator,
      b. Body of mandible,
      c. Masseter,
      d. Submandibular gland,
      e. Posterior belly of digastric, and
      f. Stylohyoid muscle.
   C. At termination, it crosses: a. Internal carotid artery, b. External carotid artery, c. Hypoglossal nerve, and d. Loop of lingual artery.

3. **Tributaries**
   A. Superior ophthalmic vein,
   B. Vein from alar nasi,
   C. Superior labial vein,
   D. Buccal vein,
   E. Deep facial vein from pterygoid plexus,
   F. Inferior labial vein,
   G. Masseteric vein,

Head, Neck and Face

H. Tonsillar vein,

   I. Submental vein, and

   J. Submandibular vein

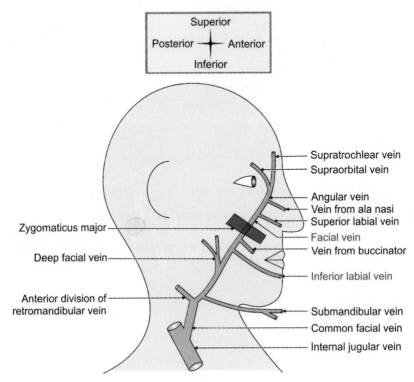

Fig. 2.8: Tributaries of the facial vein

4. **Termination:** Common facial vein terminates into internal jugular vein.

5. Applied anatomy

> Infection of the face can spread to intracranial venous sinus. Hence, the veins draining

Upper lip

Septum of nose, and

Adjoining nose lying between angular and deep facial veins forms the dangerous area of the face.

   ⚷ USA is the dangerous area of face.

> Following are the routes for the spread of infection.
   - Angular vein ✦ superior ophthalmic vein ✦ cavernous sinus.
   - Deep facial vein ✦ pterygoid venous plexus ✦ emissary vein ✦ cavernous sinus.
> The spread of septic emboli from the infected area to cavernous sinus can cause serious complications because of following reasons.

- Veins of the face do not have valves.
- Veins of the face lie on facial muscles.
- There is no deep fascia on the face.
- The movements of the facial muscles may facilitate the spread of septic emboli to cavernous sinus.

OLA-12 Why the facial muscles are called "muscles of facial expression"?

The muscles of face are not inserted on bone but in the skin. Since there is no deep fascia in the face, contraction of these muscles causes contraction of some part of skin on the face. It acts as a medium to express the emotional feelings. Hence, facial muscles are called muscles of facial expression.

OLA-13 What is the nerve supply of facial muscles?

1. All the muscles on the face are supplied by facial nerve except levator palpebrae superioris which is supplied by oculomotor nerve.
2. Majority of the muscles on the face are muscles of facial expression. However, there are exceptions. These are buccinator and platysma. They are supplied by facial nerve.
3. The muscles present on the face but included as muscles of mastication are temporalis, masseter, medial and lateral pterygoid. These are supplied by mandibular nerve, branch of trigeminal nerve (Vth cranial nerve).

SN-26 Deep facial vein

Introduction: It is a communicating channel that connects the facial vein to pterygoid venous plexus (Fig. 2.9).

1. **Course:** It leaves the facial vein before it crosses the lateral surface of masseter and to the ramus of mandible.
2. **Communications:** It is connected to the cavernous sinus by the emissary veins passing through the
   A. Foramen lacerum,
   B. Foramen ovale, and
   C. Foramen spinosum.
3. **Peculiarities:** It has no valves.
4. Applied anatomy
   ➢ The dangerous area of face lies between angular and deep facial veins.
   ➢ The infection from the upper lip and the lower part of the nose can spread through the deep facial vein and cause cavernous sinus thrombosis. The movements of the facial muscles may facilitate the spread of septic emboli.

Head, Neck and Face

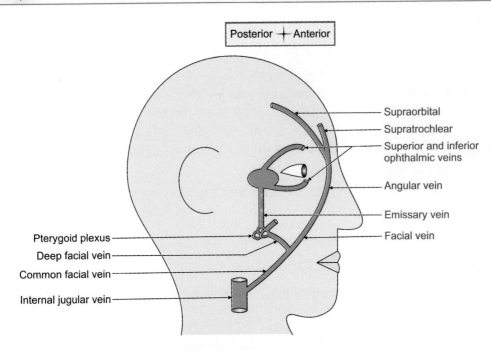

Fig. 2.9: Deep facial vein

SN-27   Dangerous area of face

Infection of the face can spread to intracranial venous sinus. Hence, the veins draining the following area is called dangerous area of face.

1. **Area:** [⚿━ USA]

   <u>U</u>pper lip.

   <u>S</u>eptum of nose.

   <u>A</u>djoining part of nose and lip lying between angular and deep facial veins forms the dangerous area of the face (Fig. 2.10).

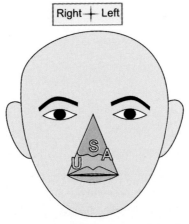

Fig. 2.10: Dangerous area of the face

2. **Following are the routes for the spread of infection.**
   A. Facial vein ✦ deep facial vein ✦ pterygoid venous plexus ✦ cavernous sinus.
   B. Angular vein ✦ superior ophthalmic vein ✦ cavernous sinus.
3. The spread of septic emboli from the infected area to cavernous sinus can cause serious complications because of following reasons.
   A. Veins of the face do not have valves.
   B. Veins of the face directly lie on the muscles of face.
   C. There is no deep fascia on the face.
   D. The movements of the facial muscles may facilitate the spread of septic emboli to cavernous sinus.

OLA-14 What are the constituents of lacrimal apparatus?

It consists of
1. Lacrimal gland
   A. Orbital part, and
   B. Palpebral part
2. Conjunctival sac
3. Punctum
4. Canaliculus
   A. Superior, and
   B. Inferior canaliculus
5. Lacrimal sac
6. Nasolacrimal duct

OLA-15 What are the structural differences between lacrimal gland and serous salivary gland?

Table 2.4: Structural differences between lacrimal gland and serous salivary gland

Particulars	Lacrimal gland	Serous salivary gland
• **Shape of acini**	• Larger • Irregular and elongated	• ▲ lar in shape • Apical cytoplasm is eosinophilic due to the presence of eosinophilic granules called zymogen granules • Cytoplasm at the base of each cell is basophilic. • The secretion of serous acini is watery
• **Lumina**	• Wider	• Small
• **Myoepithelial cells**	• Present between glandular epithelium and basement membrane	• Spindle ⬤ shaped cells with oval ⬤ nuclei • They are located within the basal lamina of the secretory acini and

Contd.

Head, Neck and Face

Table 2.4: Structural differences between lacrimal gland and serous salivary gland (Contd.)

Particulars	Lacrimal gland	Serous salivary gland
		the ducts of the glands. Contraction in these cells propels the secretions from the acini and the duct.
• **Lining epithelium of smaller duct (intralobular excretory duct)**	• Cuboidal epithelium	• Intercalate (inserted or placed between) Simple cuboidal epithelium. • Striated: Simple cuboidal epithelium; cells have basal striations.
• **Lining epithelium of bigger duct (interlobular excretory duct)**	• Columnar or pseudostratified	• Simple columnar epithelium in small ducts and stratified columnar epithelium in large ducts

OLA-16 D/L microscopic structure of serous demilune

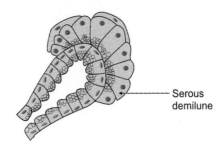

Serous demilune

Fig. 2.11: Serous demilune

OLA-17 Enumerate the difference between serous and mucus acini.

Table 2.5: Difference between serous and mucus acini

Particulars	Serous acini	Mucous acini
• **Cells**	• ▲ lar	• Tall
• **Nucleus**	• Round nucleus at base	• Flat nucleus at the base
• **Cytoplasm at the apex**	• Eosinophilic due to the presence of eosinophilic granules	• Cells appear pale as the cytoplasm does not stain well. Cells appear empty.
• **Cytoplasm at the base**	• Basophilic	—
• **Lumen**	• Small	• Larger as compared to serous acini.
• **Type of secretion**	• Watery	• Thick

OLA-18 What are serous demilunes?

1. Some of mucous acini are capped with serous cells.
2. They are arranged as a half moon.
3. Hence, they are called serous demilunes.

OLA-19 **Where do we get myoepithelial cells in the body? How will you identify them?**

1. Site
   A. **Ducts:** Between the epithelium and the basement membrane of the ducts.
   B. **Sweat gland:** There are cuboidal secretory cells of the sweat gland. At the base of the secretory cells, there are numerous myoepithelial cells.
   C. **Identifying features** (Fig. 2.12):
      a. The cells are thin and spindle ⬭ shaped.
      b. They are located at the base of the secretory cells.

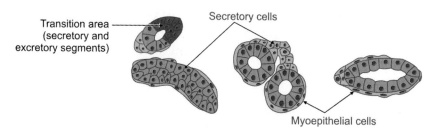

Fig. 2.12: Cross-section and three-dimensional appearance of an eccrine sweat gland. Stain: hematoxylin and eosin. Low magnification

OLA-20 **What are the functions of saliva?**

1. The saliva lubricates the luminal surface of the upper digestive and respiratory tracts.
2. It moistens the food to help in deglutination.
3. It initiates digestion of carbohydrates by the enzyme salivary amylase.
4. It contains lysozyme and immunoglobulin. They are bactericidal in nature.

LAQ-4 **Describe lacrimal apparatus under the following heads:**
1. Components,
2. Blood supply,
3. Nerve supply, and
4. Applied anatomy

1. **Components:** Lacrimal gland with ducts, conjunctival sac, lacrimal caruncle, lacrimal punctate, lacrimal canaliculus, lacrimal sac and nasolacrimal duct.
   A. **Lacrimal gland:** Table 2.6 shows different parts of lacrimal gland.

Table 2.6: Orbital and palpebral parts of lacrimal gland

Particulars	Orbital part	Palpebral part
• Location	• Medial surface of frontal process of zygomatic bone (lacrimal fossa)	• Below levator palpebrae superioris
• Shape	• Almond 🥜	• Flat
• No. of ducts	• 4–5	• 8

Head, Neck and Face

a. **Functions of lacrimal fluid (tears):** $\boxed{\text{⦿━ TEARS}}$

Maintains Transparency of cornea

Expresses emotion,

Acts as bactericidal,

Renders nourishment to cornea,

Keeps the orbital Surface of conjunctiva moist.

B. **Conjunctiva**

a. **Gross features:** It is transparent membrane covering sclera and lining the inner surface of eyelid.

b. **Conjunctival sac:** It is a potential space between two eyelids and cornea/sclera in the closed position of eyelids. It consists of

   I. *Orbital part* which is in contact with the sclera and cornea.

   II. *Palpebral part:* It is highly vascular, adherent to tarsal plate. It lines the eyelid.

c. **Nerve supply**

   I. Ophthalmic division of trigeminal nerve.

   II. Maxillary division of trigeminal nerve.

d. **Blood supply**: Palpebral branch of ophthalmic artery.

C. **Puncta with lacrimal canaliculi:** Each lacrimal canaliculus begins with punctum.

a. Length of canaliculus:10 mm. It has

   I. Vertical part—2 mm

   II. Horizontal part—8 mm

b. It is lined by stratified squamous non-keratinized epithelium. It opens in the lateral wall of lacrimal sac behind medial palpebral ligament.

D. **Lacrimal sac:** It is a membranous sac, continues with nasolacrimal duct. It is a blind pouch. Superiorly, it measures 12 × 5 mm. It continues inferiorly with nasolacrimal duct.

E. **Relations of lacrimal sac** (Fig. 2.13)

a. **Anterior**

   I. Medial palpebral ligament.

   II. Orbicularis oculi muscle.

b. **Medially:** Lacrimal groove.

c. **Laterally:** Lacrimal fascia and lacrimal part of orbicularis oculi.

F. **Nasolacrimal duct:** It is a membranous passage of 18 mm long. It runs from the lower end of lacrimal sac and opens in the inferior meatus of nose. The lower end of the duct is guarded by valve of Hasner. It prevents backward flow of fluid.

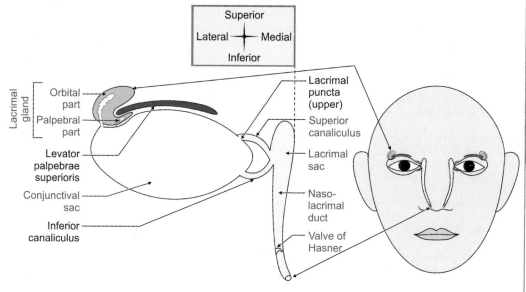

Fig. 2.13: Right lacrimal apparatus

2. **Blood supply**

A. Arterial supply: Lacrimal artery, branch of ophthalmic artery.

B. Venous drainage: Lacrimal vein drains into ophthalmic vein.

3. Nerve supply

A. **Sensory:** The sensations are carried by lacrimal branch of ophthalmic division of trigeminal nerve.

B. **Sympathetic:** It is vasomotor in function (Fig. 2.14).
   a. Preganglionic fibres arise from spinal cord (T1–T5 segments) and goes to superior cervical sympathetic ganglion.
   b. Postganglionic fibres are the plexus around internal carotid artery and around ophthalmic artery.

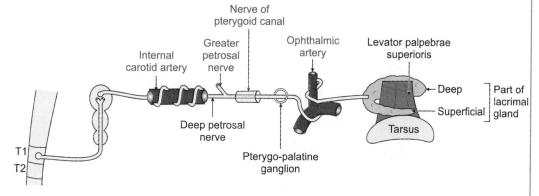

Fig. 2.14: Sympathetic fibres of lacrimal gland

Head, Neck and Face

C. **Parasympathetic nerve** is secretomotor in function (Fig. 2.15). It is carried by facial nerve → pterygopalatine ganglion → maxillary nerve (VII— pterygopalatine ganglion—V2).

   a. Preganglionic fibres arising from lacrimatory nucleus present in the pons, pass via facial nerve, greater petrosal nerve and joins with deep petrosal nerve to form nerve to pterygoid canal. The fibres are relayed in the pterygopalatine ganglion.

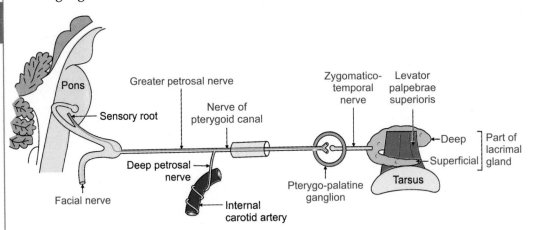

Fig. 2.15: Secretomotor fibres of lacrimal gland

   b. Postganglionic fibres pass through maxillary nerve (zygomaticotemporal)— lacrimal nerve—lacrimal gland.

4. **Applied anatomy**

   ➤ **Dacryoadenitis** (*dacryo*—tear) is the inflammation of lacrimal gland.
   ➤ **Dacryocystitis** is inflammation of lacrimal sac and presents with pain, oedema and redness.
   ➤ **Dacryocystectomy** is removal of lacrimal sac.
   ➤ Removal of palpebral part is equal to the removal of entire gland because the ducts of the orbital part pass through palpebral part.
   ➤ **Epiphora** (*Epiphora*—sudden burst)—overflow of tears.

OLA-21 **What is dacryocystitis?**

Inflammation of the lacrimal sac is called dacrocystitis.

OLA-22 **What is nature of lacrimal gland?**

It is serous gland.

OLA-23 **What are the parts of lacrimal gland?**

1. Orbital part
2. Palpebral part

SN-28   **Orbicularis oculi**

(*Orbiculus*—orbit, *oculi*—eyeball)

Introduction: It is a muscle of face, the sphincter of orbital fissure.

1. **Attachments:** It has three parts:

    A. **Palpebral part:** It is confined to the lids. It arises from medial palpebral ligament. It is inserted into lateral palpebral raphe.

    B. **Orbital part:** It extends beyond orbit. It arises from

       a. Nasal part of frontal bone

       b. Anterior lacrimal crest

       c. Frontal process of maxilla: It forms concentric rings and return to the point of origin.

    C. **Lacrimal part** (deeper part): It is attached medially to the

       a. Posterior lacrimal crest, and

       b. Lacrimal sac,

       c. They are inserted into upper and lower eyelids.

2. **Nerve supply**

    A. Mainly by zygomatic branch of facial nerve.

    B. It is also supplied by temporal branch of facial nerve.

3. **Actions**

    A. Palpebral part closes the eyelid gently.

    B. Orbital and palpebral parts together closes the eyelid forcibly.

    C. Levator palpebrae superioris is the opponent of upper palpebral fibres of orbicularis oculi.

    Occipitofrontalis opposes the orbital part.

4. **Development:** They are developed from the mesoderm of the 2nd pharyngeal arch.

5. **Applied anatomy:** Infranuclear lesion of the facial nerve leads to paralysis of orbicularis oculi. Hence, the patient cannot close the eyelid tightly. Frequent closure of eyelids is required for the normal drainage of tears through the lacrimal ducts. Due to paralysis of orbicularis oculi, there is overflowing of tears through the eyelid and expose keratitis.

OLA-24   **Enumerate the branches of facial artery on the face**

1. Inferior labial,

2. Superior labial,

3. Lateral nasal, and

4. Angular artery.

LAQ-5 **Describe facial nerve under the following headings:**

1. Course and relations

2. Branches

3. Applied anatomy

It is a nerve of 2nd pharyngeal arch.

1. **Course and relations**

A. **Intraneuronal** (Fig. 2.16)

a. Motor root arises from motor nuclei of facial nerve situated in deep part of pons. It winds around abducent nucleus. It forms a bulging in the floor of IVth ventricle called facial colliculus. It is due to the phenomenon of neurobiotaxis. The nerve fibres have a tendency to migrate in the direction from which they receive their stimuli.

b. Sensory root (nervus intermedius) is formed by

I. Superior salivatory nucleus and lacrimatory nucleus.

II. Nucleus tractus solitarius.

Both the roots emerge at the junction of pons and olive.

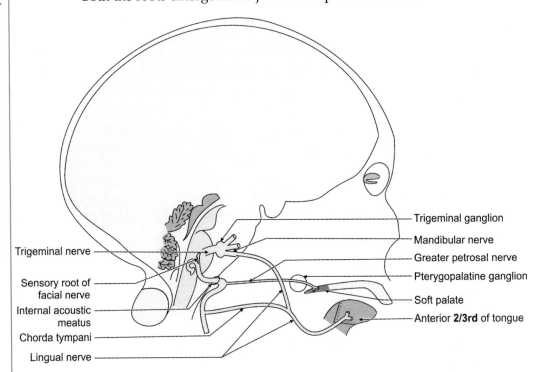

Fig. 2.16: Facial nerve showing taste sensation fibres of anterior two-thirds of tongue

B. **Extraneuronal:** Divided into three parts (Fig. 2.17)

a. First part: It passes through the internal acoustic meatus. It reaches anterosuperior angle of the medial wall of the middle ear cavity. It bends to form second part. It forms a bulging at the bend called geniculate ganglion.

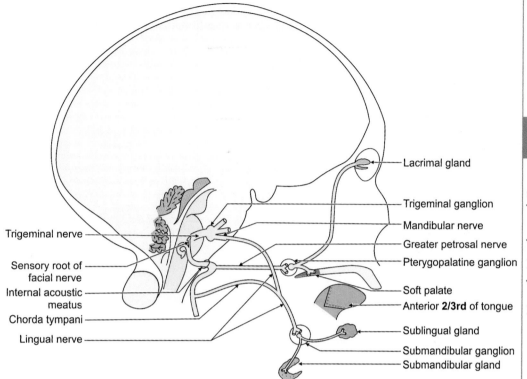

Lacrimal gland

Trigeminal ganglion

Mandibular nerve

Greater petrosal nerve

Pterygopalatine ganglion

Trigeminal nerve

Sensory root of facial nerve

Internal acoustic meatus

Chorda tympani

Lingual nerve

Soft palate

Anterior **2/3rd** of tongue

Sublingual gland

Submandibular ganglion

Submandibular gland

Fig. 2.17: Facial nerve showing secretomotor fibres to the glands

    b. Second part: It runs horizontally backwards along medial wall of tympanic cavity. It lies above promontory and fenestra vetibuli and runs to the posterior part of medial wall.

    c. Third part: It is posterior to posterior wall of middle ear cavity. Runs vertically downwards and comes outside the cranium through stylomastoid foramen.

  C. **Extracranial:** It turns anteriorly and pierces the posteromedial surface of parotid gland. It emerges from anteromedial surface of parotid gland.

  D. **Terminates in the parotid gland:** By dividing into terminal branches.

2. Branches

  A. **Intracranial**

    a. First part: No branches:

    b. At the junction of 1st and 2nd parts, greater petrosal nerve arises. It carries secretomotor fibres to the lacrimal gland.

    c. Second part:

      I. Sympathetic branches to middle meningeal artery.

      II. Branch to lesser petrosal nerve, by which it reaches the otic ganglion.

    d. Third part:

      I. Stapedial branch: It passes through small canal and supplies stapedius muscle.

II. **Chorda tympani nerve:** It joins lingual nerve and carries taste fibres from anterior 2/3rd of tongue. It also carries secretomotor fibres to submandibular gland (Figs 2.18 and 2.19).

III. **Communicating branch to vagus.**

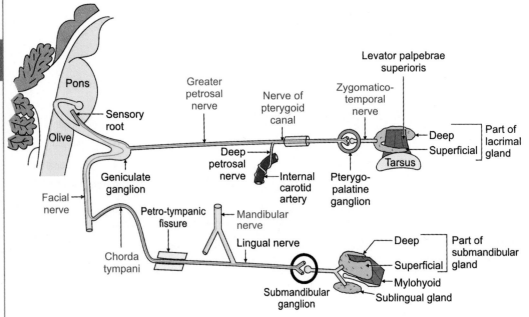

Fig. 2.18: Secretomotor fibres of facial nerve

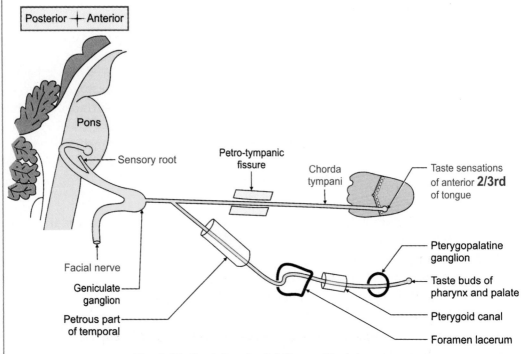

Fig. 2.19: Gustatory (taste) fibres of facial nerve

B. **Extracranial**

a. Posterior auricular branch gives communicating branch to great auricular and lesser occipital. It divides into

I. Auricular branch to auricularis posterior.

II. Occipital branch to occipital belly of occipitofrontalis.

b. Digastric branch to posterior belly of digastric.

c. Stylohyoid branch to stylohyoid muscle.

C. **Terminal**

a. Temporal branch to

I. Frontal belly of occipitofrontalis,

II. Muscles of external ear

i. Auricularis superior

ii. Auricularis anterior

III. Corrugator supercilii.

b. Zygomatic branch to orbicularis oculi

c. Buccal

I. Upper (lower zygomatic)

i. Zygomaticus major

ii. Zygomaticus minor

iii. Levator labii superioris

iv. Levator labii superioris alaequae nasi

v. Levator anguli oris

II. Lower

i. Buccinator

ii. Orbicularis oris

d. Mandibular branch to risorius.

e. Cervical branch to platysma (Fig. 2.20)

D. **Pes anserinus** (*pes*—foot, *anser*—goose)[NEET]: Branches of the facial nerve in the substance of parotid gland form a network called pes anserinus. This divides the parotid gland into superficial and deep parts.

Box 2.2

Pes anserinus

1. Branches of facial nerve
2. Muscles attached to upper part of medial surface of tibia.

---

3. Applied anatomy : Upper and lower motor neuron lesion of facial nerve (Fig. 2.21). Refer SN-29, 30 and 31.

Head, Neck and Face

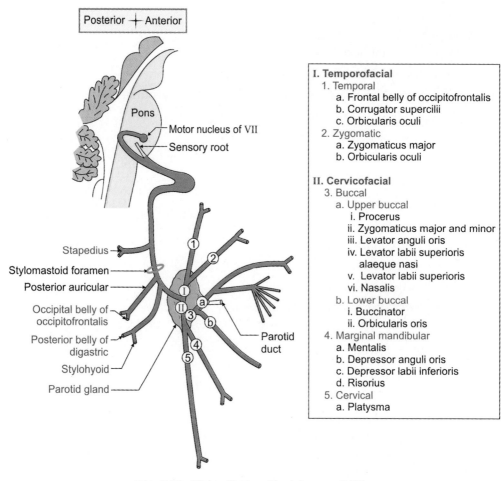

Posterior — Anterior

Pons
Motor nucleus of VII
Sensory root

Stapedius
Stylomastoid foramen
Posterior auricular
Occipital belly of occipitofrontalis
Posterior belly of digastric
Stylohyoid
Parotid gland

Parotid duct

I. **Temporofacial**
  1. Temporal
    a. Frontal belly of occipitofrontalis
    b. Corrugator supercilii
    c. Orbicularis oculi
  2. Zygomatic
    a. Zygomaticus major
    b. Orbicularis oculi

II. **Cervicofacial**
  3. Buccal
    a. Upper buccal
      i. Procerus
      ii. Zygomaticus major and minor
      iii. Levator anguli oris
      iv. Levator labii superioris alaeque nasi
      v. Levator labii superioris
      vi. Nasalis
    b. Lower buccal
      i. Buccinator
      ii. Orbicularis oris
  4. Marginal mandibular
    a. Mentalis
    b. Depressor anguli oris
    c. Depressor labii inferioris
    d. Risorius
  5. Cervical
    a. Platysma

Fig. 2.20: Motor fibres of facial nerve (VIII)

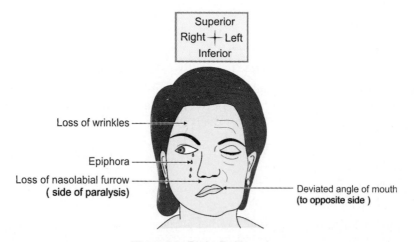

Superior
Right — Left
Inferior

Loss of wrinkles
Epiphora
Loss of nasolabial furrow (side of paralysis)
Deviated angle of mouth (to opposite side)

Fig. 2.21: Right Bell's palsy

Note: While attempting to close the right eye (paralyzed side), the eye does not close and the eyeball rotates superiorly and laterally

SN-29 Upper and lower motor neuron lesions of facial nerve

The difference in the upper and lower motor neuron lesions is displayed in Table 2.7.

Table 2.7: Upper and lower motor neuron lesions of facial nerve

Particulars	Upper motor neuron lesion (supranuclear palsy)	Lower motor neuron lesion (LMNL) (intranuclear palsy)
• Site	• Above the facial nerve nucleus.	• Below the facial nerve nucleus
• Cause of lesion	• Lesion in the genu of internal capsule is due to cerebral haemorrhage	• Damage in the parotid gland • Bell's palsy • Lesion in the middle ear • Tumours in the internal acoustic meatus
• Muscles paralysed	• Muscles of the lower half of the face on opposite side are paralysed	• All the muscles of the same side of the face are paralysed

SN-30 Lower motor neuron lesion of facial nerve

The causes, and manifestation of lower motor lesion are described below.

1. **Lesion of facial nerve distal to stylomastoid foramen:** The lesion of facial nerve is due to vertical incision of the parotid gland.

2. **Lesion of facial nerve at the stylomastoid foramen:** It results in Bell's palsy. The 'Bell's palsy' is the lower motor neuron type of facial palsy (paralysis of muscles of facial expression). It occurs due to inflammation of facial nerve in the facial canal at the stylomastoid foramen. The exact cause of inflammation is not known, but it is thought to be due to viral infection. It causes inflammation and oedema of facial nerve. It results in compression of facial nerve in the facial canal.

   Pain of variable intensity behind the ear precedes facial weakness which develops over 48 hours period.

3. **Characteristic features** (All muscles of whole face are affected on the side of paralysis.)

   A. **Facial asymmetry:** Due to unopposed action of muscles of opposite side.

   B. **Loss of wrinkles on forehead:** Due to paralysis of fronto-occipitalis.

   C. **Inability to close the eye (wide palpebral fissure):** Due to paralysis of orbicularis oculi.

   D. **Inability to move the angle of the mouth upwards** and laterally during laughing due to paralysis of zygomaticus major.

   E. **Loss of nasolabial furrow** due to paralysis of levator labii superioris alaeque nasi.

   F. **Accumulation of food** in the vestibule of the mouth due to paralysis of the buccinator.

   G. **Dribbling of saliva:** Due to paralysis of orbicularis oris.

   H. **Inability to inflate the cheek properly:** Due to paralysis of buccinator muscle.

Head, Neck and Face

4. **Lesion in the vertical course of the facial nerve within the mastoid bone** results in the

   A. Loss of taste sensation on the anterior two-thirds of the tongue on the side of the lesion.

   B. There is loss of secretion from submandibular salivary gland; however, lacrimation and the stapedius reflex would be normal.

   C. A lesion in the middle ear segment of the nerve (tympanic) does not affect lacrimation but results into ipsilateral **hyperacusis** due to paralysis of stapedius.

5. **Lesion at or proximal to the geniculate ganglion (translabyrinthine)** produces diminished lacrimation on the same side, as well as disturbance in function of the other branches. After regeneration, the parasympathetic secretomotor fibres intended for salivary glands grow, and join the secretomotor fibres intended to supply the lacrimal gland; the anticipation of food then produces lacrimation, instead of salivation (**syndrome of crocodile tears or Bogard syndrome**)[NEET]. The specific feature of this syndrome is paroxysmal lacrimation during eating.

6. Exact cause of lesion is not known. Most often it is due to viral infection leading to oedema and inflammation of the nerve.

SN-31   Upper motor neuron lesion

1. **Causes:** It is due to damage of corticonuclear fibres. The lesion may be

   A. Facial nerve nucleus in the pons or

   B. Above the nucleus.

   The main cause is lesion in the internal capsule.

2. **Manifestations:**

   A. Supranuclear lesions produce upper motor neuron type of paralysis. The muscles of the lower half of the face of opposite side are paralysed. The muscles of the upper half of the face are normal because they are bilaterally innervated.

   B. Effects of upper motor neuron lesion: *The patient is able to wrinkle the skin of his forehead, but he is not able to perform the actions of the muscles of lower 1/2 of the face (as they have unilateral innervation from the cerebral hemisphere hence paralyzed).*

OLA-25   What are the functions of buccinator muscle?

1. It flattens cheek against gums and teeth.
2. It prevents accumulation of food in the vestibule.
3. This is the whistling muscle.

Side of the Neck

LAQ-6 Describe investing layer of deep cervical fascia under the following heads:

1. Attachments

2. Features

3. Applied anatomy

It is connective tissue like a cervical collar. It keeps all the structures of the neck in position (Figs 3.1 and 3.2).

1. **Attachments**

   A. **Superiorly**

   a. External occipital protuberance

   b. Superior nuchal line

   c. Mastoid process

   d. Base of mandible

   B. **Inferiorly**

   a. Spine of scapula

   b. Acromion process

   c. Clavicle

   d. Manubrium.

   C. **Anteriorly**

   a. Symphysis menti

   b. Hyoid bone

   c. Oblique line of thyroid cartilage.

2. **Features** (Fig. 3.3)

   A. **Thickness varies**

   a. It is thick over.

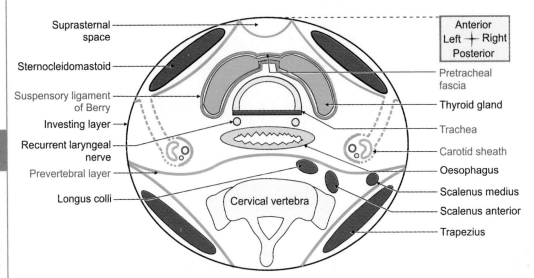

Fig. 3.1: Investing layer of deep cervical fascia

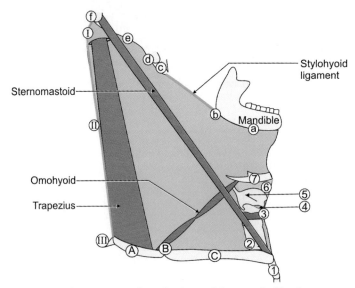

Route of tracings of attachment of investing layer of deep cervical fascia
Anterior inferior ⟶ anterior superior ⟶ posterior superior ⟶ posterior inferior ⟶ anterior inferior

Anteroinferior
1. Manubrium sternum
2. Trachea
3. Cricoid cartilage
4. Cricothyroid membrane
5. Oblique line of thyroid cartilage
6. Thyrohyoid membrane
7. Body of hyoid bone

Posterior
I. External occipital crest
II. Ligamentum nuchae
III. Spine of 7th cervical vertebra

Superior
a. Base of mandible
b. Angle of mandible
c. Styloid process
d. Mastoid process
e. Superior nuchal line
f. External occipital protuberance

Inferior
A. Spine of scapula
B. Acromioclavicular joint
C. Clavicle

Fig. 3.2: Schematic representation of investing layer of deep cervical fascia

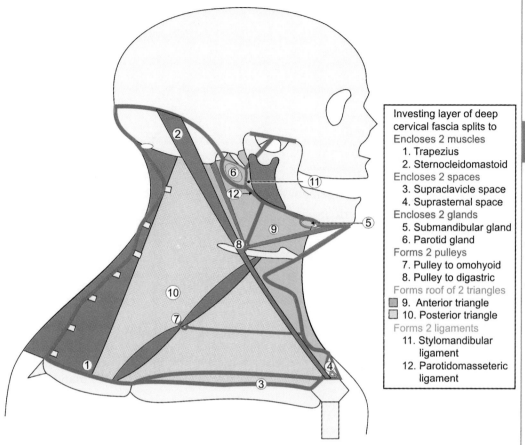

Investing layer of deep
cervical fascia splits to
Encloses 2 muscles
　1. Trapezius
　2. Sternocleidomastoid
Encloses 2 spaces
　3. Supraclavicle space
　4. Suprasternal space
Encloses 2 glands
　5. Submandibular gland
　6. Parotid gland
Forms 2 pulleys
　7. Pulley to omohyoid
　8. Pulley to digastric
Forms roof of 2 triangles
　9. Anterior triangle
　10. Posterior triangle
Forms 2 ligaments
　11. Stylomandibular
　　　ligament
　12. Parotidomasseteric
　　　ligament

Head, Neck and Face

Fig. 3.3: Features of investing layer of deep cervical fascia

　　I. Over parotid gland, called *parotid fascia*.
　　II. Between styloid process and angle of mandible called *stylomandibular* ligament.
　b. It is thin on
　　I. Styloid process,
　　II. Mandible, and
　　III. Tympanic plate.
B. **Magic of** 🔑 **"2"**
　a. Encloses **2** muscles
　　I. Trapezius and
　　II. Sternocleidomastoid.
　b. Encloses **2** salivary glands
　　I. Parotid and
　　II. Submandibular.
　c. Forms **2** laminae

I. Pretracheal and

II. Prevertebral.

d. Forms roof of 2 triangles

I. Anterior and

II. Posterior.

e. Forms 2 spaces

I. Suprasternal and

II. Supraclavicular.

f. Forms 2 structures

I. Stylomandibular ligament and

II. Parotidomasseteric fascia.

g. Forms 2 slings

I. Intermediate tendon of digastric and

II. Omohyoid.

3. Applied anatomy

> **Ludwig's angina:** It is a ▲ lar swelling primarily due to infection of the submandibular with sublingual and submental space. It is limited laterally by two halves of mandible and posteriorly by hyoid bone. This is because of the attachments of investing layer of deep cervical fascia to the base of mandible and hyoid bone.

> **Collar stud abscess:** The abscess is formed deep to deep fascia. The main cause is tuberculosis of deep cervical lymph nodes. It leads to caseation of lymph nodes. The abscess accumulates in deeper layer and penetrates deep fascia and points in the superficial layer called collar stud abscess.

> **Mumps:** Viral infection of the parotid gland is called *mumps*. The fascia over parotid gland is thick and closely adherent. The inflammation or abscess of the gland does not have space for expansion. The capsule is stretched and the nerves are stimulated. Hence, the infection of the parotid gland is painful.

SN-32   Applied anatomy of deep fascia of neck

1. The investing layer of deep cervical fascia is fixed to hyoid bone. Any collection of blood, pus, serum or abscess in the subcutaneous tissue of the suprahyoid area does not descend below the hyoid bone.

2. Pus collected from caries of cervical vertebrae may travel

   A. Axillary sheath: First it appears in the axilla and then in the arm.

   B. Pharyngeal wall: It travels in the superior mediastinum and appears as a midline swelling. It is seen when the mouth is opened.

   C. In the thorax: It presents as a swelling in the superior mediastinum.

3. Carotid sheath is frequently exposed in block dissection of the neck during surgical removal of deep cervical lymph nodes.

4. When the neck is extended, the carotid sheath retracts backwards. Hence, suicidal attempt by sharp cutting weapons often fails to reach the carotid arteries.
5. **Thyroid Swelling moves with Swallowing but does not Swift (move) on protrusion of tongue.**
6. The abscess in the floor of mouth is drained by a deep incision below the mandible by dividing the mylohyoid muscle.
7. The blood vessels in the deep fascia do not contract and tend to bleed profusely.
8. Injury in the suprasternal space of Burn ruptures anterior jugular vein and results into air embolism which may be fatal.

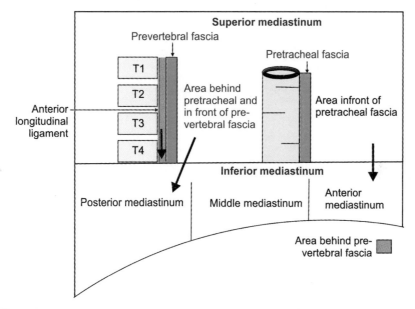

Fig. 3.4: Pathology in the superior mediastinum has three roots: (1) Anterior to pretracheal fasica leads to anterior mediastinum; (2) Posterior to pretracheal fascia and anterior to prevertebral fascia leads to posterior mediastium; (3) Posterior to prevertebral fascia leads to superior mediastinum

SN-33   Suprasternal space (space of Burns)

Introduction: It is the space above the sternum (Fig. 3.5).
1. **Formation:** It is formed by two laminae of investing layer of deep cervical fascia (Fig. 3.6).
2. **Attachments:** It is attached to anterior and posterior borders of jugular notch.
3. **Contents**
   A. *Muscles:* Sternal heads of right and left sternomastoid.
   B. *Veins*
      a. Jugular venous arch and
      b. Anterior jugular vein
   C. *Suprasternal lymph nodes*
   D. *Interclavicular ligaments*

Head, Neck and Face

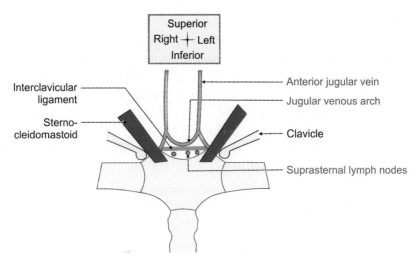

Fig. 3.5: Suprasternal space

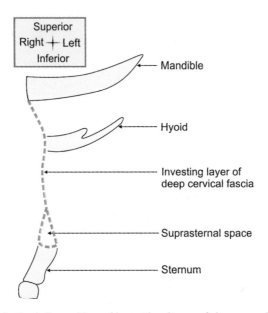

Fig. 3.6: Vertical disposition of investing layer of deep cervical fascia

SN-34   Pretracheal fascia

The condensed deep cervical fascia in front of trachea is called pretracheal fascia.

1. **Attachments** (Fig. 3.7)

    A. **Superiorly**

        a. Hyoid bone in the median plane,

        b. Oblique line of thyroid cartilage, and

        c. Cricoid cartilage, more laterally.

B. **Inferiorly**

a. Below the thyroid gland, it encloses the inferior thyroid veins. It passes behind the brachiocephalic veins, and finally blends with the arch of the aorta.

b. On either side, it fuses with the carotid sheath deep to the sternomastoid.

2. **Other features**

A. On either side, it sends septa which connect the thyroid gland to the cricoid cartilage and form a suspensory ligament of the thyroid gland. It is called ligament of Berry. Hence, the thyroid gland moves with deglutition.

B. The ligaments are attached chiefly to the cricoid cartilage and may extend to thyroid cartilage.NEET

C. It supports the thyroid gland and do not let it sink into the mediastinum.

D. The capsule of the thyroid gland is very weak along the posterior borders of the lateral lobes. Hence, the thyroid gland can enlarge posteriorly and compress oesophagus and produces dysphagia.

3. **Functions**

A. The fascia provides a slippery surface for free movements of the trachea during swallowing.

B. It forms neurovascular sheath to carotid vessels.

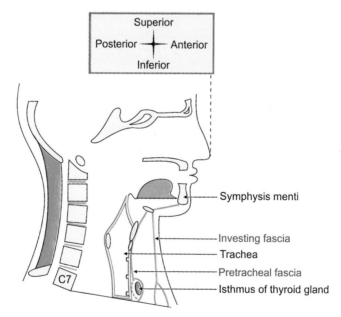

Fig. 3.7: Vertical disposition of pretracheal fascia

4. **Applied anatomy**

➤ Thyroid swelling moves with swallowing but does not shift on protrusion of tongue.

➤ The abscess present in front of pretracheal fascia descends in the anterior mediastinum.

➤ The abscess present behind the pretracheal fascia descends to the posterior mediastinum.

Head, Neck and Face

SN-35   Prevertebral fascia

It is a deep fascia of neck, present in front or anterior to the cervical and 1st four thoracic vertebrae (Fig. 3.8).

1. **Attachments**
    A. **Superiorly:** Base of skull.
    B. **Posteriorly:** Anterior longitudinal ligament of body of 3rd and 4th thoracic vertebrae.
    C. **Laterally:** Gets lost deep to trapezius.

2. **Features**
    A. It splits into anterior and posterior layers.
        a. Anterior layer is called alar fascia. It fuses with buccopharyngeal fascia.
        b. Posterior layer is firmly attached to anterior longitudinal ligament.
    B. It encloses vertebral muscles.
    C. It forms the floor of posterior triangle.
    D. It contributes axillary sheath (cervicoaxillary canal).
    (*It does not invest subclavian and axillary veins which lie in the loose areolar tissue*).

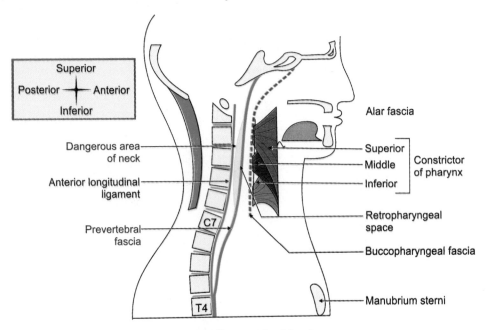

Fig. 3.8: Prevertebral fascia

3. **Structures piercing**
    A. Great auricular nerve (**C2, C3**). ⎤
    B. Lesser occipital nerve (**C2**).   ⎬ Cutaneous branches of cervical plexus
    C. Transverse cervical nerve and   ⎟
    D. Supraclavicular nerves.   ⎦
    Ref. LAQ-7, Fig. 3.10

Head, Neck and Face

4. **Relations**

   A. **Anteriorly:** Retropharyngeal space.

   B. **Superficial**

      a. Accessory nerve (**XIth** cranial nerve)

      b. Lymph nodes of posterior triangle.

   C. **Deep**

      a. Muscles forming floor of triangle.

      b. Cervical plexus.

      c. Trunks of brachial plexus.

      d. 3rd part of subclavian artery.

5. **Functions:** To provide a smooth base for gliding movements of pharynx, oesophagus and carotid sheath during movements of neck and during swallowing.

6. Applied anatomy

   ➤ There is dangerous area of the neck. It is bounded anteriorly by anterior layer of alar fascia and posteriorly by posterior layer of prevertebral fascia.

   ➤ The abscess formed behind the prevertebral fascia travel down into superior mediastinum up to **T3–T4.**

   ➤ The abscess formed infront of prevertebral fascia travel to superior mediastinum and then the posterior mediastinum.

SN-36   Carotid sheath

It is a condensation of deep cervical fascia around carotid artery and internal jugular vein (Fig. 3.9).

1. **Extent:** It extends from base of skull to the arch of the aorta.

2. **Formation:** It is formed by all the layers of deep cervical fascia.[NEET]

   A. Anterior wall is formed by pretracheal fascia.

   B. Posterior wall is formed by prevertebral fascia, and

   C. Investing layer of deep cervical fascia.

3. **Thickness:** It is thick around artery and thin around vein to allow free expansion during increased venous return.

4. **Relations**

   A. Anteriorly: Ansa cervicalis within the wall of the sheath.

   B. Posteriorly: Sympathetic trunk behind the sheath.

5. **Contents**

   A. Internal carotid artery in the upper part of sheath.

   B. Common carotid artery in the lower part of sheath.

   C. Internal jugular vein behind the internal or common carotid artery.

   D. Vagus nerve posteriorly and in between artery and vein.

   E. Deep cervical lymph nodes.

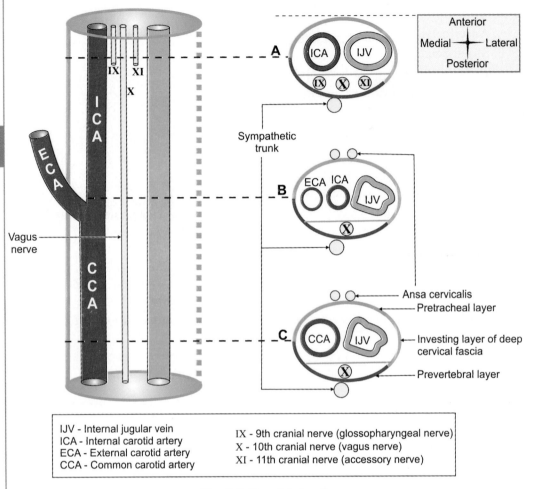

IJV - Internal jugular vein
ICA - Internal carotid artery
ECA - External carotid artery
CCA - Common carotid artery

IX - 9th cranial nerve (glossopharyngeal nerve)
X - 10th cranial nerve (vagus nerve)
XI - 11th cranial nerve (accessory nerve)

Fig. 3.9: Carotid sheath

6. Applied anatomy

> Carotid sheath frequently exposed in block dissection of the neck during surgical removal of deep cervical lymph nodes.
> Infection or inflammation of adjacent structures may involve carotid sheath. It may produce symptoms of
> • Thrombosis of internal jugular vein.
> • Compression of 11th to 12th cranial nerves.
> Carotid body tumour (potato tumour) arises from carotid body.[NEET]

OLA-26 Name the muscles forming floor of the posterior triangle.

1. Splenius capitis.
2. Levator scapulae.
3. Scalenus medius.
4. Semispinalis capitis—occasionally

OLA-27 Name the boundaries of posterior triangle of neck

1. **Anteriorly:** Posterior border of sternocleidomastoid.
2. **Posteriorly:** Anterior border of trapezius.
3. **Base:** Middle one-third of clavicle.
4. **Apex:** Meeting point of sternocleidomastoid and trapezius at superior nuchal line.

LAQ-7 Describe posterior triangle under the following headings:
1. **Boundaries,**
2. **Subdivisions,**
3. **Roof,**
4. **Floor,**
5. **Contents, and**
6. **Applied anatomy.**

1. **Boundaries**
    A. **Anteriorly:** Posterior border of sternocleidomastoid.
    B. **Posteriorly:** Anterior border of trapezius.
    C. **Base:** Middle one-third of clavicle.
    D. **Apex:** Meeting point of sternocleidomastoid and trapezius at superior nuchal line.
2. **Subdivisions:** It is subdivided by inferior belly of omohyoid into
    A. **Occipital triangle**
    B. **Subclavian or supraclavicular triangle**
3. **Roof**
    A. Skin.
    B. Superficial fascia.
    C. Investing layer of deep cervical fascia.
    D. Platysma forms the lower and anterior part of roof.
    E. Roof is pierced by
        a. Nerve: The arrow in front of nerves indicates the direction of nerves (Fig. 3.10)
            I. Lesser occipital, ←
            II. Great auricular, ↑
            III. Transverse cutaneous nerve of neck, →
            IV. Supraclavicular nerves. ↓
        b. Veins: External jugular vein and its tributaries.
        c. Lymph vessels.

Head, Neck and Face

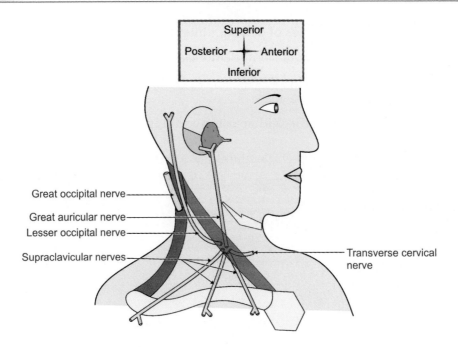

Fig. 3.10: Nerves in roof of posterior triangle of neck

4. **Floor:** Mainly formed by 2nd layer of muscles of neck (above downwards). These muscles are carpeted by deep fascia of neck. They are grouped as

A. Obliquely placed

a. Splenius capitis,

b. Levator scapulae,

B. Vertically placed

a. Scalenus medius, and

b. Scalenus posterior.

C. **Muscles** present occasionally are carpeted by prevertebral fascia.

a. Semispinalis capitis at the apex;

b. 1st digitations of serratus anterior.

Note: Scalenus anterior usually does not form the floor. It is overlapped by the sternomastoid.

5. **Contents:** The spinal accessory nerve and the lymph nodes are the true contents of the posterior triangle and all others are behind or infront of the fascial floor.

A. **Muscle:** Inferior belly of omohyoid.

B. Nerves ○━▶ ABC

a. **A**ccessory nerve: It is hooked by lesser occipital nerve. The nerve divides the triangle into **upper care free triangle** and **lower careful triangle**. The important structures lie below the spinal root of accessory nerve.

b. Roots, trunks of **b**rachial plexus and their **b**ranches.

I. Nerve to rhomboids.

II. Nerve to serratus anterior.

III. Nerve to subclavius.

IV. Suprascapular nerve.

V. Muscular branches to

    i. Scalenus muscles.

    ii. Longus colli.

c. Cervical nerves

I. Greater occipital nerve emerges from the apex of the triangle and reaches the scalp.

II. Great auricular nerve.

III. Lesser occipital nerve.

IV. Transverse cervical nerve of neck.

V. Supraclavicular nerve.

VI. 3rd and 4th cervical nerves supplying trapezius.

C. **Arteries**

a. Occipital artery, a dorsal branch of external carotid artery emerges from the apex of the occipital triangle.

b. Transverse cervical artery is a branch of thyrocervical trunk (branch of 1st part of subclavian artery). *It is one of the contents of occipital triangle.* It divides into ascending and descending branches at anterior border of sternocleido-mastoid.

c. Suprascapular artery

d. Transverse cervical artery has to reach anterior border of trapezius to distribute the same and to anastomose around scapula. It needs to travel through subclavian triangle.

D. **Veins:** External jugular vein and its tributaries.

a. Transverse cervical

b. Suprascapular

c. Anterior jugular veins.

d. *Subclavian vein is lower down and is not included in the triangle.*

E. **Lymph nodes**

a. Supraclavicular lymph nodes are present along the posterior border of sternomastoid.

b. Occipital lymph nodes.

6. Applied anatomy

➤ Left supraclavicular (Virchow's) lymph nodes are enlarged in malignancy of testis, stomach and other abdominal organs.

➤ The pressure in the external jugular vein can be recorded in the recumbent position. It is increased in right-sided heart failure and in the obstruction of the superior vena cava.

➤ The retropharyngeal abscess may extend in the lower part of posterior triangle.

Head, Neck and Face

> Spinal root of accessory nerve is the important content. It is plastered to the investing layer of deep fascia at the roof of triangle. Hence, a superficial incision to open a subcutaneous abscess at the posterior border of sternocleidomastoid should be made carefully to avoid injury to nerve.

> Sometimes nerve to subclavius gives a branch to join the phrenic nerve. This is called accessory phrenic nerve. In surgery of phrenic avulsion from the root of the neck, the accessory phrenic nerve, if present, might tear the subclavian vein with alarming symptom. This is because the main trunk loops around the vessel.

Important nerve to unimportant muscle—Tip

Box 3.1

The accessory phrenic nerve, branch of nerve to subclavius is an important nerve of unimportant muscle.

> **Subclavian steal syndrome:** It takes place in obstruction of the subclavian artery proximal to the origin of vertebral artery. The blood from the brain is diverted to the limb via subclavian artery.

LAQ-8 **Describe the subclavian triangle under the following headings:**

1. Boundaries,

2. Contents, and

3. Applied anatomy.

1. **Boundaries:** A subclavian triangle is lower part of posterior triangle. It has following boundaries (Fig. 3.11).

   A. **Anteriorly** by lower part of posterior border of sternocleidomastoid.

   B. **Posteriorly** by anterior border of inferior belly of omohyoid.

   C. **Base** by middle one-third of clavicle.

   D. **Apex** is meeting point of inferior belly of omohyoid with sternocleidomastoid

   E. **Roof** by

       a. Skin containing platysma,

       b. Superficial fascia,

       c. Investing layer of deep cervical fascia, and

       d. Structures piercing deep fascia. They are

           I. External jugular vein

           II. Supraclavicular nerve

           III. Unnamed cutaneous vessels and lymphatics.

   F. **Floor** contains

       a. 1st rib,

       b. Scalenus medius, and

       c. 1st digitation of the serratus anterior.

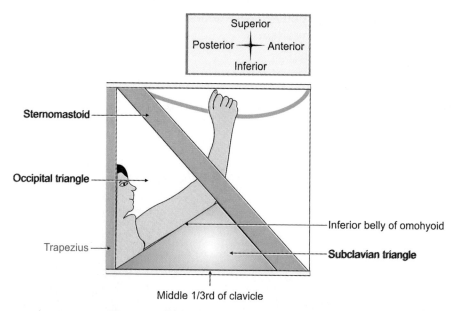

Fig. 3.11: Boundaries of subclavian triangle

2. **Contents** (Fig. 3.12)

   A. **Third part of subclavian artery:** It curves laterally and downwards between the scalenus anterior and scalenus medius. It runs along the brachial plexus. It passes through the cervicoaxillary canal.

   B. **Dorsal scapular artery (branch of 3rd part of subclavian artery):** This artery is also called descending scapular artery. It passes laterally through or in front of brachial plexus.

   C. **Suprascapular artery (branch of thyrocervical trunk):** It is one of the three branches of thyrocervical trunk. It passes in front of

   a. Scalenus anterior and phrenic nerve and behind

   b. Sternomastoid and internal jugular vein.

   D. **Superficial (transverse) cervical artery (branch of thyrocervical trunk):** It crosses in front of phrenic nerve and scalenus anterior before it enters posterior triangle.

   E. **Terminal part of external jugular vein:** It pierces deep fascia and drain into subclavian vein.

   F. **Trunks of brachial plexus:** The upper and middle trunks lie above and lower trunk lies below the 3rd part of subclavian artery.

   G. **Branches of roots of brachial plexus**

   a. Dorsal scapular nerve: It supplies rhomboids major and minor.

   b. Long thoracic nerve: It supplies serratus anterior.

   H. **Branches from trunks of brachial plexus**

   a. Nerve to subclavius: It supplies subclavius.

   b. Suprascapular nerve: Near the posteroinferior angle, it accompanies suprascapular artery. It supplies supraspinatus and infraspinatus.

Head, Neck and Face

I. **Supraclavicular lymph nodes:** These nodes also called posteroinferior group of deep cervical nodes. They drain
   a. Occipital region of scalp,
   b. Back of the neck,
   c. Axillary and
   d. Deltopectoral nodes of the superior extremity, and also the
   e. Upper deep cervical lymph nodes.

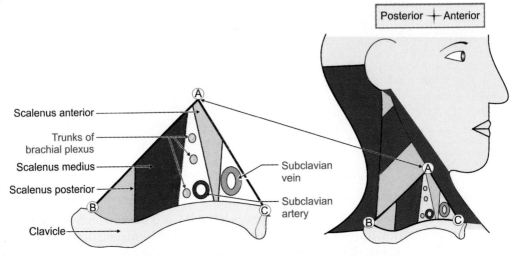

Posterior ━ Anterior

Scalenus anterior

Trunks of brachial plexus

Scalenus medius

Scalenus posterior

Clavicle

Subclavian vein

Subclavian artery

Fig. 3.12: Important contents of subclavian triangle

True contents of posterior triangle—Tip

Box 3.2
Note: Spinal accessory nerve and lymph nodes are the true contents of the posterior triangle as they lie between fascial roof and the floor of the triangle. All others are either behind the fascial floor or in front of the fascial roof.

3. **Applied anatomy**
   ➢ Subclavian triangle is an important clinical area for following reasons.
     • It is better inspected from front but palpated from behind.
     • The pulsations of the great veins may be seen, if the central venous pressure is raised. The external jugular vein, a prominent feature, may be distended due to
       ▪ Kinking,
       ▪ Raised venous pressure or
       ▪ Obstruction of the veins.
   ➢ Subclavian vein is used to keep the venous catheter for long-term intravenous injections.
   ➢ The subclavian artery can be felt pulsating as it crosses the 1st rib.

> The trunks of brachial plexus may be felt above and behind it. The brachial plexus block is given by injecting anaesthetic agent around the trunk just above the midpoint of clavicle.
> **Troisier's sign**: Enlargement of the left supraclavicular lymph nodes in cancer of the stomach.
> The cancer of the lung and breast spreads to the supraclavicular nodes of the side of lesion.

SN-37   Omohyoid

Omohyoid (*omos*—pertaining to shoulder)
1. **Attachments**
   A. **Origin:** Lateral part of inferior border of hyoid bone.
   B. **Insertion**
      a. Superior border of scapula
      b. Suprascapular ligament.
2. **Features:** It has
   A. Superior belly,
   B. Inferior belly, and
   C. Intermediate tendon.
      The two bellies are pulled by fibrous pulley, a band of deep cervical fascia and attached to clavicle.
      It divides the posterior triangle into two parts. The part above the muscle is called occipital triangle and the part below the muscle is called subclavian triangle.
3. **Nerve supply**
   A. **Superior belly:** Superior root of ansa cervicalis.
   B. **Inferior belly:** Inferior root of ansa cervicalis.
4. **Applied anatomy**: It overlaps internal jugular vein near hyoid bone. Hence, it acts as a useful guide during operation of the underlying vein.

SN-38   Great auricular nerve

1. **Root value:** Ventral ramus of **C2** and **C3** (branches for cervical plexus). **C2** is more important. It is a large trunk passing obliquely upwards over sternocleidomastoid.
2. **Distribution**
   A. **Skin over**
      a. Angle of mandible,
      b. Parotid gland,
      c. Lower and lateral surface of ear lobule,
      d. Mastoid region, and
      e. Skin of scalp posterior to ear.
   B. **Parotid fascia**

Head, Neck and Face

3. **Applied anatomy**: It is palpable and visibly thickened in tuberculoid leprosy.[NEET]

SN-39   Sternocleidomastoid

Table 3.1: Origin and insertion of sternocleidomastoid.

Parts	Proximal attachments	Distal attachments
• Sterno-occipitalis	• Upper part of manubrium sternum	• Lateral 2/3rd of superior nuchal line of occipital bone.
• Sternomastoid		• Mastoid process
• Cleidomastoid	• Upper part of medial surface of clavicle	• Mastoid process
• Cleido-occipitalis		• Lateral 2/3rd of superior nuchal line of occipital bone.

1. **Relations**

   A. **Superficial:** Skin containing

      a. Cutaneous nerves

         I. Great auricular,

         II. Transverse cervical, and

         III. Medial supraclavicular.

      b. Vein: External jugular vein

   B. **Deep**

Table 3.2: Deep relations of sternocleidomastoid at origin and insertion

Structure	At origin	In the middle	At insertion
• Muscles	• Sternohyoid • Sternothyroid • Omohyoid	• Scalenus medius • Scalenus posterior • Levator scapulae • Splenius capitis • Inferior belly of omohyoid	• Splenius capitis, • Longus capitis and posterior belly of digastric } Deep muscles of neck
• Vessels	• Anterior jugular vein	• Common carotid artery	• Occipital artery
• Nerves	—	• Cervical plexus • Brachial plexus • X and XII nerves • Inferior root of ansa cervicalis	—
• Glands	—	• Thyroid gland and lymph nodes	—

2. **Nerve supply**

   A. **Motor:** Spinal root of accessory nerve (**11th** cranial nerve).

   B. **Proprioceptive:** 2nd and 3rd ventral rami of cervical nerves.

3. **Action**

A. The chief purpose of the muscle is to *protract* the head (it is a combination of flexion of cervical spine and extension of atlantoaxial joint simultaneously). Protraction is brought by the contraction of muscles of both sides.

B. Contraction of muscle of one side tilts the head towards the same side of shoulder and turns the chin towards the opposite side.[NEET]

4. **Testing of the muscle**

A. The chin is turned to the opposite side against resistance. The muscle of one side is palpated.

B. The chin is bent downwards to test the sternocleidomastoid of both sides.

5. Applied anatomy

➤ **Congenital torticollis:** During difficult labour, undue pulling of the head of the baby causes tearing of the fibres of the sternocleidomastoid. The subsequent fibrosis and contracture is called congenital torticollis (wry neck).

➤ **Torticollis:** (*torti*—twisted, *collum*—neck): The head is bent to one side (to the side of spasm) and the chin points towards the opposite side of lesion. It is because of spasm of sternomastoid on the other side.

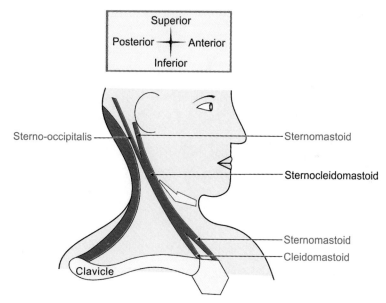

Fig. 3.13: Attachments of sternocleidomastoid

SN-40 External jugular vein

1. **Formation:** It is formed by union of posterior division of retromandibular and posterior auricular vein.

2. **Site:** It begins just below the angle of the mandible or within the parotid gland.

3. **Peculiarity:** It is provided with no valves in its entire course of the vein.

Head, Neck and Face

4. **Course**

 A. Begins in the lower part of parotid gland.

 B. Descends almost vertically between platysma and the deep fascia.

 C. Pierces the fascial roof of the supraclavicular triangle of the neck at the posterior border of sternocleidomastoid.

 D. Runs in the subcutaneous tissue superficial to sternocleidomastoid.

 E. It pierces the anteroinferior angle of the posterior triangle and opens into subclavian vein.

5. **Tributaries (Fig. 3.14)**

 A. Transverse cervical,

 B. Supraclavicular,

 C. Anterior jugular vein, and

 D. Posterior external jugular vein.

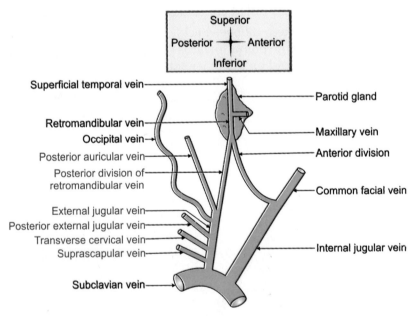

Fig. 3.14: External jugular vein and its tributaries

6. **Termination:** It drains into subclavian vein behind clavicle.

7. **Applied anatomy**

 ➤ The level of the blood column in the external jugular vein is an indication of the right atrial pressure.

 ➤ Puncture of external jugular vein is fatal because of following reasons:
  • It pierces deep fascia above the clavicle to drain into subclavian vein.
  • Its lumen is held open by the deep fascia which is attached to its margin.
  • Leads to sucking of air into the lumen due to negative intrathoracic pressure. Thereby, it produces an air embolism which is a fatal condition.

LAQ-9 **Describe accessory nerve under the following headings:**
1. Origin, course and distribution,
2. Branches, and
3. Applied anatomy.

1. Origin, course and distribution (Figs 3.15 and 3.16)
   A. **Cranial root**
      a. It emerges by 4 to 5 rootlets, attached to posterolateral sulcus of the medulla.
      b. It runs with 9th and 10th cranial nerves and the spinal root of accessory root. They reach the jugular foramen.
      c. In the jugular foramen, the cranial root unites with the spinal root and again separates.
      d. The cranial root, fuses with the vagus nerve and supplies the muscles of pharynx and larynx.

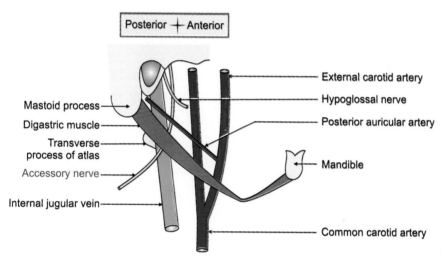

Fig. 3.15: Course of accessory nerve at the base of skull

   B. **Spinal root**
      a. It arises as small rootlets between the ventral and dorsal rami of spinal nerves, from upper 5 segments of spinal cord.
      b. In the vertebral canal, the filaments unite to form a single trunk and enter the cranium through foramen magnum.
      c. It runs along with cranial root of accessory and joins in the jugular foramen. They get separated and emerged independently.
      d. It descends vertically, between the internal jugular vein and internal carotid artery.
      e. It reaches a point midway between the angle of the mandible and the mastoid process.
      f. It runs downwards and backwards superficial to internal jugular vein and deep to sternomastoid.

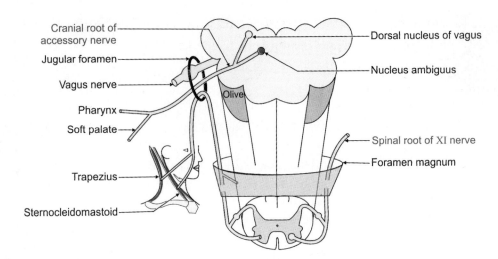

Fig. 3.16: Nuclear origin of spinal and cranial roots of accessory nerve

g. It pierces the anterior border of sternomastoid at the junction of upper 1/4th with the lower 3/4th and emerges through the posterior border of sternomastoid a little above its middle.

h. It enters the posterior triangle and lies over the levator scapulae muscle.

i. It leaves the posterior triangle by passing deep to the anterior border of trapezius and ends by supplying it.

2. **Branches**

A. **Cranial root supplies muscles of**

a. Palate (except tensor palati which is supplied by mandibular nerve),

b. Pharynx (except stylopharyngeus which is supplied by glossopharyngeal nerve), and

c. Larynx.

B. **Spinal root supplies**

a. Sternocleidomastoid, and

b. Trapezius.

3. Applied anatomy

➤ The accessory nerve is tested clinically

• By asking the patient to shrug his shoulders (trapezius) against resistance and comparing the power on the two sides, and

• By asking the patient to turn the face to the opposite side (sternomastoid) against resistance and again comparing the power on the two sides.

➤ The effects of damage of the spinal part of accessory nerve is as follows:

• The face is turned towards the side of injury.[NEET]

• There is an inability to shrug the shoulder towards the side of injury. It is due to paralysis of trapezius muscle.

➢ The pus accumulated near the posterior border of sternocleidomastoid is drained by taking incision across the sternomastoid. A note of caution, the incision is not taken along the posterior border of sternocleidomastoid to avoid injury of the spinal part of accessory nerve.

➢ Spinal root of accessory nerve is crossed by lesser occipital nerve at the middle of posterior border of sternocleidomastoid.

Head, Neck and Face

4

Back of the Neck

OLA-28 | What is the cause of neck rigidity in meningitis?

Neck rigidity is seen in cases with meningitis. It is due to spasm of the extensor muscles. This is caused by irritation of the nerve roots. The nerve roots pass through the subarachnoid space which is infected. The passive flexion of neck and straight leg raising test cause pain as the nerves are stretched.

LAQ-10 | Describe suboccipital triangle under the following heads:
1. Boundaries,
2. Floor,
3. Roof,
4. Contents, and
5. Applied anatomy.

1. **Boundaries** (Fig. 4.1)
   A. **Superolaterally:** Superior oblique. It extends from the back of lateral mass of the atlas to the lateral part of occipital bone between superior and inferior nuchal line.
   B. **Superomedially**
      a. **Rectus capitis posterior major**
         I. It is wrongly named.
         II. It is not vertical.
         III. It arises from outer surface of the bifid spinous process of the 2nd cervical vertebra.
         IV. It is attached to the lateral part of area below inferior nuchal line.
         V. It extends and rotates the head toward the same side.
      b. **Rectus capitis posterior minor**
         I. It is the only muscle attached to the posterior arch of atlas.

II. It arises from small fossa near the midline and passes vertically upwards to be inserted into the medial part of the area below the inferior nuchal line.

III. It extends the head.

C. **Inferiorly by** oblique capitis inferior. It is attached between the

  a. Outer surface of bifid spine of the axis, and

  b. Back of the lateral mass of the atlas.

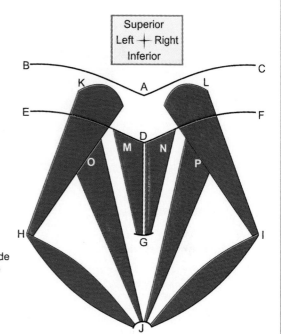

A - External occipital protuberance
G - Posterior arch of atlas
H - Left transverse process of atlas
I - Right transverse process of atlas
J - Bifid spine of axis

Lines representing structures.
AB, AC - Superior nuchal line on left and right side
ED, DF - Inferior nuchal line on left and right side
HK, IL - Superior oblique on left and right side
HJ, JI - Inferior oblique on left and right side
GM, GN - Rectus capitis posterior minor
JO, JP - Rectus capitis posterior major

Fig. 4.1: Boundaries of suboccipital triangle

2. **Floor**

  A. Posterior arch of the atlas, and

  B. Posterior atlanto-occipital membrane.

3. **Roof** is formed by

  A. Semispinalis capitis medially, and

  B. Longissimus capitis laterally.

    Both muscles are separated by dense fibrous tissue. The structures crossing the roof are

    a. Greater occipital nerve which crosses inferomedially.

    b. Occipital artery which crosses superolaterally.

4. **Contents** (Fig. 4.2A to C)

  A. Third part of vertebral artery runs across the floor of the triangle.

  B. Dorsal ramus of 1st cervical nerve (suboccipital nerve) and its muscular branches emerge through the floor of suboccipital triangle.

  C. Suboccipital venous plexus.

  D. Lymphatic plexus.

  E. Fibrofatty tissue.

Head, Neck and Face

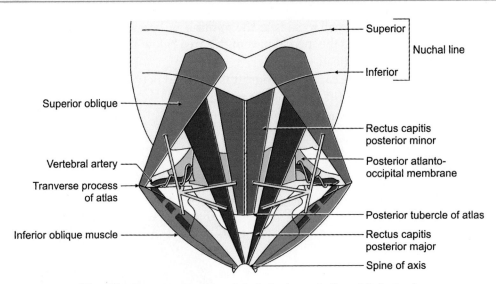

Fig. 4.2: Contents of suboccipital trianlge—A, B and C (below)

A. 3rd part of vertebral artery

1. Emissary vein
2. Occipital vein
3. Muscular vein
4. Internal vertebral venous plexus
5. Vertebral venous plexus

B. Formation of suboccipital venous plexus

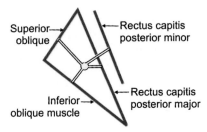

C. Left suboccipital triangle showing muscular branches of dorsal ramus of 1st cervical nerve

5. **Applied anatomy**

> **Neck rigidity** is an important sign of meningitis. It is due to spasm of extensor muscles (muscles of suboccipital triangle), caused by irritation of nerve roots, present in the subarachnoid space.
> **Cisternal puncture** is done through suboccipital triangle. It is done to collect CSF from cisterna magna. The needle is introduced just above the spine of axis in forward and upward direction.
> Posterior cranial fossa can be approached through the suboccipital triangle.

SN-41   Suboccipital nerve

Introduction: It supplies all the muscles forming boundaries and roof of the suboccipital triangle.
1. **Root value: C1**—1st cervical nerve.
2. **Peculiarity:** It does not have cutaneous branches.

Head, Neck and Face

3. **Course:** Suboccipital nerve is one of the contents of suboccipital triangle. It lies between vertebral artery and bone, i.e. atlas vertebra.

| ⚷━ N lies between A and B. |

A. **Branches**

a. **Ventral ramus:** It winds around lateral side of atlanto-occipital joint and passes forward to join the cervical plexus. It forms superior root of ansa cervicalis. It supplies
I. Geniohyoid
II. Thyrohyoid

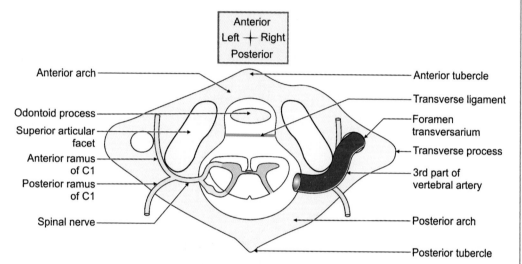

Fig. 4.3: Lateral view of atlas

b. **Dorsal ramus:** It has
I. Muscular branches supplying two recti, two oblique muscles and semispinalis capitis
i. Rectus capitis posterior major,
ii. Rectus capitis posterior minor,
iii. Superior oblique (oblique capitis superior),
iv. Inferior oblique (oblique capitis inferior), and
v. Semispinalis capitis.
II. Sensory branch to meninges of brain

4. **Applied anatomy :** Neck rigidity: It is caused by irritation of the nerve roots that are passing through the infected subarachnoid space.

SN-42   Greater occipital nerve

Introduction: Large medial branch of dorsal ramus of **C2**.
1. **Root value:** Dorsal ramus of **C2**.
2. **Peculiarities:** Thickest cutaneous nerve of body.

3. **Distribution**

   A. **Sensory:** Skin of scalp over posterior part of ear.

   B. **Motor:** Semispinalis capitis.

4. **Course and relations**

   A. Crosses suboccipital triangle.

   B. Pierces semispinalis capitis and trapezius.

   C. Runs on back of head and reaches vertex.

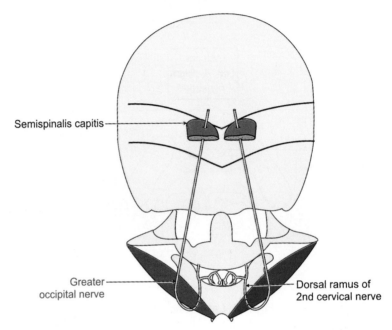

Semispinalis capitis

Greater
occipital nerve

Dorsal ramus of
2nd cervical nerve

Fig. 4.4: Origin, course and distribution of greater occipital nerve

5. **Applied anatomy**

   ➢ In meningitis, there is irritation of nerve root. This manifests as neck rigidity.

   ➢ The nerve is palpable and thick in leprosy. It is palpated along the posterior border of sternocleidomastoid.

   ➢ Greater occipital neuralgia: It is a syndrome of pain and paraesthesia felt in the distribution of greater occipital nerve. The nerve is caught as it pierces the semispinalis capitis and trapezius.

Contents of Vertebral Canal

SN-43 Ligamentum denticulatum

1. **Definition:** The pia mater on each side forms a narrow vertical ridge, called the ligamentum denticulatum (Fig. 5.1).
2. **Features**
   A. It is extension of pia mater to dura mater. It pierces arachnoid mater.
   B. It is present between the ventral and dorsal nerve roots.
   C. It gives a series of ▲ lar tooth-like processes which project from its lateral free border.
   D. Each ligament has 21 processes;
      a. 1st at the level of the foramen magnum, and
      b. Last between 12th thoracic and 1st lumbar spinal nerves.
   E. The processes suspend the spinal cord in the middle of the subarachnoid space.

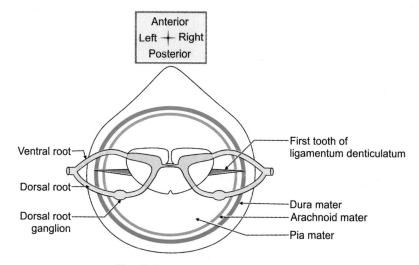

Fig. 5.1: Ligamentum denticulatum

3. **Applied anatomy**

➤ Its identification helps the surgeon in locating the 1st lumbar nerve during operation.
➤ Surgical sectioning of the lateral spinothalamic tract is called anterolateral cordotomy. It is necessary to relieve intractable pain. In this procedure, the incision is placed in front of the ligamentum denticulatum to access the lateral spinothalamic tract.

SN-44   Lumbar puncture

Introduction: It is performed to obtain samples of cerebrospinal fluid for laboratory analysis.

1. **Location:** Spinal cord ends at lower border of **L1** vertebra. Hence, lumbar puncture is done between **L3** and **L4** spine.
2. **Landmark:** A line tangential to the highest points of the iliac crests passes through the lower border of the 4th lumbar vertebra or the interspace between the 4th and 5th lumbar vertebra.
3. **Procedure:** Local anaesthetic drug is injected in the space between the 4th and 5th lumbar vertebrae and a spinal needle is inserted. Needle passes successively through
   A. Skin,
   B. Superficial fascia,
   C. Supraspinous ligament,
   D. Interspinous ligament (between the paired ligamentum flava),
   E. Epidural space, and
   F. Dura and arachnoid to enter the subarachnoid space.

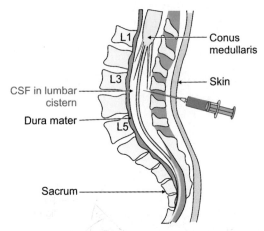

Fig. 5.2: Sagittal section passing through vertebral column to show lumbar puncture

4. **Applied anatomy**: Lumbar puncture is done for the

➤ Biochemical analysis of cerebrospinal fluid to diagnose type of meningitis.
➤ To differentiate extradural and subdural haemorrhage.
➤ For epidural and subdural anaesthesia (spinal anaesthesia).

SN-45   Enumerate the cranial nerves

1. **Olfactory nerve (1st cranial nerve):** It is the smallest cranial nerve.[NEET] It is a nerve of smell. It carries smell sensation from upper part of
   A. Lateral wall of nose, and
   B. Nasal septum.

2. **Optic nerve (2nd cranial nerve)**
   A. It is the nerve of vision.
   B. It is the thickest cranial nerve, hence whatever you see you rarely forget.
   C. It is not a true cranial nerve. It is prolongation of brain since it is covered by meninges.
   D. It is not covered by neurolemmal sheath. Hence, it does not regenerate.
   E. It is supplied by central artery of retina which is an end artery. Rupture of this artery results into blindness.

3. **Oculomotor (*Oculo*—eyeball, *motor*—movement) (3rd cranial nerve)**
   A. It is nerve of the muscles of eyeball.
   B. **It supplies all the following muscles of eyeball except lateral rectus and superior oblique. The muscles supplied by oculomotor nerve are**
      a. Levator palpebrae superioris,
      b. Superior rectus,
      c. Medial rectus,
      d. Inferior rectus, and
      e. Inferior oblique.

4. **Trochlear (*Trochlea*—pulley) (4th cranial nerve):** It has the longest intracranial course.[NEET] It is the motor nerve which supplies the superior oblique muscle. The superior oblique muscle winds around trochlea and gets inserted into eyeball. Hence, the nerve is called trochlear.

5. **Trigeminal (5th cranial nerve):** It is the largest sensory cranial nerve.[NEET] It has three roots
   A. Ophthalmic
   B. Maxillary
   C. Mandibular
   A. Ophthalmic, and
   B. Maxillary divisions are purely sensory. They are sensory to scalp and area of face excluding lower jaw.
   C. **Mandibular** division is mixed. It carries the sensation of
      a. Skin of
         I. Scalp,
         II. Lower jaw, and
         III. External ear.
      b. General sensations of anterior two-thirds of tongue,
      c. Temporomandibular joint,

Head, Neck and Face

  d. Secretomotor fibres to parotid gland.
  e. It supplies the
      I. Muscles of mastication
          i. Masseter,
          ii. Temporalis,
          iii. Medial, and
          iv. Lateral pterygoid
      II. Tensor tympani,
      III. Tensor palatini,
      IV. Anterior belly of digastric, and
      V. Mylohyoid.
6. **Abducent** (*abducent*—abduction) (6th cranial nerve) **LR6**. It is motor nerve, supplying lateral rectus. It rotates the eyeball laterally. It is nerve having intradural course. [NEET]
7. **Facial (7th cranial nerve):** It has the largest intraosseous course.[NEET] It is motor to the muscles of
  A. Facial expression,
  B. Muscles of scalp,
  C. Muscles of external ear,
  D. Muscle of middle ear, i.e. stapedius,
  E. Buccinator,
  F. Posterior belly of digastric, and
  G. Stylohyoid.
  H. It carries special sensation of taste from anterior two-thirds of tongue.
  I. It carries secretomotor fibres to
      a. Lacrimal gland
      b. Submandibular, and
      c. Sublingual glands

> Use of one's hand to recollect distribution of facial nerve—Tip

Box 5.1

To recollect the distribution of muscles of facial nerve
- Slide your palm on the face and say muscles of facial expression
- Slide on scalp and say muscles of scalp
- Slide on external ear and say muscles of external ear, i.e. auricularis anterior auricularis posterior, auricularis superior
- Slide in front of tragus of ear and say muscle of middle ear, i.e. stapedius
- Slide on the cheek and say buccinator
- Slide at the base of mandible and say platysma
- Slide from angle of mandible to styloid process and say posterior belly of digastric
- Slide from styloid process to hyoid and say stylohyoid

8. **Vestibulocochlear (8th cranial nerve):** It has two parts.

   A. Vestibular nerve is the nerve of balance.

   B. Cochlear nerve is the nerve of hearing.

9. **Glossopharyngeal (9th cranial nerve):** It is

   A. Sensory part: It is sensory of

   　　a. Posterior one-third of tongue,

   　　b. Middle ear cavity,

   　　c. Carotid body,

   　　d. Carotid sinus, and

   　　e. Palatine tonsil

   B. It carries special sensation from posterior one-third of tongue

   C. Motor nerve of muscle of pharynx, i.e. stylopharyngeus.

   D. It is secretomotor to parotid gland.

10. **Vagus (10th cranial nerve).** Cranial nerve having largest extracranial course.[NEET]

    A. It is motor nerve of the

    　　a. Muscles of larynx,

    　　b. Soft palate, and

    　　c. Pharynx.

    B. It is sensory nerve of

    　　a. Most posterior part of tongue, and

    　　b. Mucous membrane of larynx.

11. **Accessory (11th cranial nerve):** It has spinal part and cranial part.

    A. The spinal part is motor to muscles of neck, i.e. trapezius and sternocleidomastoid.

    B. The cranial part takes part in the pharyngeal plexus which supplies muscles of pharynx and soft palate.

12. **Hypoglossal (12th cranial nerve):** It is motor nerve to the muscles of tongue.

SN-46　Trapezius

1. **Proximal attachments**

   A. Medial one-third of superior nuchal line

   B. External occipital protuberance

   C. Ligamentum nuchae

   D. Spines of 7th cervical to 12th thoracic vertebrae

   E. Corresponding supraspinous ligaments

2. **Distal attachments:** It is inserted into

   A. Upper fibres into the posterior border of lateral one-third of clavicle.

   B. Middle fibres into the medial margin of the acromion and upper lip of the crest of spine of the scapula.

Head, Neck and Face

C. Lower fibres on the apex of ▲ lar area at the medial end of the spine, with a bursa intervening.

3. **Nerve supply**

A. **Motor:** Spinal root of accessory nerve (XIth cranial nerve)

B. **Sensory:** Proprioceptive by **C3** and **C4**

C. **Actions:**

a. The principal action of the trapezius is to rotate the scapula during abduction of the arm beyond 90°.

b. Upper fibres act with levator scapulae and elevate the scapula as in shrugging.

c. Middle fibres with rhomboids retract the scapula.

d. Upper and lower fibres with serratus anterior rotate the scapula forwards round the chest wall and play an important role in abduction of the arm beyond 90°.

D. **Testing the muscle:** Clinically, the muscle is tested by asking the patient to shrug his shoulder against resistance.

SN-47   Important events taking place at C6 vertebra

1. Structures end

   A. Larynx

   B. Laryngopharynx

2. Structures begin

   A. Trachea

   B. Oesophagus

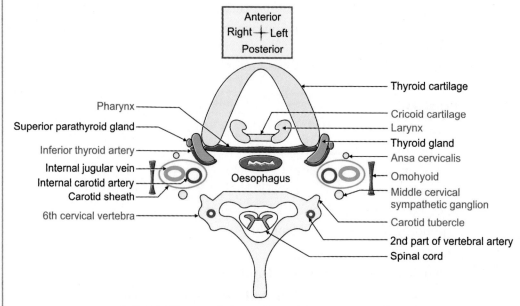

Fig. 5.3: Events of structures at 6th cervical vertebra

3. Structures present
   A. Carotid tubercle (anterior tubercle of transverse process of C6 vertebra).
   B. Middle cervical sympathetic ganglion.
   C. Superior parathyroid gland.
   D. Ansa cervicalis
   E. Widest breadth of spinal cord
4. Structure enters: Vertebral artery enters foramen transversarium of C6.
5. Apex of triangle
   A. Scalenovertebral triangle (longus colli and scalenus anterior meet).
6. Inferior thyroid artery loops medially
7. Meeting of two bellies of omohyoid

Head, Neck and Face

Cranial Cavity

OLA-29 Why the bleeding or pus collection beneath the pericranium is not extensive?

Pericranium is attached to sutures and does not cross the sutural line. Therefore, it is restricted to underlying bone.

OLA-30 Why is it not advisable to feel both the carotid pulsations simultaneously?

Feeling the pulsations of both carotid arteries simultaneously may block the blood supply to the brain. This can prove to be fatal. Hence, pulsations of both common carotid arteries are not palpated simultaneously.

OLA-31 Cephalohydrocoele

Cephalohydrocoele: Serous or watery accumulation under the pericranium. The CSF accumulates beneath the pericranium due to tear of dura and arachnoid mater. It is called traumatic meningocoele. Such swellings are restricted to the bones of vault and take the shape of underlying bone.

OLA-32 Cephalhaematoma

Definition: It is the collections of pus or blood beneath the pericranium. Dura mater is firmly attached to the sutural lines. Therefore, it takes the shape of underlying bone.

It is particularly seen in birth injuries as a result of trauma.

SN-48 Define venous sinuses and enumerate different venous sinuses.

1. Venous **⚷** SINVS ARE

These are the spaces in the cranium lined by endothelium, present

In between two layers of dura mater (endosteal and meningeal) except inferior sagittal and straight sinuses which are in between two meningeal layers.

Non-compressive in nature, without

<u>V</u>alves and

<u>S</u>mooth muscles,

<u>A</u>bsorbs cerebrospinal fluid through arachnoid granulations,

<u>R</u>eceives valveless emissary veins, which

<u>E</u>qualize venous pressure within and outside the skull.

2. **Classification**

   A. **Paired** (Fig. 6.1)

   B. **Unpaired** (Fig. 6.2)

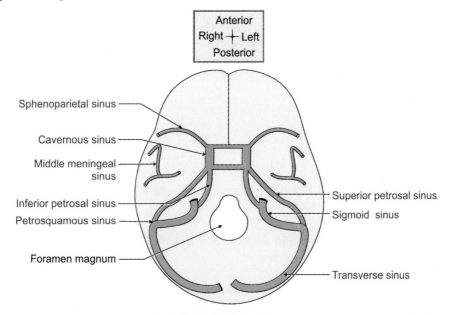

Fig. 6.1: Paried dural venous sinuses

Visualisation of paired dural venous sinuses—Tip

Box 6.1

The paired sinuses can be recollected by visualizing interior of skull and starting in the middle cranial fossa as the sequence below and take the help of the diagram (Fig. 6.1)

Table 6.1: Paired and unpaired venous sinuses

Paired venous sinuses	Unpaired venous sinuses
• Middle meningeal vein	• Anterior intercavernous
• Sphenoparietal	• Posterior intercavernous
• Cavernous	• Basilar venous plexus
• Superior petrosal	• Occipital
• Petrosquamous	• Straight
• Inferior petrosal	• Inferior sagittal
• Sigmoid	• Superior sagittal
• Transverse	

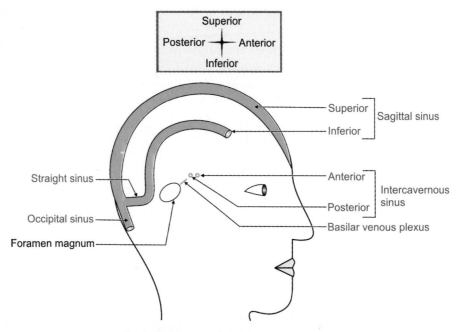

Fig. 6.2: Unpaired dural venous sinuses

LAQ-11	Describe cavernous sinus under the following heads:
	1. Formation,
	2. Relations,
	3. Extent,
	4. Contents,
	5. Communications, and
	6. Applied anatomy

1. **Formation**
   A. **Roof and lateral wall:** Meningeal layer of dura mater.
   B. **Floor:** Endosteal layer of dura mater.
   C. **Medial wall**
      a. Meningeal layer of dura mater, and
      b. Endosteal layer of dura mater.
2. **Relations** (Table 6.2)
3. **Extent:** Apex of orbit to the apex of petrous part of temporal bone.
4. **Contents** (Fig. 6.3): True content is blood.
   A. Other structures are separated by a layer of endothelium.
   B. Structures passing through the sinus
      a. Internal carotid artery with sympathetic nerve and venous plexus.

Table 6.2: Relations of structure of cavernous sinus

Features	Structures related
• **Superiorly**	• Optic tract • Internal carotid artery • Anterior perforated substance
• **Inferiorly**	• Foramen lacerum
• **Medially**	• Sphenoidal air sinus • Hypophysis cerebri
• **Laterally**	• Uncus of temporal lobe of cerebral hemisphere • Cavum trigeminale with trigeminal ganglion

> Internal carotid artery in the cavernous sinus is only artery lined inside and outside by endothelium—Tip

Box 6.2

Note: This is only artery in the body lined inside and outside by endothelium.

b. Abducent (VI) nerve (below and lateral to internal carotid artery).

C. Structures in the lateral wall (from below upwards) ⚷ **MOTO.**

Maxillary nerve—2nd division of trigeminal nerve—5th cranial nerve

Oculomotor nerve—3rd cranial nerve

Trochlear nerve—4th cranial nerve

Ophthalmic nerve—1st division of trigeminal nerve—5th cranial nerve.

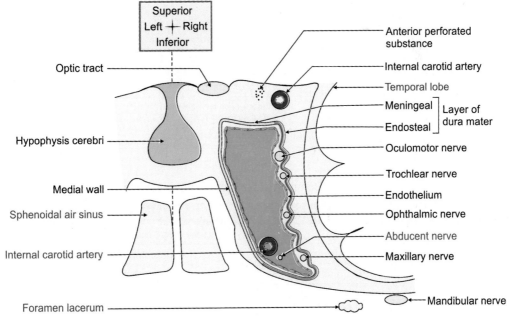

Fig. 6.3: Boundaries and contents of the cavernous sinus

Head, Neck and Face

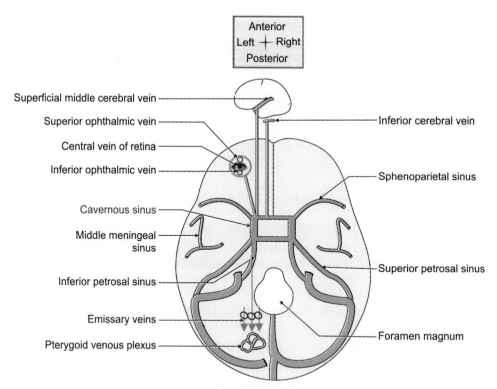

Fig. 6.4: Tributaries and outgoing channels of cavernous sinus

D. **Incoming channel:** From [🔑 **3B**]

Table 6.3: Tributaries of cavernous sinus

• **B**rain	• Superficial middle cerebral vein • Inferior cerebral vein
• **B**one	• Sphenoparietal sinus • Middle meningeal vein • Petrosquamous sinus.
• **E**yeball	• Superior ophthalmic vein • Inferior ophthalmic vein • Central vein of retina

5. **Communications**

Table 6.4: Communications of cavernous sinus

Region	To	Through
• Anterior	• Facial vein	• Superior ophthalmic vein
• Posterior	• Transverse sinus	• Superior petrosal sinus
	• Internal jugular vein	• Inferior petrosal sinus
• Superior	• Superior sagittal sinus	• Superficial middle cerebral vein

Contd.

Table 6.4: Communications of cavernous sinus (Contd.)

Region	To	Through
• Inferior	• Pterygoid venous plexus	• Emissary vein passing through • Foramen ovale • Foramen lacerum • Foramen spinosum
• Opposite	• Cavernous sinus	• Anterior intercavernous sinus • Posterior intercavernous sinus

6. **Applied anatomy**

➤ **Thrombosis of cavernous sinus** is caused by septic infections of the dangerous area of face. These areas are ☞ USA

<u>U</u>pper lip.

<u>S</u>eptum of nose and nasal cavities.

<u>A</u>djoining area of cheek and paranasal air sinus.

➤ **Clinical manifestations of thrombosis** in cavernous sinus are
  • Ophthalmoplegia and diplopia, if III, IV and VI nerves are involved.
  • Severe pain in the area of distribution.
  • Oedema of eyelids, and
  • Papilloedema
  • Exophthalmos.
  • There will be loss of vision, if central vein and artery are involved.

➤ **Arteriovenous aneurysm** is caused by rupture of internal carotid artery and results in
  • Loud systolic thrill.
  • Unilateral pulsatile exophthalmos.

SN-49   Superior sagittal sinus

Venous sinus situated at convex margin of falx cerebri between its two layers.

1. **Extent:** Crista galli (*crista*—crest or tuft of hair on an animal's head, *galli*—cock) to internal occipital protuberance (Fig. 6.5).

2. **Course:** Above the foramen caecum > crista galli > inner surface of frontal sagittal margins of parietal and squamous part of occipital.

3. **Size:** It becomes progressively larger as it passes backward to internal occipital protuberance.

4. **Fate:** Usually ends in right transverse sinus.

5. **Shape:** ▲lar in cross-section.

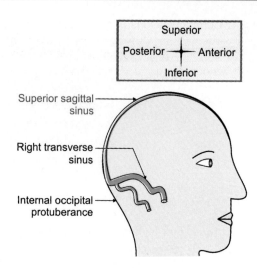

Fig. 6.5: Extent and termination of superior sagittal sinus

6. **Features**

A. Arachnoid granulations are projected in superior sagittal sinus.

B. There are numerous fibrous strands at inferior angle.

7. **Tributaries**

A. Veins from nose.

B. Superior cerebral veins which are 8 to 12 in number and collects blood from

a. Superolateral, and

b. Medial surface of cerebral hemisphere.

C. Diploic and emissary veins through venous lacunae.

8. **Communicates with**

A. Veins of scalp through parietal emissary vein.

B. Veins of nose passing through foramen caecum.

C. Cavernous sinus through

a. Superior anastomotic vein (Trolard's vein).

b. Superficial middle cerebral vein.

9. **Applied anatomy**

Thrombosis of superior sagittal sinus is caused by infection of nose, scalp and diploe. The manifestations are

➢ Signs and symptoms of increased intracranial tension.

➢ Paraplegia (due to involvement of paracentral lobule).

➢ Convulsions due to compression of motor area.

OLA-33 **What is the clinical importance of sigmoid sinus?**

1. The infection of the scalp behind the ear can spread through the mastoid emissary vein to the sigmoid venous sinus. It can be dangerous or fatal.

2. Infections from posterior cranial fossa can reach internal jugular vein through sigmoid sinus.

3. The sigmoid and transverse sinuses are often together termed the lateral sinus by clinicians. The sigmoid sinus is closely related to the mastoid air cells and middle ear cavity. Hence, these sinuses liable to infective thrombosis secondary to otitis media.

SN-50   Sigmoid sinus

Introduction: It is a space lined by endothelium present in cranium. It is between two folds of dura mater (endosteal and meningeal layers), which are non-compressive in nature. It devoids smooth muscles and valves.

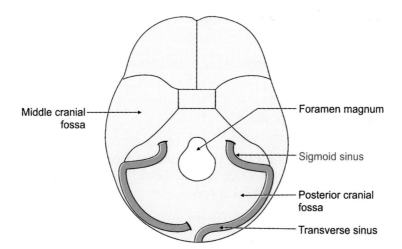

Fig. 6.6: Sigmoid sinus

1. **Site:** Posterior cranial fossa on parietal, temporal and occipital bones.
2. **Shape:** "S" shape.
3. **Termination:** It continues as internal jugular vein through the jugular foramen.
4. **Extent:** Extends from anterior end of transverse sinus to posterior end of jugular foramen.
5. **Tributaries:** Connects to
   A. Pericranial veins through mastoid and condylar foramen.
   B. Cerebellar vein.
   C. Internal auditory vein.
6. Applied anatomy
   ➤ Infections from posterior cranial fossa can reach internal jugular vein through sigmoid sinus.
   ➤ It is closely related to mastoid air cells. Hence, the infection from middle ear or mastoid antrum can spread to sigmoid sinus and other venous sinuses.

Head, Neck and Face

OLA-34 State the types of cells in adenohypophysis and their secretions.

Table 6.5: Cells in adenohypophysis and their secretions

Type of cell		Hormone
• Acidophil	• Somatotropes • Thyrotropes • Mammotropes	• Growth hormone—GH • Thyroid stimulating hormone—TSH • Prolactin
• Basophil	• Corticotropes • Gonadotropes	• Adrenocorticotropic hormone—ACTH • Follicle stimulating hormone—FSH • Luteinising hormone—LH

SN-51   Development of hypophysis cerebri

1. **Development** (Fig. 6.7)

   A. **Chronological age:** It develops in the middle of the 4th week of intrauterine life (IUL).

   B. **Germ layer:** Ectoderm.

   C. **Site:** Roof of the stomodeum.

   D. **Source**

   a. **Rathke's pouch:** It is a blind pouch arising from surface ectoderm of the stomodeum. It grows upwards and comes in contact with the diverticulum arising from the floor of diencephalon.

   b. **Neuroectoderm:** 🔑 3D downward diverticulum from floor of diencephalon.

   c. **Derivatives**

      I. Rathke's pouch gives rise to

         i. Pars distalis (pars anterior): Anterior lobe

         ii. Pars intermediate lobe

         iii. Pars tuberalis

      II. Neuroectoderm gives rise to

         i. Pars nervosa (posterior lobe), and

         ii. Stalk.

   E. **Anomalies**

   a. **Craniopharyngiomas:** It is a tumour growing from the hypophyseal stalk or Rathke's pouch. The Rathke's pouch may persist, forming a benign cystic tumour in the body of sphenoid. It is associated with increased intracranial pressure and showing deposition of calcium in the capsule. Compression causes hypopituitarism, hydrocephaly and personality changes.

   b. **Hyperplasia:** More than normal growth.

   c. **Aplasia**

   d. **Hypoplasia:** Less than normal growth of the gland.

   e. **Accessory pharyngeal hypophysis:** It is present in the roof of nasopharynx.

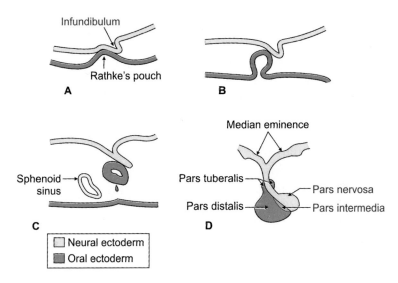

Fig. 6.7: Development of pituitary gland

2. **Applied anatomy**

➢ Pituitary tumour gives rise to two main types of symptoms.

   • General symptoms: Due to pressure over the surrounding structures.

   • Specific symptoms: Pressure over optic chiasma. It causes bilateral hemianopia.

➢ Acidophilic adenoma causes acromegaly in adult and gigantism in young individual.

➢ Basophilic adenoma causes Cushing's syndrome. The damage of the posterior lobe causes diabetes insipidus.

➢ Pressure over hypothalamus gives rise to hypothalamic symptoms.

LAQ-12 | **Describe hypophysis cerebri under the following heads:**
1. Gross anatomy,
2. Blood supply,
3. Histology, and
4. Applied anatomy

---

1. **Gross anatomy**

   A. **Situation:** It is an endocrine gland situated in the pituitary fossa of the body of sphenoid bone.

   B. **Shape:** Oval ⬭

   C. **Size:** 8 mm × 12 mm

   D. **Weight:** 500 mg

E. **Relations**

   a. Superior

      I. Diaphragma sellae,

      II. Optic chiasma,

      III. Tuber cinereum (grey coloured), and

      IV. Infundibular recess of 3rd ventricle.

   b. Inferior

      I. Body of sphenoid, and

      II. Sphenoidal air sinus

   c. **Lateral:** Cavernous sinus.

2. **Blood supply:** It is site of portal circulation.

   A. Arterial supply : Arterial supply is divided into arteries of (Fig. 6.8)

      a. Neurohypophysis, and

      b. Adenohypophysis.

      a. **Neurohypophysis**

         I. Superior hypophyseal artery

         II. Inferior hypophyseal artery } Internal carotid artery

         I. Each superior hypophyseal artery supplies

            i. Ventral part of hypothalamus

            ii. Upper part of infundibulum through trabecular artery

         II. Each inferior hypophyseal artery divides into

            i. Medial branch and

            ii. Lateral branch.

               They form an arterial ring around posterior lobe. Branches of these circles supply posterior lobe.

      b. **Adenohypophysis:** It is supplied exclusively by portal system. They arise from capillary tufts formed by the superior hypophyseal arteries.

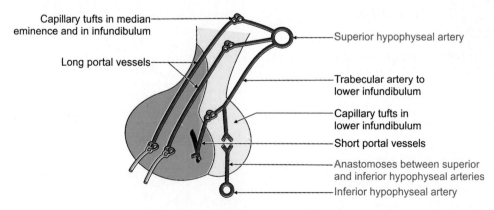

Fig. 6.8: Arterial supply of the hypophysis cerebri

I. The long portal vessels drain the

    i. Median eminence, and

    ii. Upper infundibulum.

II. The short portal vessels drain the lower infundibulum.

The portal vessels carry hormone releasing factors.

B. **Venous drainage**: Short veins emerge on the surface of gland and drain into cavernous sinuses.

3. **Histology** (Fig. 6.9):

A. **Anterior lobe:** It forms 3/4th of the gland. It consists of

    a. Chromophil cells (50% of the cells have affinity to colours).

      I. Acidophils (alpha cells, about 43% of cells).

      II. Basophils (beta cells, about 7% of cells).

    b. Chromophobe cells (50% of the cells do not take colour).

B. **Intermediate lobe:** It is made up of numerous basophil cells and chromophobe cells. They surround colloid material.

C. **Posterior lobe:** It consists of

    a. Large number of non-myelinated nerve fibres.

    b. Modified neuroglial cells, called pituicytes.

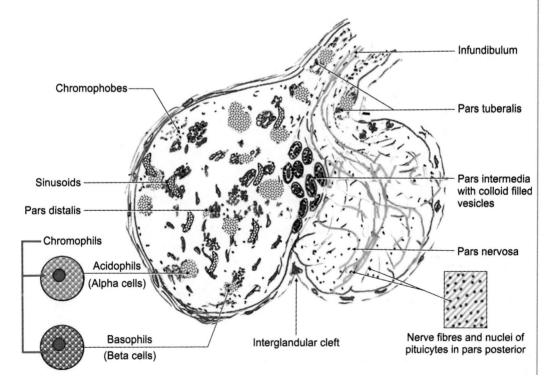

Fig. 6.9: Histology of pituitary gland

Head, Neck and Face

4. **Applied anatomy** : Pituitary tumours produce signs and symptoms of both pressure effects and disturbances in endocrine function.
   ➢ **Pressure effects**
     • Pressure on the optic chiasma causes bitemporal hemianopia.
     • Pressure on nerves in the cavernous sinus and its contained nerves produces ophthalmoplegia and may cause exophthalmos.
     • Pressure on the 3rd ventricle causes increased intracranial tension.
   ➢ **Endocrine effects**
     • Acromegaly or gigantism in case of adenoma of acidophil cell.
     • Cushing's syndrome in case of adenoma of basophil cells.

OLA-35   Lesions of optic chiasma

1. Pressure over the central part of optic chiasma causes bitemporal hemianopia.
2. Lesion in peripheral part of optic chiasma leads to binasal hemianopia.

SN-52   Diaphragma sellae

(*Diaphragm*—partition, *sellae*—saddle)

Introduction: It is the inner layer of dura mater covering the pituitary fossa (Fig. 6.10).

1. **Features**
   A. It forms the roof of the pituitary fossa.
   B. It is fibrous in nature.
2. **Attachments**
   A. **Anteriorly:** Tuberculum sellae
   B. **Posteriorly:** Dorsum sellae
   C. On both sides, it is continuous with dura mater of middle cranial fossa.
3. **Perforations:** It is perforated
   A. Centrally by pituitary gland
   B. Anteriorly by optic nerve.
4. **Blood supply:** It has little blood supply by
   A. Middle meningeal artery
   B. Accessory meningeal artery } branch of 1st part of maxillary artery)
   C. Meningeal branch of ascending pharyngeal artery (branch of external carotid artery).
5. **Nerve supply** : Meningeal branch of maxillary nerve.

SN-53   Falx cerebelli

(*Falx*—sickle ⸑ shaped)

Introduction: It is a fold of dura mater projecting into posterior cerebellar notch (Fig. 6.11).

1. **Formation:** It is formed by duplication of inner dural layer.

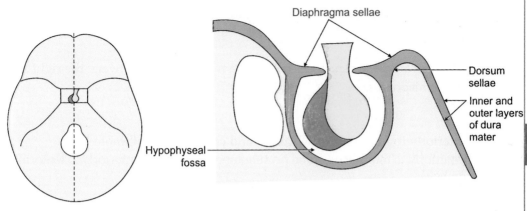

Fig. 6.10: Diphragma sellae

2. **Extent:** It extends from internal occipital protuberance along the internal occipital crest to the posterior margin of the foramen magnum.
3. **Content:** Occipital sinus[NEET]
4. **Features:** It has
   A. **Base:** It is attached to the posterior part of inferior surface of the tentorium cerebelli in the median plane.
   B. **Apex** has two parts which surround the foramen magnum.
   C. **Posterior margin:** It is convex and attached to internal occipital crest. It encloses the occipital venous sinus.
   D. **Anterior margin** is free.

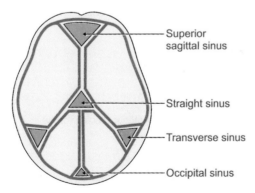

Fig. 6.11: Folds of dura mater and the venous sinuses in the posterior cranial fossa

5. **Functions**
   A. It partly separates two cerebellar hemispheres.
   B. It minimizes the rotator displacement of the brain.

Box 6.3
Note: The tentorium cerebelli is an insensitive structure.

Head, Neck and Face

SN-54   Falx cerebri

(*Falx*—L. sickle)

Introduction: It is sickle ⌠ shaped fold of dura mater present between the right and left cerebral hemispheres.

1. **Features**
   A. **Attachments**
      a. Anteriorly to frontal crest of frontal and crista galli of ethmoid bone.
      b. Posteriorly to internal occipital protuberance and posteroinferiorly to tentorium cerebelli
      c. Superiorly to the sagittal sulcus.
      d. Inferiorly it has free margin.
   B. **Surfaces:** It has two surfaces and related to medial surface of cerebral hemisphere.
   C. **Contents**[NEET]
      a. Superior sagittal sinus
      b. Inferior sagittal sinus
      c. Straight sinus

SN-55   Tentorium cerebelli

(*Tentorium*—tent)

Introduction: It is **tent**-like fold of dura mater separating occipital lobe of cerebrum from cerebellum (Fig. 6.12).

1. **Features**
   A. **Surfaces**
      a. Upper surface supports the occipital lobe.
      b. Lower surface roofs the cerebellum.

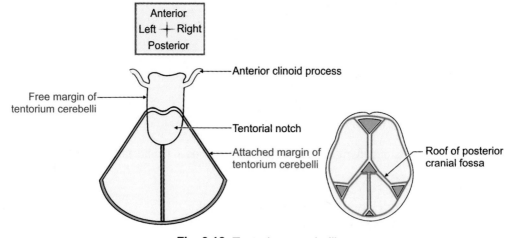

Fig. 6.12: Tentorium cerebelli

   B. **Margins**
      a. Attached margin: It is convex. At periphery, it is attached to
         I. Lips of transverse sulci,

II. Superior border of petrous part of temporal bone.

III. Posterior clinoid process.

b. **Free margin:** It is **U** shaped and free. It is attached to anterior cranial fossa.

2. **Structures piercing**

A. Great cerebral vein pierces the dura mater and joins the inferior sagittal sinus to form the straight sinus.

B. Trochlear nerve pierces before crossing the free and attached margin of tentorium cerebelli.

C. Oculomotor nerve pierces after crossing the free and attached margin of tentorium cerebelli.

3. **Contents**

A. The following venous sinuses are enclosed in the tentorium cerebelli. (There is no venous sinus in the free margin of tentorium.)[NEET]

   a. Transverse sinus,

   b. Superior petrosal sinus, and

   c. Straight sinus.

B. Other contents

   a. Trigeminal ganglion

   b. Sensory and motor root of trigeminal nerve with covering of pia mater and arachnoid mater that contains CSF.

4. **Recess:** Trigeminal cave is formed by the folds of dura mater.

A. Above by 2 meningeal layers of dura mater

B. Below by 1 meningeal and one endosteal layer of dura mater.

5. **Blood supply**

A. **Arterial:** Meningeal branches of

   a. Ascending pharyngeal artery ⎫
   b. Occipital artery   ⎬ branch of external carotid artery
                                  ⎭

   c. Vertebral artery (branch of 1st part of subclavian artery).

B. **Venous:** Drain into meningeal vein and the dural venous sinus.

6. Nerve supply : **Sensory nerve supply:** Recurrent meningeal branch of ophthalmic division of trigeminal nerve.

7. **Functions**

A. **Stabilization of brain:** They play important role in stabilizing the brain in case of sudden movements of head.

B. It absorbs the stress.

C. It bears the weight of occipital lobe without transmitting to cerebellum.

8. Applied anatomy

➢ Supratentorial and infratentorial compartments are communicated through the narrow space around midbrain and tentorial notch. In case of obstruction of the

Head, Neck and Face

communication, there is dilatation of ventricles and subarachnoid space of posterior cranial fossa.

➤ Inflammation of the supratentorial compartment gives rise to frontal or parietal headache since it is innervated by ophthalmic division of trigeminal nerve.

SN-56 Middle meningeal artery

Introduction: It is the main source of blood to the bones of vault of the skull.

1. **Origin:** It is the 1st branch of the 1st part of maxillary artery given in the infratemporal fossa.
2. **Relations:** It is superficial to sphenomandibular ligament and deep to lateral pterygoid muscle. It is accompanied by
   A. Plexus of sympathetic nerves.
   B. Middle meningeal vein, a loyal friend.
3. **Branches** (Fig. 6.13): The major branches of middle meningeal artery run between periosteal and meningeal layers of dura mater. The small branches are within periosteal layers.
   A. Ganglionic branches to trigeminal ganglion,
   B. Petrosal branch,
   C. Superior tympanic branch,
   D. Temporal branch, and
   E. Anastomosing branch.

> Branches of meningeal artery justifies the name by coursing through two layers of dura mater—Tip

Box 6.4

Note: The major branches of middle meningeal artery run between periosteal and meningeal dura layers. The small branches are within periosteal layers.

4. **Course** (Fig. 6.13)
   A. Ascends between two roots of auriculotemporal nerve.
   B. Enters the middle cranial fossa through foramen spinosum.
   C. Runs upwards and forwards on greater wing of sphenoid bone and divides into anterior and posterior divisions.
   D. Anterior division is closely related to motor area of brain.
   E. Posterior division runs backwards on superior temporal sulcus of brain. It ends at posteroinferior angle of parietal bone by dividing into frontal and parietal branches.

5. **Applied anatomy**

   ➤ **Fracture of the skull** may cause injury to the middle meningeal artery producing extradural haemorrhage. The resultant extradural haematoma compresses the motor area of the cerebral cortex and causes paralysis of the muscles of opposite

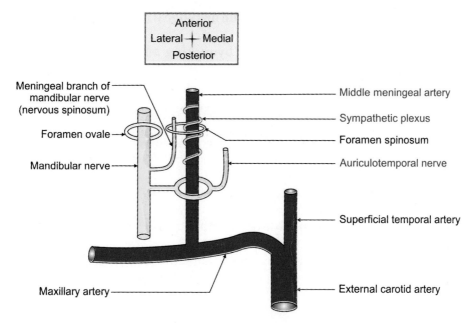

A. Extracranial course of middle meningeal artery.

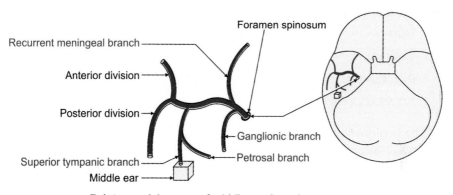

B. Intracranial course of middle meningeal artery.

Fig. 6.13: Extra- and intracranial course and branches of middle meningeal artery

Head, Neck and Face

side of body. The paralysis of muscles depends upon the extent of compression by haematoma.

➤ **Talk and die syndrome**: Injury at pterion by small stone results in rupture of middle meningeal artery. The patient gets transient unconsciousness. He becomes conscious, talks for sometime and again becomes unconscious. The duration of consciousness between two unconsciousness periods is called lucid interval. Patient dies before the condition is diagnosed. So in case of any head injury, the patient should be kept 24 hours for observation to rule out extradural haemorrhage.

➤ The **rupture of middle meningeal artery** is a **surgical emergency**. The symptoms of brain compression occur within 3 hours. It should be explored immediately to arrest the bleeding and to remove the blood clot.

➤ **Rupture of posterior division of middle meningeal artery** results in contralateral deafness.

➤ The **anterior division is approached by making** a hole at pterion (4 cm above midpoint of zygomatic arch).

> ### Intracranial haemorrhage
> ### Arterial–venous–arterial

Box 6.5

Note: Intracranial haemorrhage may be arterial or venous. It is remembered as *arterial–venous–arterial*

A. Between bone and endosteal layer of dura mater (extradural or epidural haemorrhage—arterial)

B. Between dura mater and arachnoid mater (subdural haemorrhage—venous)

C. Between arachnoid mater and pia mater (subarachnoid haemorrhage—usually arterial)

D. Intracranial haemorrhage never separates the 'two layers' of the dura mater and it never separates pia mater from the underlying cortex.

LAQ-13 **Describe oculomotor nerve under the following heads:**

1. Origin,

2. Course,

3. Distribution, and

4. Applied anatomy

---

1. **Origin:** The oculomotor nerve arises from oculomotor nucleus, present in the grey matter of midbrain at the level of superior colliculus.

2. **Course** (Fig. 6.14)

   A. **Nuclei:**

   a. Median unpaired central nucleus for

   I. Convergence, and

   II. Accommodation.

   b. Paired lateral motor nucleus for all extraocular muscles of eyeball except lateral rectus and superior oblique.

   c. Paired small nucleus (Edinger-Westphal nucleus) for parasympathetic pupillary fibres for pupil constriction and ciliary body.

   B. **Intraneuronal:** Oculomotor nucleus ⟶ tegmentum ⟶ red nucleus ⟶ medial part of substantia nigra and emerges out of brainstem on medial side of crus cerebri through oculomotor sulcus.

   C. **Extraneuronal:** It pierces the pia mater and lies in the subarachnoid space in the posterior cranial fossa.

a. **Posterior cranial fossa:** It passes between posterior cerebral artery and superior cerebellar artery.

    I. It lies posterior to posterior cerebral artery and

    II. Superior and anterior to superior cerebellar artery and passes

    III. Lateral and parallel to posterior communicating artery.

    IV. It pierces

        i. Arachnoid mater and lies in the interval between free and attached margin of tentorium cerebelli.

        ii. Dura mater lateral to posterior clinoid process.

        iii. Cavernous sinus and traverses the roof and descends in the lateral wall of cavernous sinus.

    V. It receives a few filaments from internal carotid artery and communicates with ophthalmic division of trigeminal nerve.

b. **Cavernous sinus:** The relations from above downwards are 3rd and 4th cranial nerves, ophthalmic and maxillary division of trigeminal nerve.

    I. The nerve divides into upper and lower divisions at anterior end of cavernous sinus.

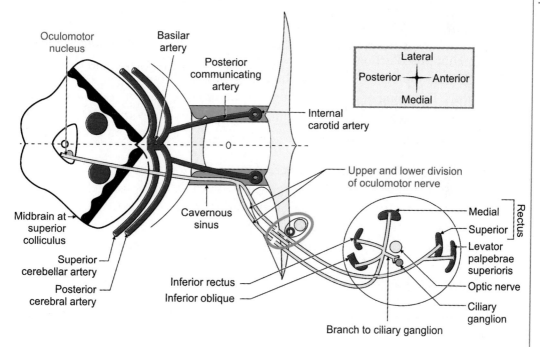

Fig. 6.14: Course and relations of oculomotor nerve

D. **Superior orbital fissure:** It divides in two divisions.

3. **Distribution**

    A. **Motor**

        a. Upper division

            I. Levator palpebrae superioris

Head, Neck and Face

II. Superior rectus
Note: Superior rectus only has crossed innervation.
b. Lower division
I. Inferior rectus
II. Inferior oblique
III. Medial rectus
B. Parasympathetic branch to ciliary ganglion. It supplies sphincter pupillae and ciliaris muscle, through the branch of inferior oblique.

4. **Applied anatomy**

➤ Infranuclear paralysis of oculomotor nerve results into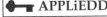
Loss of accommodation.
Ptosis.
Protrusion of eyeball—proptosis
Lateral squint.
Embolus in cavernous sinus is one of the causes of paralysis of 3rd nerve.
Diplopia.
Dilatation of pupil.
➤ Complete division of oculomotor nerve is manifested as[NEET]
- Eyeball is depressed and abducted. "Down and out". External strabismus: Due to unopposed action of lateral rectus.
- Ophthalmoplegia > Diplopia where false image is higher than true image.
- Ptosis: Drooping of eyelid due to involvement of levator palpebrae muscle.
- Sphincter pupillae is not functioning. It results into dilatation of pupil (mydriasis)
- Dilated and fixed pupil.
- Loss of accommodation reflex because of paralysis of three muscles.
  - Medial rectus—medial convergence of eyeball is lost.
  - Sphincter pupillae—pupillary constriction is lost.
  - Ciliaris muscle—thickness of lens will increase.
- Apparent protrusion of eyeball due to flaccid paralysis of most of ocular muscles.
- Patient finds difficulty in getting down the staircase and reading the books. He gets diplopia while doing these activities.
➤ In paralysis of oculomotor nerve, patient cannot look upwards, downwards or medially.
➤ 3rd nerve is usually affected due to syphilitic periarteritis of posterior cerebral and superior cerebellar arteries as the nerve passes between the arteries.
➤ **Weber's syndrome**: Ipsilateral paralysis of oculomotor nerve with contralateral hemiplegia.
➤ **Benedikt's syndrome** (tegmental mesencephalic paralysis): It involves lesion of oculomotor nerve and red nucleus. There is damage of corticospinal tract. It manifests as

Head, Neck and Face

- Ipsilateral
  - Paralysis of the muscles supplied by oculomotor nerve, and
  - Ataxia
- Contralateral
  - Hyperkinesia
  - Tremor of the arm and leg.

➤ In meningitis[NEET], one of the dreadful complication is uncal herniation that affects oculomotor nerve.

➤ **In uncal herniation or compression by the aneurysm of posterior communicating artery**[NEET], the peripheral fibres of oculomotor nerve are first compressed. Theses are parasympathetic fibres going to pupil. They are first affected and results in dilatation of pupil. As the compression progresses, the extrinsic muscles of eyeball are also affected.

➤ Unexplained fixed pupil with headache[NEET] is a dictum of rupture of aneurysm of posterior communicating artery in circle of Willis. It produces compression of peripheral fibres of oculomotor nerve.

➤ Paralysis of oculomotor nerve in diabetic patient, there is paralysis of muscles of eyeball. There is no affection of parasympathetic fibres which spares pupillary reaction.

➤ Internuclear ophthalmoplegia[NEET] is due to lesion in medial longitudinal bundle (fasciculus). There is weakness of adduction on the same side and contralateral abduction nystagmus.

➤ One and half syndrome[NEET]: It is lesion in parapontine reticular formation (PPRF) on same side.

SAQ-1   Weber's syndrome

1. **Condition which includes**
   A. Upper motor neuron lesion of corticospinal tract in crus cerebri of the midbrain, and
   B. Lower motor neuron lesion of third nerve, supplying the muscles of eyeball.
2. **Clinical features:** It results in
   A. Contralateral hemiplegia, and
   B. Ipsilateral paralysis of muscles of eyeball supplied by oculomotor nerve.

LAQ-14   Describe trochlear nerve under the following heads:
1. Course and distribution
2. Applied anatomy

1. **Course and distribution** (Fig. 6.15)
   A. **Peculiarity: It is only cranial nerve emerging from dorsal aspect of brainstem.**
   B. The trochlear nerve emerges from the superior medullary velum near the frenulum veli just below the inferior colliculus. It winds two peduncles.

a. Superior cerebellar peduncle, and the

b. Cerebral peduncle just above the pons.

C. It passes between two arteries

a. Posterior cerebral artery, and

b. Superior cerebellar artery. It appears ventrally lateral to the cerebral peduncle.

D. It enters the cavernous sinus by piercing the posterior corner of its roof.

E. It runs forwards in the lateral wall of the cavernous sinus between the

a. Oculomotor, and

b. Ophthalmic nerves. In the anterior part of the sinus, it crosses over the 3rd nerve.

F. It enters the orbit through the lateral part of the superior orbital fissure.

G. In the orbit, it passes medially above the origin of levator palpebrae superioris and ends by supplying the superior oblique muscle through its orbital surface.

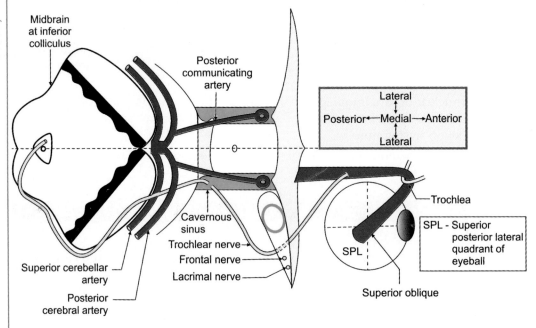

Fig. 6.15: Course of trochlear nerve

2. **Applied anatomy** : When the trochlear nerve is damaged, diplopia occurs on looking downwards, vision is single, as long as the eyes look above the horizontal plane.

LAQ-15 Describe abducent nerve under the following heads:

1. Origin and nuclei

2. Course and distribution

3. Applied anatomy

This is the 6th cranial nerve. It supplies the lateral rectus muscle of the eyeball.

1. **Origin and nuclei:**

   A. The abducent nerve has a motor nucleus. It belongs general somatic efferent column supplying lateral rectus muscle. It also belongs to general somatic afferent carrying proprioceptive sensations of lateral rectus to mesencephalic nucleus of trigeminal nerve.

   B. It arises from motor nucleus present in the dorsal part of lower part of pons. It lies deep to axons of facial nerve. The motor nucleus of abducent nerve and axons of facial nerve collectively form a bulging in the floor of fourth ventricle. The bulging is called facial colliculus.

2. **Course and distribution** (Fig. 6.16)

   A. The nerve emergs from brainstem at the pontomedullary junction.

   B. It passes between labyrinthine artery and anterior inferior cerebellar artery. It runs upwards, forwards and laterally through the cisterna pontis.

   C. It passes deep to petrosphenoidal ligament, and bends sharply forwards.

   D. It passes through Dollero's canal.[NEET] The canal is situated at the junction of apex of petrous part of temporal bone and clivus of occipital bone.

   E. It passes through the substance of cavernous sinus along with internal carotid artery.

   F. The entry of abducent nerve in the cavernous sinus is at a point

      a. Lateral to the dorsum sellae, and

      b. Superior to the apex of the petrous temporal bone.

   G. It enters the orbit through the middle part of the tendinous ring of superior orbital fissure. Here it lies inferolateral to the oculomotor and nasociliary nerves.

   H. In the orbit, it ends by supplying the lateral rectus muscle. It enters the ocular surface of the muscle.

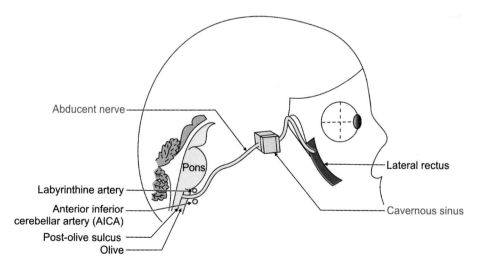

Fig. 6.16: Course of abducent nerve

3. **Applied anatomy**: Paralysis of the abducent nerve results in:

> Medial (internal or convergent) squint, and
> **Diplopia:** Change in the visual axis of the two eyes leading to double vision due to paralysis of lateral rectus muscle.

SN-57 Meckel's cave (trigeminal cave)

Introduction: It is a diverticulum of inner layer of dura mater and arachnoid mater.

1. **Site:** Anterior surface of apex of the petrous temporal bone in the middle cranial fossa.
2. **Contents:** Trigeminal ganglion.
3. **Formation:** It is formed by evagination of sensory and motor roots of trigeminal nerve. Since these layers pierce subarachnoid space, they are bathed by CSF.
4. **Applied anatomy**

> In trigeminal neuralgia, alcohol is injected into the trigeminal ganglion to alleviate the pain.
> The approach to sensory root of trigeminal nerve is avoided in the Meckal's cave. Failure of this approach may result into transient facial palsy.
> - **It is explained as**
>   - The greater petrosal nerve lies deep to trigeminal ganglion. The stripping of the dura mater exerts pressure on facial nerve—geniculate ganglion—motor fibres of facial nerve that causes transient paralysis of muscles of face.

SN-58 Trigeminal neuralgia (tic douloureux)

Introduction: It is a sensory disorder of the sensory root of trigeminal nerve, 5th cranial nerve. It occurs most often in middle-aged and elderly persons.

1. **Manifestations**
   A. It is characterized by sudden attacks of excruciating, lightening-like jabs (penetrating) of facial pain.
   B. A *paroxysm* (sudden sharp pain) can last for 15 min or more.
   C. The pain may be so intense that the person winces; hence the common term *tic* (twitch).
   D. In some cases, the pain may be so severe that psychological changes occur, leading to depression and even suicide attempts.
2. **Nerves involved:** Frequency of the nerves involved
   A. Maxillary—most common
   B. Ophthalmic—less common
   C. Mandibular—least common
3. The paroxysms of sudden stabbing pain are often set off by touching the face, brushing the teeth, shaving, drinking, or chewing. The pain is often initiated by touching a sensitive *trigger zone.*

4. **Cause** is not known.
5. **Treatment:** In maxillary nerve involvement, the temporary relief is given by blocking the infraorbital nerve. The nerve is blocked at the infraorbital foramen by using alcohol. This treatment usually relieves pain temporarily.

OLA-36 Inferior sagittal sinus

1. It is unpaired dural venous sinus.
2. Situation: Posterior two-thirds of the lower, concave free margin of the falx cerebri.
3. Termination: It ends in the straight sinus.

OLA-37 Confluence of sinuses

1. It is meeting point of 5 sinuses[NEET]—1 paired and 3 unpaired sinuses.
2. Site: Internal occipital protuberance
3. Sinus opening
   A. Paired sinus—transverse sinus
   B. Unpaired sinuses:
      a. Superior sagittal sinus
      b. Straight sinus
      c. Occipital sinus
   C. Tributaries:
      a. Cerebral vein
      b. Cerebellar vein

SN-59 Trigeminal ganglion (semilunar or gasserian ganglion)

Introduction: It is sensory ganglion present in the course of trigeminal nerve.

1. **Site:** The trigeminal ganglion lies within a pouch of dura mater called the trigeminal cave. It is present on trigeminal impression present on the anterior surface of petrous part of temporal bone.
2. Homologous to dorsal root ganglion of the spinal nerve. It consists of pseudo-unipolar nerve cells with **T** shaped arrangement of their processes. One process arises from the cell body which then divides into a central and a peripheral process.

   The ganglion is semilunar ◖ in shape. The three divisions of the trigeminal nerve emerge from the ganglion. The posterior concavity of the ganglion receives the sensory root of the nerve.
3. **Relations**
   A. *Medially*
      a. Internal carotid artery.
      b. Posterior part of cavernous sinus.
   B. *Laterally:* Middle meningeal artery.
   C. *Superiorly:* Parahippocampal gyrus.

Head, Neck and Face

D. *Inferiorly*
   a. Motor root of trigeminal nerve.
   b. Greater petrosal nerve.
   c. Apex of the petrous temporal bone.
   d. Foramen lacerum.

4. **Associated roots:** The central processes of the trigeminal ganglion cells enter the lateral aspect of the pons and divide into ascending and descending branches which terminate in one or another component of the sensory nucleus of V.

   A. The peripheral processes of the ganglion cells form three divisions of the trigeminal nerve, namely the *ophthalmic, maxillary and mandibular.*

5. **Blood supply:** The ganglion is supplied by twigs from:

   A. Internal carotid artery, one of two terminal branches of common carotid artery.
   B. Middle meningeal, branch of 1st part of maxillary artery.
   C. Accessory meningeal arteries, branch of 1st part of maxillary artery.
   D. By the meningeal branch of the ascending pharyngeal artery, medial branch of external carotid artery.

6. **Surface anatomy**: A little in front of pre-auricular point at a depth of 4.5 cm.

7. **Applied anatomy**

   ➤ Trigeminal neuralgia is relieved by injecting 90% alcohol in the affected division of trigeminal ganglion.
   ➤ A *herpes zoster virus infection* may produce a lesion in the trigeminal ganglia. This occurs in 20% of cases. It is manifested of vesicles in one of the divisions of trigeminal nerve.
   ➤ Removal of trigeminal ganglion results in temporary loss of taste sensations of anterior two-thirds of the tongue.

❖ **Treatment**
   ➤ Medical
   ➤ Surgical treatment.
      • In maxillary nerve involvement
         ▪ For temporary relief: Block the infraorbital nerve at the infraorbital foramen by using alcohol. This treatment usually relieves pain temporarily.
         ▪ Avulsion or cutting of the branches of the nerve at the infraorbital foramen.
         ▪ *Radiofrequency selective ablation of parts of the trigeminal ganglion* by a needle electrode passing through the cheek and the foramen ovale.
         ▪ Rhizotomy: Sensory root of the trigeminal nerve may be partially cut between the ganglion and the brainstem *(rhizotomy).*
         ▪ Tractotomy: Sectioning the spinal tract of fifth cranial nerve *(tractotomy).* After this operation, the sensation of pain, temperature and simple (light) touch is lost over the area of skin and mucous membrane supplied by the affected component of the trigeminal nerve.

Contents of the Orbit

SN-60   **Nasociliary nerve**

Introduction: It is the branch of ophthalmic division of trigeminal nerve. It is sensory nerve to the

A. Whole eyeball (eye, cornea, iris and ciliary body but not conjunctiva),

B. Paranasal air sinus, mucous membrane of the nasal cavity, and

C. Skin of the external nose.

1. **Course and relations**

   A. Runs through the tendinous ring between the two divisions of oculomotor nerve.

   B. Passes by sitting on optic nerve $\boxed{\text{ON} \, \text{⊶} \, \text{(optic nerve)}}$ and below superior rectus.

   C. Enters anterior ethmoidal foramen as anterior ethmoidal nerve.

   D. Runs in the roof of middle and anterior ethmoidal air cells.

2. **Branches of nasociliary nerve**[NEET] (Fig. 7.1)

   A. **Communicating branches to** ciliary ganglion: It forms sensory root to ciliary ganglion.

   B. **Collateral branches**

      a. Long ciliary nerve:

         I. It is sensory to

            i. Cornea,

            ii. Iris, and

            iii. Ciliary body.

         II. It is sympathetic to dilator pupillae.

      b. Posterior ethmoidal nerve: It is sensory to following air sinuses

         I. Posterior ethmoidal sinus, and

         II. Sphenoidal air sinus.

C. **Terminal branches**

    a. Infratrochlear nerve (smaller terminal branch): It is sensory to

        I. Conjunctiva,

        II. Lacrimal sac,

        III. Caruncle,

        IV. Medial end of eyelids, and

        V. Upper half of the external nose.

    b. Anterior ethmoidal nerve (larger terminal branch): It is sensory to

        I. Anterior ethmoidal sinus,

        II. Middle ethmoidal sinus.

        III. Dura mater of anterior cranial fossa

        IV. Mucosa of nose, and

        V. Skin of the lower half of the nose.

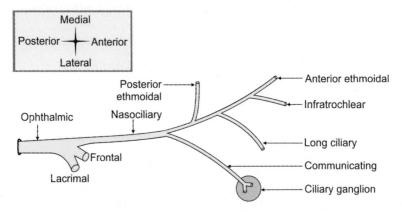

Fig. 7.1: Branches of nasociliary nerve

3. **Applied anatomy**: A lesion of the nasociliary nerve at the superior orbital fissure causes

  ➢ Paraesthesia in the forehead and nose, and

  ➢ Loss of corneal blink reflex.

SN-61   Short ciliary nerves

1. **Origin:** Arise from ciliary ganglion. They are 15 to 20 in number.

2. **Course:** They pass with the optic nerve to the back of the eyeball.

3. **Distribution:** They supply

    A. Ciliary body (oculomotor nerve fibres), which is concerned with accommodation.

    B. Circular muscle of iris (oculomotor nerve fibres), which constricts the pupil.

    C. Radial fibres of iris (sympathetic nerve fibres), which dilate the pupil.

OLA-38 What is squint (strabismus)?

1. It is weakness or paralysis of muscles of eyeball.
2. It may be concomitant or paralytic.
   A. Concomitant squint is congenital. Movements are not affected and there is no diplopia.
   B. In paralytic squint, movements are limited. There is diplopia and vertigo. The head is turned in the direction of the function of paralysed muscle. There is a false orientation of the field of vision.

SN-62 What is Tenon's capsule?

1. **Definition:** It forms a thin, loose membranous sheath around the eyeball.
2. **Extent:** It extends from the optic nerve to the sclerocorneal junction.
3. **Function:** Free movement of eyeball within the sheath.
4. **Structures piercing**
   A. Tendons of the various extraocular muscles.
   B. Ciliary vessels.
   C. Ciliary nerves.
5. **Expansions**
   A. A tubular sheath covers each orbital muscle.
   B. The medial check ligament is a strong ▲ lar expansion of medial rectus muscle. It is attached to the lacrimal bone.
   C. The lateral check ligament is a strong ▲ lar expansion from the sheath of the lateral rectus muscle. It is attached to zygomatic bone.
   D. The lower part of Tenon's capsule is thickened and is named the suspensory ligament of the eye or the suspensory ligament of Lockwood.
      a. It is expanded in the centre and narrows at its extremities and is slung like a hammock below the eyeball.
      b. It is formed by union of margins of sheaths of
         I. Inferior rectus and
         II. Inferior oblique muscles with
         III. Medial and lateral check ligaments.

OLA-39 What is the mode of blood supply of optic nerve?

It is divided into arterial supply and venous return.
1. **Arterial supply:** The arteries form plexus. They are derived from two sources
   A. Plexus formed by the
      a. Superior hypophyseal artery, branch of internal carotid artery,
      b. Ophthalmic artery,
      c. Posterior ciliary artery (branch of ophthalmic artery), and

d. Extraneural branches of central artery.

B. Branches of the central artery.

2. **Venous return:** Central vein.

SN-63   Palpebral (canthal) ligaments

These ligaments connect the tarsal plates to the orbits. They are medial and lateral palpebral ligaments (Fig. 7.2).

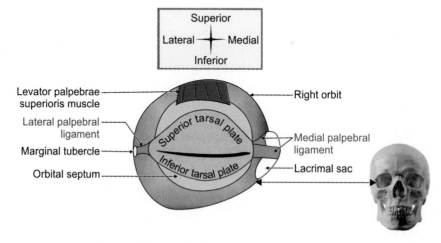

Fig. 7.2: Right orbit showing palpebral ligaments

A. **Medial palpebral ligament**
   a. It is well developed.
   b. It is superficially situated.
   c. It connects medial ends of two tarsal plates to the anterior lacrimal crest and frontal process of maxilla.
   d. At its insertion, it splits into tarsal plates to surround lacrimal canaliculi. It lies in front of nasolacrimal sac and the orbital septum.

B. **Lateral palpebral ligament**
   a. It is poorly developed.
   b. It extends from the lateral ends of tarsal plates to small tubercle on the zygomatic bone (Whitnall's tubercle).
   c. It is deeply situated.
   d. It lies deep to orbital septum and lateral palpebral raphe of orbicularis oculi.

LAQ-16   Describe extraocular muscles under the following heads:

1. Attachments (origin and insertion),

2. Action,

3. Nerve supply, and

4. Applied anatomy

The extraocular muscles are voluntary and involuntary.

A. Voluntary muscles are
   a. Four recti,
   b. Two obliqui, and
   c. Levator palpebrae superioris.

   a. Four recti:
      I. Superior rectus,
      II. Inferior rectus,
      III. Medial rectus, and
      IV. Lateral rectus.

   b. Obliqui
      I. Superior oblique
      II. Inferior oblique

   c. Levator palpebrae superioris

B. Involuntary: Orbitalis

1. **Attachments**

   A. **Origin of recti:** The recti muscles arise from the respective positions of a common tendinous ring. The ring is attached to the orbital surface of the apex of the orbit. The lateral rectus has an additional small tendinous head, which arises from the orbital surface of greater wing of sphenoid bone.

   B. **Insertion of recti:** The recti are inserted into the sclera in front of the equator. They are inserted few mm posterior to the sclerocorneal junction. The approximate distances of the insertion are (Fig. 7.3)

   | 🔑 5, 6, 7, 8 mm **MILS** |

   • <u>M</u>edial rectus: <u>5</u> mm behind the sclerocorneal junction.
   • <u>I</u>nferior rectus: <u>6</u> mm behind the sclerocorneal junction.
   • <u>L</u>ateral rectus: <u>7</u> mm behind the sclerocorneal junction.
   • <u>S</u>uperior rectus: <u>8</u> mm behind the sclerocorneal junction.

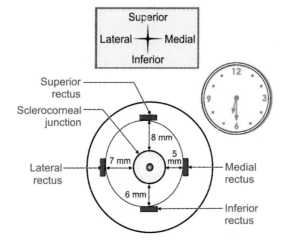

Fig. 7.3: Insertion of recti muscle

Head, Neck and Face

Clue to remember the distance of insertion of recti
from sclerocorneal junction—Tip

Box 7.1

Note: Visualise a clock. The 12 O' clock position represents superior rectus, 3 O' clock medial rectus, 6 O' clock inferior rectus and 9 O' clock positions represent lateral rectus. Now focus at 6 O' clock position, the digit 6 of 6 O' clock represents the insertion of inferior rectus behind sclerocorneal junction. The digit prior to 6 is 5 and represents the insertion of medial rectus. The digits after 6 are 7 and 8 which represent the insertion of lateral rectus and superior rectus.

a. Two obliqui:

Table 7.1: Origin and insertion of the oblique muscles and levator palpebrae superioris

Muscle	Origin	Insertion
• Superior oblique	• Body of sphenoid bone, • Superomedial to the optic canal	• SPL Superior posterior lateral quadrant of the sclera of eyeball, behind the equator.
• Inferior oblique	• Orbital surface of maxilla, • Lateral to the lacrimal groove.	• IPL Inferior posterior lateral quadrant of the sclera of the eyeball, behind the equator.
• Levator palpebrae superioris	• Orbital surface of lesser wing of the sphenoid bone	• Superior lamella • Anterior surface of the superior tarsus • Skin of the upper eyelid. • Inferior lamella: Upper margin of superior tarsus.

All extraocular muscles arise from apex of orbit except inferior oblique which arises from floor of orbit.[NEET]

C. **Involuntary muscles** (Fig. 7.4)
   a. Superior tarsal muscle is the deep part of levator palpebrae superioris. It is inserted on the upper margin of superior tarsus.
   b. Inferior tarsal muscle connects the inferior tarsus of the lower eyelid to the fascial sheath of the inferior rectus and inferior oblique. It helps in depression of lower lid.
   c. Orbitalis muscle bridges the inferior orbital fissure.

2. **Action** (Figs 7.5 and 7.6)
   A. **Action of individual muscles.**
      a. Superior rectus: Elevation, adduction, intorsion.
      b. Inferior rectus: Depression, adduction, extorsion.
      c. Inferior oblique: Elevation, abduction, extorsion.
      d. Superior oblique: Dépression, abduction, intorsion.
      e. Medial rectus: Adduction.
      f. Lateral rectus: Abduction.

Table 7.2: Yoke muscles (contralateral synergist)[NEET]

Recti muscles	Yoke muscles
Right superior rectus	Left inferior oblique
Right inferior rectus	Left superior oblique
Left superior rectus	Right inferior oblique
Left inferior rectus	Right superior oblique
Right lateral rectus	Left medial rectus
Left lateral rectus	Right medial rectus

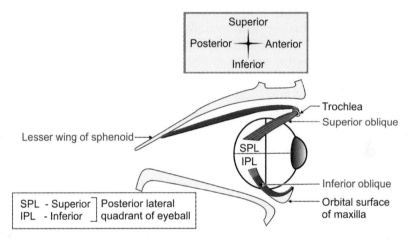

Fig. 7.4: Origin and insertion of the oblique muscle

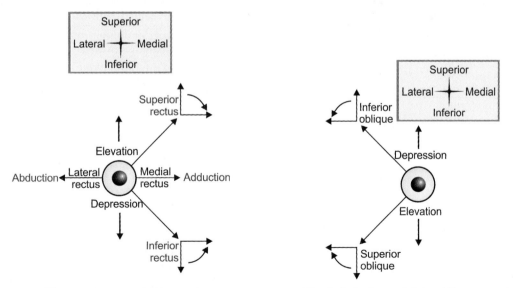

Fig. 7.5: Actions of right recti   **Fig. 7.6:** Actions of right oblique muscles

B. **Muscles bringing particular action.**

    a. Adduction: Medial rectus, superior rectus and inferior rectus.

    b. Abduction: Lateral rectus, inferior oblique and superior oblique.

    c. Elevation: Superior rectus and inferior oblique.

    d. Depression: Inferior rectus and superior oblique.

    e. Intorsion: Superior rectus and superior oblique.

    f. Extorsion: Inferior rectus and inferior oblique.

3. **Nerve supply**

    A. All the extraocular muscles of the eyeball are supplied by oculomotor nerve except **SO4** superior oblique, supplied by trochlear nerve (4th cranial nerve) and **LR6** lateral rectus supplied by abducent nerve (6th cranial nerve) (superior, inferior and medial recti, inferior oblique and levator palpebrae superioris are supplied by oculomotor nerve). SO4, LR6 and R3—superior oblique by 4th (trochlear nerve), lateral rectus by 6th (abducent) and rest all muscles by 3rd cranial nerve (oculomotor).

    B. Tarsal muscles are supplied by carotid nerve. The fibres of the nerve are post-ganglionic sympathetic fibres arising from superior cervical sympathetic ganglion.

4. **Applied anatomy**

    ➤ The muscles of eyeball are tested in following ways (Table 7.3).

Table 7.3: Testing of recti and oblique muscles

Muscle	Initial position of eyeball	Movement to be carried
• Recti	• Laterally	• For testing of the superior rectus muscle, ask to move the eyeball upward. • For the testing of inferior rectus muscle, ask to move eyeball downward.
• Oblique	• Medially	• For testing superior oblique muscle, ask to move the eyeball downward. • For the testing inferior oblique muscle, ask to move the eyeball upward.

    ➤ *Oculomotor nerve* lesion produces

      • Lateral strabismus,

      • In complete ophthalmoplegia

        ▪ There is paralysis of the muscles of the eyeball.

        ▪ Ptosis of the eyelid.

        ▪ Pupil is dilated (mydriasis).

        ▪ Loss of accommodation reflex.

    ➤ *Trochlear nerve* lesion produces diplopia (double vision) when looking downwards. Individuals with diplopia usually experience difficulty and apprehension on descending staircase.

➢ *Abducent nerve* lesion produces medial strabismus {*squint* (to have eyes that look in different direction)}. In this condition, the two eyes appear to look in different directions. Diplopia is minimal when looking to the opposite side of the lesion.

- Nystagmus is characterized by involuntary, rhythmical oscillatory movements of the eyes. This is due to incoordination of the ocular muscles. It may be either vestibular or cerebellar in origin.

SN-64   Ciliary ganglion

Introduction: It is collection of cell bodies of parasympathetic nerve. It supplies the sphincter pupillae muscle.

1. **Size:** Pinhead.
2. **Content:** Cell bodies of multipolar neuron.
3. **Situation:** Apex of the *orbit* in the angle made by optic nerve and lateral rectus muscle.
4. **Relations**
   A. **Medially:** Optic nerve.
   B. **Laterally:** Lateral rectus muscle.
5. **Connections:** Three roots
   A. **Motor (parasympathetic)** (Fig. 7.7)
      a. Preganglionic fibres arise from Edinger-Westphal nucleus > lower division of 3rd nerve > ciliary ganglion > fibres are relayed into ciliary ganglion.
      b. Postganglionic fibres carried by short ciliary nerve and supply
         I. Sphincter pupillae, and
         II. Ciliaris muscle.

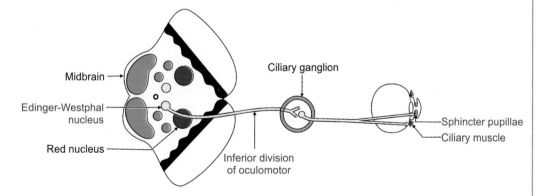

Fig. 7.7: Parasympathetic root of ciliary ganglion

   B. **Sensory:** Nasociliary fibres pass through ciliary ganglion without relay (Fig. 7.8).
   C. **Sympathetic** fibres pass through the ciliary ganglion without relay.
      a. Preganglionic fibres arise from spinal nerve and reach to superior cervical sympathetic ganglion.

(vertical margin text) Head, Neck and Face

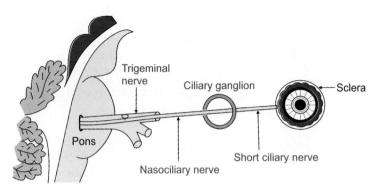

Fig. 7.8: Sensory root of ciliary ganglion

    b. Postganglionic fibres arise from the plexus around ophthalmic artery pass through short ciliary nerve and supply dilator pupillae.

6. **Branches:** 8 to 10 short ciliary nerves.

7. **Peculiarity:** The postganglionic parasympathetic fibres of ciliary ganglion are myelinated.

8. **Applied anatomy**

   ➤ Complete division of oculomotor nerve is manifested as [NEET]

     • Eyeball is depressed and abducted. "Down and out". External strabismus: Due to unopposed action of lateral rectus.

       Ophthalmoplegia >Diplopia where false image is higher than true image.

     • Ptosis: Drooping of eyelid due to involvement of levator palpebrae muscle.

     • Sphincter pupillae is not functioning. It results into dilatation of pupil (mydriasis)

     • Dilated and fixed pupil.

     • Loss of accommodation reflex because of paralysis of three muscles.

       ▪ Medial rectus—medial convergence of eyeball is lost.

       ▪ Sphincter pupillae—pupillary constriction is lost.

       ▪ Ciliaris muscle—thickness of lens.

     • Apparent protrusion of eyeball due to flaccid paralysis of most of ocular muscles.

   ➤ Neurosyphilis causes inflammation of posterior cerebral and superior cerebellar arteries. This compresses oculomotor nerve.

   ➤ Weber's syndrome: Contralateral hemiplegia (upper motor neuron lesion) and ipsilateral paralysis of muscles supplied by oculomotor nerve.

OLA-40 **What happens in case of unilateral ocular muscle paralysis?**

1. Paralysis of a muscle will cause limitation of movement of the eyeball. One will have double vision when one attempts to use the muscle.

Head, Neck and Face

A. When the abducent nerve supplying the lateral rectus is paralyzed, the individual cannot abduct the eyeball on the affected side. The eyeball is fully adducted by the unopposed pull of the medial rectus.

B. In complete 3rd nerve paralysis, the
  a. Eye cannot be moved upward, downward or inward.
  b. At rest, the eye looks laterally (external strabismus) because of the activity of the lateral rectus, and
  c. Downward because of the activity of the superior oblique.
  d. The patient has double vision (diplopia).
  e. Drooping of the upper eyelid (ptosis) occurs because of paralysis of the levator palpebrae superioris.
  f. The pupil is widely dilated and non reactive to light because of the paralysis of the sphincter pupillae and the unopposed action of the dilator pupillae (supplied by the sympathetic).
  g. Accommodation of the eye is lost.

C. In 4th nerve paralysis, the patient complains of double vision on looking straight downward. This is because the superior oblique is paralyzed and the eye turns medially as the inferior rectus pulls the eye downward.

D. In 6th nerve paralysis, the patient cannot
  a. Turn the eyeball laterally.
  b. When looking straight ahead, the lateral rectus is paralyzed, and
  c. Unopposed medial rectus pulls the eyeball medially, causing internal strabismus.

OLA-41 **Why the paralysis of extraocular muscles causes diplopia?**

1. The perception of two images of a single object is called diplopia.
2. The objects lying in different parts of the visual field produce images over different spots on the retina.
3. The brain judges the position of an object by the position at which its image is formed on the retina.
4. Normally, the movements of the right and left eyes are in perfect alignment, and an object casts an image on corresponding spots on the two retinae so that only one image is perceived by the brain.
5. When a muscle of the eyeball is weak, and a movement involving that muscle is performed, the movement of the defective eye is slightly less than that of the normal eye.
6. As a result, images of the object on the two retinae are not formed at corresponding points but over two points near each other. The brain, therefore, 'sees' two images, one from each retina.

OLA-42 **What is conjugate movements of eyes?**

Normally, movements of the two eyes are harmoniously coordinated. Such coordinated movements of both eyes are called conjugate ocular movements.

Head, Neck and Face

OLA-43 What is nystagmus?

1. An involuntary rhythmical, oscillatory movement of eyeball is called nystagmus.
2. This is due to incoordination of the ocular muscles. It may be either
   A. Vestibular or
   B. Cerebellar, or even
   C. Congenital.

SN-65 Orbital nerve

It is a branch of pterygopalatine ganglion. It is actually branch of maxillary nerve. It also carries parasympathetic and sympathetic fibres which pass through the ganglion.

1. **Course:** It passes through the inferior orbital fissure.
2. **Distribution:** It supplies the
   A. Periosteum of the orbit, and
   B. Orbitalis muscle.
   C. Mucous membrane of sphenoidal and ethmoidal air sinuses.

Anterior Triangle of the Neck

SN-66   Platysma

It is a broad, flat muscle, remnant of panniculus carnosus.[NEET]
It lies superficial to deep fascia of neck (Fig. 8.1).

1. **Proximal attachments** are fascia over the
    A. Pectoralis major, and
    B. Deltoid.
2. **Distal attachments:** They are divided into anterior and posterior fibres.
    A. Anterior fibres are inserted to the base of mandible.
    B. Posterior fibres to the skin of the lower part of face and lip.
3. **Action:** Depresses the skin. It pulls the angle of the mouth downwards as in horror.
4. **Development:** It is developed from the mesoderm of 2nd pharyngeal arch hence supplied by cervical branch of facial nerve.

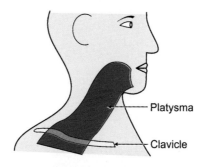

Fig. 8.1: Platysma

SN-67   Muscular triangle

1. **Boundaries** (Fig. 8.2)
    A. **Anteriorly:** Anterior median line of the neck from the hyoid bone to the sternum.
    B. **Posterosuperiorly:** Superior belly of the omohyoid muscle.
    C. **Posteroinferiorly:** Anterior border of the sternocleidomastoid muscle.

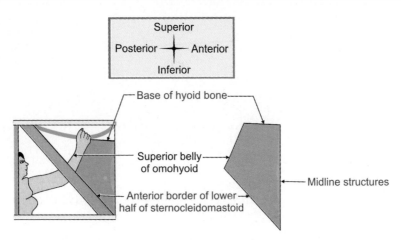

Fig. 8.2: Boundaries of muscular triangle

2. **Contents:** Infrahyoid muscles are the chief contents of the triangle. These are

    a. Sternohyoid,

    b. Sternothyroid,

    c. Thyrohyoid, and

    d. Omohyoid.

SN-68   **Occipital artery**

Introduction: It is the artery supplying the posterior aspect of scalp. It gives muscular branches to the sternocleidomastoid and stylohyoid.

1. **Origin:** It is the 1st dorsal branch of external carotid artery arising opposite facial artery. It emerges at the apex of posterior triangle of neck. It goes along with GON greater occipital nerve.

2. **Course and relations**

    A. Courses deep to the lower border of posterior belly of digastric.

    B. Grooves the base of skull at the occipitomastoid suture.

    C. Lies deep to the digastric notch.

3. **Peculiarities**

    A. At its origin, it is crossed superficially by hypoglossal nerve.

    B. Its upper branch acts as a guide to the accessory nerve.

    C. It has a tortuous course in the superficial fascia of scalp.

4. **Branches** (Fig. 8.3)

    A. Muscular branch to stylohyoid and sternocleidomastoid.

    B. Meningeal branch

    C. Bony branch to mastoid process.

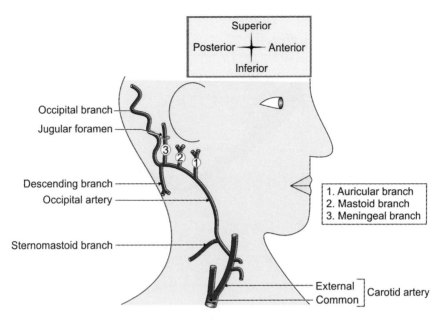

Fig. 8.3: Branches of occipital artery

LAQ-17	Describe digastric triangle under the following headings:

1. **Boundaries,**
2. **Roof,**
3. **Floor,**
4. **Contents, and**
5. **Applied anatomy**

1. **Boundaries** (Fig. 8.4)
   A. Anteroinferior: Anterior belly of digastric.
   B. Posteroinferior: Posterior belly of digastric and stylohyoid.
   C. Superior (base) is by
      a. Base of the mandible, and
      b. Line joining the angle of the mandible to the mastoid process.
2. **Roof**
   A. Skin
   B. Superficial fascia containing ◄━ 3C
      Cutaneous vein (tributaries of external jugular vein).
      Cutaneous branches of great auricular nerve
      Cervical branch of facial nerve.
   C. Deep fascia encloses submandibular salivary gland.

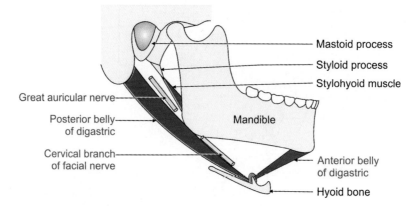

Fig. 8.4: Boundaries and roof of digastric triangle

3. **Floor:** From anterior to posterior
    A. Mylohyoid,
    B. Hyoglossus, and
    C. Middle constrictor of pharynx.
4. **Contents** (Fig. 8.5): They are grouped as structures in the
    A. Anterior part of the triangle.
        a. Structures superficial to mylohyoid are superficial part of submandibular gland and related structures. The relations can be visualized.

> Visualize the relations of submandibular gland with the fingers of your hands—Tip

Box 8.1

- Submandibular gland hugs the mylohyoid by laying its major superficial part anteriorly and small deep part posteriorly.
- Semiflex your left wrist in such a way that the 4 fingers are placed anteriorly and thumb posteriorly. Tip of fingers and thumb referred as anterior ends of the superficial part of submandibular gland.
- The number of fingers indicates size of the gland.
- Four fingers of left hand refer the larger superficial part ⟨⚷ IMRL⟩
- Index finger of left hand represents the facial vein.
- Middle finger of left hand represents the mylohyoid vessels and nerve.
- Ring finger of left hand represents submental vessels and nerve.
- Little finger of left hand represents submandibular lymph node, and
- Thumb of left hand refers smaller deep part. Position of the wrist indicates that superficial part of gland is continuous with deep part of the submandibular gland.

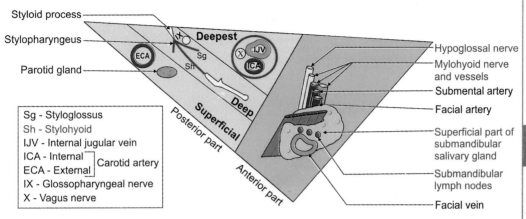

Styloid process
Stylopharyngeus
Parotid gland

Deepest
Sg
Sh
Deep
Superficial
Posterior part
Anterior part

Hypoglossal nerve
Mylohyoid nerve and vessels
Submental artery
Facial artery
Superficial part of submandibular salivary gland
Submandibular lymph nodes
Facial vein

Sg - Styloglossus
Sh - Stylohyoid
IJV - Internal jugular vein
ICA - Internal ⎤
ECA - External ⎦ Carotid artery
IX - Glossopharyngeal nerve
X - Vagus nerve

Fig. 8.5: Contents of right diagstric triangle

B. Posterior part of triangle.

Table 8.1: Structures present in the posterior part of the digastric triangle

Superficial	Deep (styloid)	Deepest (carotid sheath)
• Parotid gland • External carotid artery	• Styloid process • Styloglossus • Stylopharyngeus • Glossopharyngeal (9th cranial nerve) and pharyngeal branch (10th cranial nerve)	• Internal carotid artery • Internal jugular vein and 10th cranial nerve.

5. Applied anatomy

Ludwig's angina: It is a ▲ lar swelling due to the infection of the submandibular region. It is bounded
- Posteriorly by the hyoid bone, and
- Anterolaterally on each side by the two halves of base of mandible. This is so because the investing layer of deep cervical fascia is attached to these bones. Collection of pus may push the tongue upwards.

SN-69   Digastric muscle

Introduction: It is suprahyoid muscle of the neck (Fig. 8.6).

1. **Origin:** It has two bellies.

   A. Anterior belly arises from digastric fossa of mandible.

   B. Posterior belly arises from digastric notch, present medial to mastoid process.

2. **Insertion:** Both heads meet at the intermediate tendon which is held by a fibrous pulley attached to the hyoid bone.

Head, Neck and Face

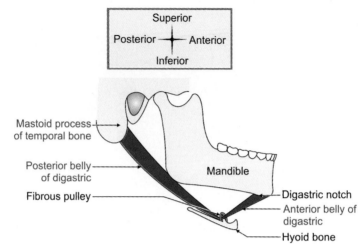

Fig. 8.6: Digastric muscle

3. Nerve supply

A. Anterior belly is supplied by nerve to mylohyoid, a branch of inferior alveolar nerve, branch of anterior division of mandibular nerve.

B. Posterior belly is supplied by facial nerve.

4. **Action**

A. It depresses mandible when mouth is opened widely.

B. It elevates the hyoid bone.

5. **Development**

A. Anterior belly develops from mesenchyme of the first pharyngeal arch.

B. Posterior belly develops from mesenchyme of the second pharyngeal arch.

LAQ-18	Describe carotid triangle under the following headings:
	1. Boundaries,
	2. Roof,
	3. Floor,
	4. Contents, and
	5. Applied anatomy

1. **Boundaries** (Fig. 8.7)

A. **Superiorly:** Posterior belly of the digastric muscle and the stylohyoid.

B. **Anteroinferiorly:** Superior belly of the omohyoid.

C. **Posteriorly:** Anterior border of upper half of the sternomastoid muscle.

2. **Roof**

A. Skin.

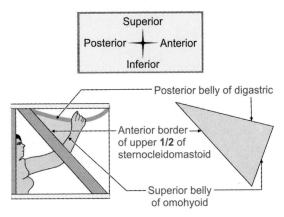

Fig. 8.7: Boundaries of right carotid triangle

B. Superficial fascia. It contains
  a. Platysma muscle,
  b. Cervical branch of the facial nerve, and
  c. Transverse cutaneous nerve of the neck.
C. Investing layer of deep cervical fascia.

3. **Floor:** It is formed by ⚷━ **HIT Mi**

<u>H</u>yoglossus.

<u>I</u>nferior constrictors of pharynx.

<u>T</u>hyrohyoid muscle.

<u>Mi</u>ddle constrictor of pharynx

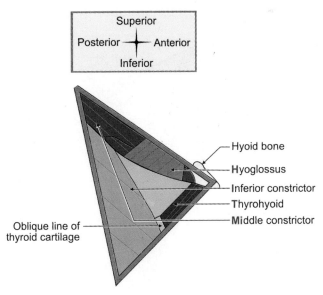

Fig. 8.8: Floor of right carotid triangle on right side—HIT Mi

4. **Contents** (Fig. 8.9)

A. **Carotid sheath**

a. **Contents**

I. Common carotid artery and its two terminal branches

i. Internal carotid artery.

ii. External carotid artery

II. Internal jugular vein.

III. Vagus nerve. It is present posteromedially.

b. **Relations of carotid sheath**

I. Anterior wall: Ansa cervicalis.

II. Posterior wall: Sympathetic trunk.

B. **Carotid body and carotid sinus.**

C. **Deep cervical lymph nodes.**

D. **Vessels and nerves.** 5, 3, 2—5 arteries, 3 veins and 2 nerves.

a. **5 branches of external carotid artery**

I. Ascending pharyngeal artery,

II. Superior thyroid artery,

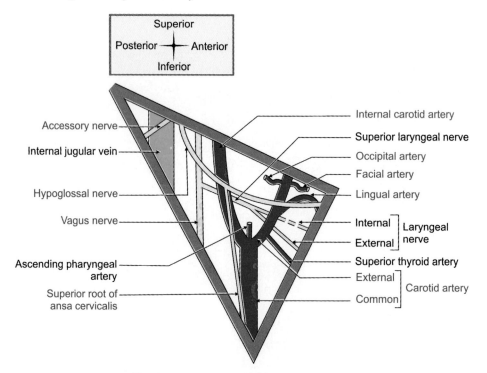

Fig. 8.9: Contents of right carotid triangle

III. Lingual artery,

IV. Facial artery, and

V. Occipital artery.

b. **3 tributaries of internal jugular vein**

I. Pharyngeal vein,

II. Lingual vein,

III. Common facial vein.

c. **2 nerves**

I. Spinal accessory nerve: It is present at the posterosuperior angle of the triangle. It passes superficial to triangle.

II. Hypoglossal nerve: It always crosses the loop of lingual artery.

5. **Applied anatomy**

➤ A strong carotid pulse is palpable in the carotid triangle inferior to the level of Adam's apple by gently pressing the common carotid artery against the underlying anterior tubercle of 6th cervical vertebra.

➤ *In the elderly, atheromatous plaques may be dislodged by palpations on left side. Hence, pulsation should be felt on the right side since a stroke induced in the right cerebral hemisphere is less devastating.*

SN-70   External carotid artery

1. **Origin:** It is one of the terminal branches of the common carotid artery given at the level of superior cornu of thyroid cartilage.
2. **Extent:** From the upper border of thyroid cartilage to the neck of mandible.
3. **Branches:** All the branches of external carotid artery lie above the level of angle of jaw, and hence, supply the face rather than neck (Fig. 8.10).

> Superior thyroid artery was too scared to climb the face—Tip

Box 8.2

The exception is superior thyroid artery, (which falls down on the job and is afraid of heights) and reaches down to grab the thyroid.

A. **Medial:** Ascending pharyngeal.
B. **Dorsal:**
   a. Occipital, and
   b. Posterior auricular.
C. **Ventral:**
   a. Superior thyroid,
   b. Lingual, and
   c. Facial.

Head, Neck and Face

D. **Terminal:**
   a. Superficial temporal, and
   b. Maxillary.

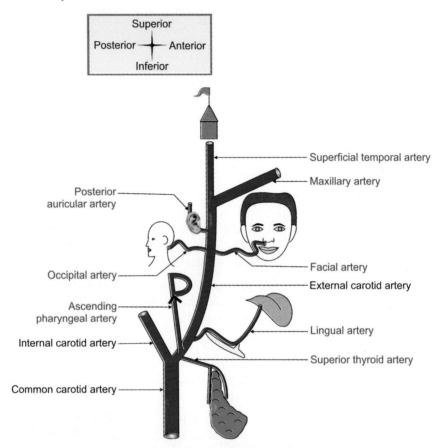

Fig. 8.10: Branches of external carotid artery

4. **Course:** It lies anterior and medial to internal carotid artery at its origin. It passes deep to the posterior belly of digastric and stylohyoid muscle, enters the parotid gland and divides into terminal branches.

5. **Relations**
   A. **Superficial**
      a. In the carotid triangle, it is overlapped by sternomastoid and crossed by hypoglossal nerve, lingual nerve and facial vein.
      b. In the digastric triangle, it is related to posterior belly of digastric and stylohyoid muscle.
      c. In parotid gland, it is overlapped by retromandibular vein.
   B. **Deep**
      a. Constrictor muscles of pharynx.
      b. Superior laryngeal nerve and its two branches: Internal and external laryngeal nerves.
      c. Internal carotid artery.

SN-71 Lingual artery

1. **Origin:** It is the 2nd ventral branch of external carotid artery, arises opposite to the tip of greater cornu of hyoid bone.
2. **Course and relations:** It is divided into three parts by hyoglossus muscle.
   A. 1st part (lateral to hyoglossus) extends from origin (external carotid artery) to the tip of greater cornu of hyoid bone. It forms upward loop to avoid rupture during the movements of hyoid bone.
   B. 2nd part lies deep to the hyoglossus muscle and on the upper border of greater cornu of hyoid bone. It lies superficial to middle constrictor.
   C. 3rd part runs along anterior border of hyoglossus muscle. It is also called deep lingual artery.
3. **Branches** (Fig. 8.11)
   A. **1st part:** Suprahyoid artery.
   B. **2nd part:** Dorsal lingual artery.
   C. **3rd part (deep lingual artery):** Sublingual artery.

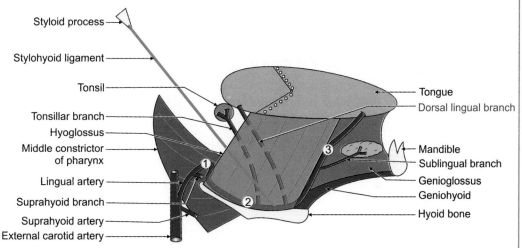

Fig. 8.11: Lingual artery and its branches

4. Applied anatomy
   ➢ In surgical removal of tongue, the 1st part of the artery is ligated before it gives any branch to tongue or tonsil.
   ➢ Bleeding from the lingual artery is arrested by pulling the tongue out.

OLA-44 Enumerate the branches of facial artery in neck.

1. Ascending palatine
2. Tonsillar branch
3. Submental
4. Glandular.

Head, Neck and Face

OLA-45 Why is facial artery tortuous?

1. Facial artery has cervical and facial parts. In both segments, the artery is tortuous.

2. The cervical part of facial artery is tortuous to adapt to the movements of pharynx during deglutition.

3. The facial part is tortuous to adapt to the movements of mandible, lips and cheek.

SN-72 Facial artery

It is the chief artery of the face.

1. **Peculiarity:** The artery is tortuous to avoid the rupture during the movements of pharynx, the contraction of the muscles of face and the movements of temporomandibular joint.

2. **Origin:** It is the 3rd ventral branch of external carotid artery arising above the level of the tip of greater cornu of hyoid bone.

3. **Course:** It is divided into cervical and facial.

   A. It runs $(⊶\text{s for s})$ superficial to superior constrictor of the pharynx and deep to posterior belly of digastric $(⊶\text{d for d})$ and to the ramus of mandible, at the anterior border of the masseter muscle. It grooves the submandibular gland.

   B. It enters the face by winding round the base of the mandible and pierces deep cervical fascia at the junction of ramus and body of mandible.

   C. It crosses the masseter at anteroinferior angle. It runs upwards half an inch lateral to angle of mouth and ascends by the side of nose and anastomoses with ophthalmic artery, branch of internal carotid artery.

4. **Branches** (Fig. 8.12)

   A. **Cervical part**

   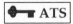 ATS

   Ascending palatine,

   Tonsillar,

   Submental, and

   Submandibular.

   B. **Facial part**

   a. Inferior labial,

   b. Superior labial, and

   c. Lateral nasal.

5. Applied anatomy: The wounds of face bleed profusely but heal quickly because of rich blood supply and profuse anastomosis.

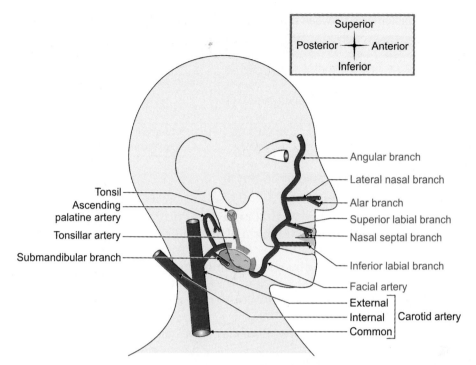

Fig. 8.12: Branches of facial artery

Head, Neck and Face

OLA-46 **Structures passing between external and internal carotid arteries.**

1. **Muscles**
   A. Styloglossus.
   B. Stylopharyngeus.
2. **Nerves**
   A. Glossopharyngeal nerve
   B. Pharyngeal branch of the vagus nerve.
3. **Bone:** Styloid process of temporal bone.
4. **Gland:** Part of the parotid gland.

SN-73 **Sites of anastomosis of external and internal carotid arteries**

Table 8.2: Anastomosis between external and internal carotid arteries

Site	Branch of external carotid	Branch of internal carotid
• Middle cranial fossa	• Deep temporal branch of maxillary artery	• Lacrimal artery, branch of ophthalmic artery
• Angle of eye	• Facial artery	• Medial palpebral artery, branch of ophthalmic artery
	• Zygomatico-orbital branch of superficial temporal artery	• Lacrimal and palpebral branches of ophthalmic artery

Contd.

Table 8.2: Anastomosis between external carotid artery and internal carotid artery (Contd.)

Site	Branch of external carotid	Branch of internal carotid
• Scalp	• Frontal branch of superficial temporal artery	• Supraorbital and supratrochlear branch of ophthalmic artery
• Maxilla	• Infraorbital branch of maxillary artery	• Branch of ophthalmic artery
• Zygoma	• Transverse facial branch of superficial temporal artery	• Lacrimal artery, branch of ophthalmic artery

SN-74   Ansa cervicalis (ansa hypoglossi)

(*Ansa*—loop, *cervicalis*—cervical)

Introduction: A loop formed by ventral rami of cervical nerves.

1. **Formation:** It is formed by ventral rami of 1st, 2nd and 3rd cervical nerves.
2. **Roots**
   A. Superior root (descending hyoglossi or anterior root) is formed by ventral ramus of **C1.**
   B. Inferior root (descending cervicalis or posterior root) is formed by ventral rami of **C2** and **C3.**
3. **Relations:** It lies on the anterior wall of carotid sheath.
4. **Distribution**
   A. **Superior root:** Superior belly of omohyoid.
   B. **Inferior root**
      a. Sternohyoid,
      b. Sternothyroid, and
      c. Inferior belly of omohyoid.

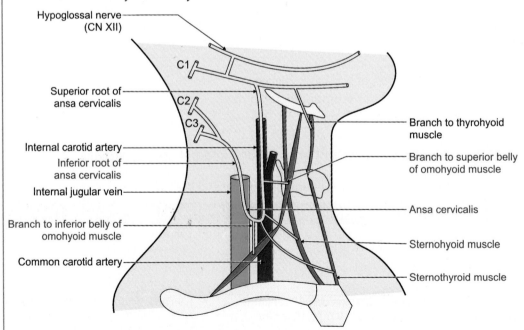

Fig. 8.13: Formation, relations and branches of ansa cervicalis

SN-75 **Superior laryngeal nerve**

1. **Origin:** It arises from inferior ganglion of the vagus.
2. **Course:**
    A. It passes downwards and forwards on the superior constrictor of pharynx. Here, it is deep to internal carotid artery.
    B. It reaches middle constrictor of pharynx and divides into branches on thyrohyoid membrane.
3. **Branches** (Fig. 8.14)
    A. **Internal laryngeal nerve**
        a. It is the larger terminal branch of superior laryngeal nerve given in the carotid sheath.
        b. It pierces the thyrohyoid membrane and passes deep to it. It passes along with superior laryngeal vessels. It is sensory to the mucous membrane of
            I. Posterior one-third of tongue, and
            II. Larynx above the vocal fold. It includes
                i. Laryngeal mucous membrane of the laryngeal vestibule,
                ii. Middle laryngeal cavity, and
                iii. Superior surface of the vocal folds.
    B. **External laryngeal nerve**
        a. It is the smaller terminal branch of superior laryngeal nerve given in the carotid sheath.
        b. It passes deep to superior thyroid artery.
        c. It is motor branch to cricothyroid, the only external muscle of larynx.

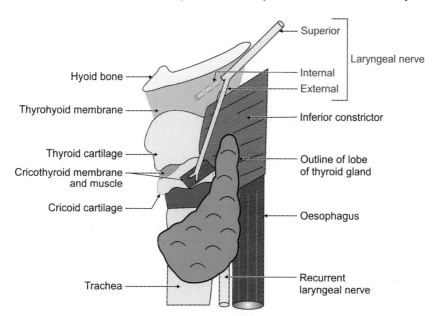

Fig. 8.14: Course, relations and branches of superior laryngeal nerve

Head, Neck and Face

4. **Relations:** Superior laryngeal nerve is accompanied by superior thyroid artery. The external laryngeal nerve has intimate and important relations with branches of superior thyroid artery supplying lateral lobe of thyroid gland. External laryngeal nerve and branches of superior thyroid artery are very close when they are away from lateral lobe of thyroid gland and go apart when they reach the gland.

5. **Development:** It is nerve of the IVth pharyngeal arch.

6. **Applied anatomy**

   ➤ During thyroidectomy, superior thyroid artery is ligated near the lateral lobe of thyroid gland to avoid the damage to superior laryngeal nerve.

   ➤ Damage to the internal laryngeal nerve causes anaesthesia of the superior laryngeal mucosa. It results into loss of protective mechanism of the larynx. Thus, the foreign bodies can easily enter the larynx.

   ➤ Injury to the external laryngeal nerve results in paralysis of cricothyroid muscle. It is unable to vary the length and tension of vocal cords. It manifests as monotonous voice. It goes unnoticed in persons who do not use wide range of tone in their speech. It is critical to singers and public speakers.

   ➤ Superior laryngeal nerve block is used with end tracheal intubation in the conscious patients.

OLA-47 **What is the effect of pressure damage to internal laryngeal nerve, external laryngeal nerve and recurrent laryngeal nerve?**

1. Pressure on internal laryngeal nerve causes loss of sensation of larynx above the vocal cords on the affected side.

2. Pressure on external laryngeal nerve causes paralysis of cricothyroid muscle. It leads to weakness of phonation due to the loss of the tightening effect of the cricothyroid muscle.

3. Pressure on the recurrent laryngeal nerve causes change in the voice.

   A. Unilateral pressure does not cause complete loss of speech.

   B. Bilateral pressure causes remarkable loss of speech.

SN-76 **Anterior jugular vein**

1. **Origin:** Begins in the submental region.

2. **Course:** It runs in the superficial fascia 1cm lateral to median plane in the anterior triangle of neck. It enters the suprasternal space by piercing investing layer of deep cervical fascia.

   It joins with its fellow of opposite side by transverse channel, the jugular venous arch and then runs deep to sternocleidomastoid .

3. **Termination:** It opens into external jugular vein.

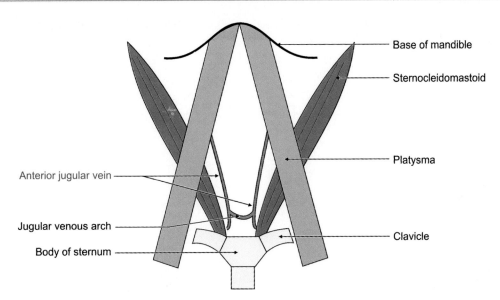

Fig. 8.15: Anterior jugular vein

4. **Applied anatomy**: It is one of the contents of suprasternal space. Injury to the vein results into air embolism.

Head, Neck and Face

Parotid Region

OLA-48 Why does opening of the jaw cause pain in mumps?

The investing layer of deep fascia is modified over the parotid gland. It forms parotid fascia. It is dense and firmly attached to parotid gland. In mumps, the parotid gland is inflamed. There is no space for the expansion of gland. As the gland enlarges, it irritates the nerves and causes pain while opening the mouth.

OLA-49 How the parotid gland is removed surgically?

Facial paralysis is one of the complications of removal of parotid gland. Hence, identification of the facial nerve is essential during surgery. The facial nerve is most distinct as it emerges from the stylomastoid foramen. In doubtful cases, electrical stimulation may be used for confirmation. The plane of clevage is defined by tracing the nerve behind forwards.

LAQ-19 Describe parotid gland under the following headings:
1. Morphology,
2. Relations,
3. Blood supply,
4. Lymphatics,
5. Nerve supply, and
6. Applied anatomy

1. **Morphology:** It is the largest salivary gland.
   A. **Weight:** 25 g.

   B. Shape is like an inverted pyramid .

   C. **Covering:** Consists of inner true capsule, formed by condensation of peripheral part of fibrous stroma of gland. It is fibrous tissue.

D. **Outer false capsule:** Formed by investing layer of deep cervical fascia. It gets thickened and form stylomandibular ligament. It extends from angle of mandible to styloid process. It divides submandibular and parotid glands.

E. Presenting parts

   a. Apex

   b. Base

   c. Borders: Anterior, medial and posterior.

   d. Surface: Superficial, anteromedial and posteromedial.

2. **Relations** (Figs 9.1 and 9.2)

Table 9.1: Relations of parotid gland

	Structures related	Structures emerging (superficial to deep)
• Apex	• Posterior belly of digastric	• Cervical branch of facial nerve • Anterior and posterior divisions of retromandibular vein
• Base	• External acoustic meatus • Posterior part of temporomandibular joint	• Temporal branch of facial nerve • Superficial temporal artery • Superficial temporal vein • Auriculotemporal nerve
• Superficial or lateral surface	• Skin • Superficial fascia • Posterior fibres of platysma • Preauricular group of lymph nodes.[NEET]	• Great auricular nerve supplying skin over the angle of mandible • Parotid fascia
• Anteromedial surface	• Masseter ⬛━ 3M • Posterior ramus of mandible • Medial pterygoid	• Maxillary artery • Maxillary vein
• Posteromedial surface	• ⬛━ 3 processes • Mastoid process and muscles attached Sternocleidomastoid, • Posterior belly of digastric. • Styloid process and structures attached to it (styloid apparatus). • Muscles—stylohyoid, stylopharyngeus, styloglossus • Ligaments—stylohyoid, stylomandibular • Transverse process of atlas: Rectus capitis lateralis	• Auriculotemporal nerve • Facial nerve • Posterior division of retromandibular vein. • External carotid artery • Occipital artery

• Borders
• Anterior
		Branches of facial nerve
		• Temporofacial
		  ▪ Zygomatic
		  ▪ Temporal
		• Cervicofacial
		  ▪ Buccal

Contd.

Head, Neck and Face

Table 9.1: Relations of parotid gland (Contd.)

	Structures related	Structures emerging (superficial to deep)
		– Upper buccal branch – Lower buccal branch • Marginomandibular • Cervical • Accessory parotid gland and its duct • Parotid duct
• Posterior	• Sternocleidomastoid • Posterior auricular branch of facial nerve • Posterior auricular vessels	
• Medial	• Pharynx	

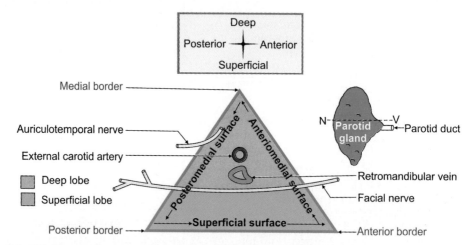

Fig. 9.1: Borders, surfaces and superficial and deep parts of parotid gland and relevant structures

3. **Blood supply**

A. **Arterial:** Branches from external carotid artery (E C A).

B. **Venous:** Tributaries of external jugular vein (E J V).

4. **Lymphatics**

A. Afferent lymphatics drain into parotid group of lymph nodes.

B. Efferent lymphatics drain to jugulodigastric group of deep cervical lymph nodes.

5. Nerve supply

A. **Gland**

a. **Sensory:**

I. Gland: Auriculotemporal nerve, a branch of mandibular nerve.

II. Parotid fascia: Great auricular nerve (**C2, C3**).

b. **Motor**

I. Secretomotor: (parasympathetic) (Fig. 9.3):

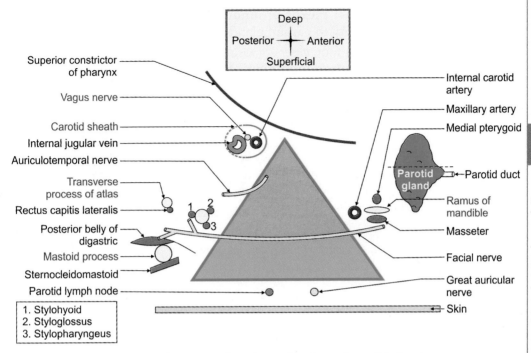

Fig. 9.2: Relations of border and surface of parotid gland

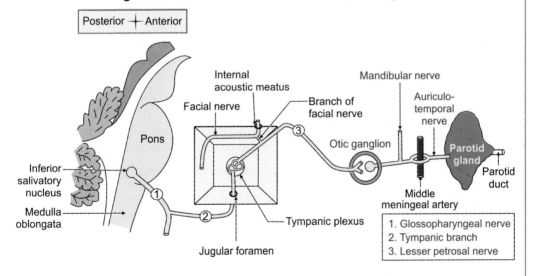

Fig. 9.3: Secretomotor fibres of parotid gland

    i. Preganglionic fibres arise from inferior salivatory nucleus. It travels via glossopharyngeal nerve—tympanic branch of glossopharyngeal nerve—tympanic plexus—lesser petrosal nerve—otic ganglion—fibres relay.

   ii. Postganglionic: Auriculotemporal nerve—parotid gland.

II. Vasomotor (sympathetic) (Fig. 9.4)

    i. Preganglionic fibres arise from thoracic segment of spinal cord>Superior cervical sympathetic ganglion.

ii. Postganglionic: Plexus around external carotid artery > middle meningeal artery to parotid gland.

Pes anserinus (*pes*—a foot, *anser*—goose): Branches of the facial nerve in the substance of parotid gland form a network called pes anserinus. This divides the parotid gland into superficial and deep parts.

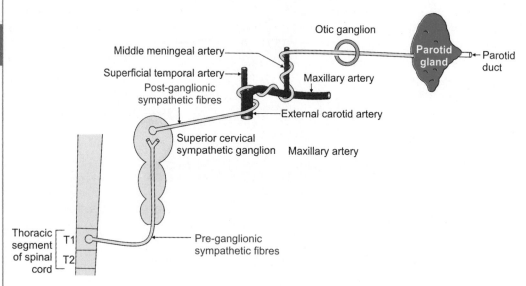

Fig. 9.4: Sympathetic fibres of parotid gland

6. **Applied anatomy**

➤ **Parotitis:** Inflammation of parotid gland is very painful due to unyielding nature of parotid fascia. Mumps is a viral infection of parotid gland, which is usually bilateral and self-limiting. There are no complications in children because gonads are not developed in children. If it occurs in adult, the complications are oophoritis in female ♀, orchitis in male ♂ and pancreatitis in both sexes.

➤ **Parotid abscess** is drained by taking **transverse** incision over parotid gland to avoid injury to the branches of facial nerve (Hilton's method).

➤ **Mixed parotid tumour:** It is most common neoplasm of parotid gland. It is slow growing, benign painless tumour and does not involve facial nerve.

➤ **Frey's syndrome:**[NEET 19] Sometimes penetrating wound of parotid gland damages auriculotemporal nerve and great auricular nerve. During regeneration, auriculotemporal nerve joins with great auricular nerve. Therefore, stimulation of auricular temporal nerve stimulates great auricular nerve. This results into sweating over the parotid region. The condition is called **Frey's syndrome.**

➤ During **partial parotidectomy**, the pes anserinus helps to distinguish between superficial and deep parts of gland.

➤ Most **common neoplasm** of the parotid is a benign tumour called **mixed parotid tumour**. It is present in the superficial lobe and consequently may be excised by superficial lobectomy.

➤ **Malignant parotid** tumours are usually present in the **deep lobe** and involve facial nerve.

➤ In removing a benign mixed salivary tumour of the parotid, the facial nerve is exposed. It is exposed posteriorly in the wedge shaped space. The space is present between the bony canal of the external auditory meatus and the mastoid process. The facial nerve is traced into the gland. The main divisions are identified and the tumour is excised with a wide margin of normal gland. The care should be taken to preserve the exposed nerves.

➤ It is interesting that giant mixed tumours can be excised with an adequate margin without even seeing the facial nerve.

SN-77   Parotid duct (Stenson's duct)

Introduction: It is thick-walled tube, which carries secretion of parotid gland to vestibule of mouth.

1. **Formation:** By union of two vertical ducts (formed by ductules).

2. **Shape** of crow quill .

3. **Length:** 5 cm, width: 3 mm.

4. **Course**

    A. **Begins** from middle of anterior border of parotid gland.

        a. Runs on masseter muscle. It has three bends.

        b. 1st bend: It directs medially at the anterior border of masseter and pierces (3B) Buccal pad of fat, Buccopharyngeal fascia and Buccinator muscle.

Box 9.1

Structures piercing buccinator are

1. Parotid duct

2. Buccal nerve, branch of mandibular nerve—sensory to the skin over buccinator

---

        c. 2nd bend: It is between Buccinator and Buccal mucous membrane of oral cavity.

        d. 3rd bend: It pierces mucous membrane and enters vestibule of mouth.

    B. **Ends by opening on the** (Fig. 9.5)

        a. Summit of raised papilla.

        b. Opposite the crown of upper 2nd molar tooth.

        c. Within vestibule of mouth.

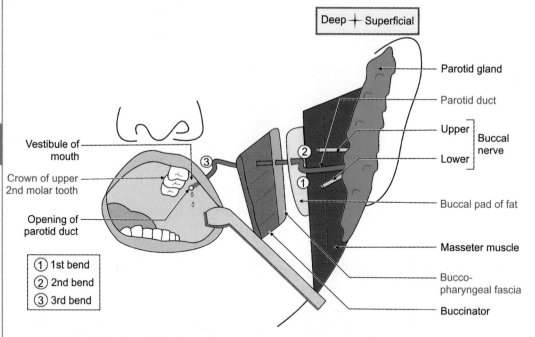

Fig. 9.5: Coronal section of the face shwoing opening of parotid ducts in the vestibule of mouth, opposite crown of upper 2nd molar tooth

Associate memory: Events at upper 2nd molar tooth—Tip

Box 9.2
Associate memory: Events at upper 2nd molar teeth
1. Opening of parotid duct, and
2. Modiolus.

5. **Structure**
    A. Outer fibroelastic coat and smooth muscle.
    B. Inner mucous membrane which is lined by stratified cuboidal epithelium.
6. **Blood supply:**
    A. **Arterial supply:**
        a. Glandular branches of transverse facial artery, a branch of superficial temporal artery.
        b. Glandular branches of posterior auricular artery.
    B. **Venous drainage:** Veins draining parotid gland drain into
        a. External jugular vein, and
        b. Internal jugular vein.

7. **Lymphatics** : Superficial and deep cervical group of lymph nodes.

8. **Nerve supply**: Auriculotemporal nerve, branch of posterior division of mandibular nerve.

9. **Development**

   A. **Germ layer:** Ectoderm[NEET]

   B. **Source:** Stomodeum.

   C. **Site:** Furrow between the mandibular and maxillary arches at the site of future angle of mouth.

10. Applied anatomy

   ➢ Oblique passage of duct between mucous membrane and the buccinator serves as a valve-like mechanism and prevents inflation of the duct during violent blowing.
   ➢ Parotid duct is palpated and rolled on the firm anterior edge of masseter muscle.

Head, Neck and Face

Temporal and Infratemporal Regions

OLA-50 Give the branches of 1st part of maxillary artery.

DAIMA

1. Deep auricular,

2. Anterior tympanic,

3. Inferior alveolar,

4. Middle meningeal, and

5. Accessory meningeal.

SN-78 **Maxillary artery**

Introduction: It is one of the two terminal branches of external carotid artery given at the neck of mandible. It is the artery of upper and lower jaws, the muscles of mastication, palate and nose.

1. **Course:** It is divided into three parts by lower head of lateral pterygoid muscle. It enters the infratemporal fossa. It lies between neck of mandible and sphenomandibular ligament. Here the auriculotemporal nerve is above the artery and maxillary vein lies below the artery. It enters the pterygopalatine fossa through pterygomaxillary fissure.

   A. It is divided conveniently into three parts by lateral pterygoid muscle (Fig. 10.1)

      a. 1st part lies proximal to the lower head of lateral pterygoid.

      b. 2nd part lies in relation to lateral pterygoid. It lies either superficial or deep to lower head of lateral pterygoid.

      c. 3rd part lies in the pterygopalatine fossa distal to the upper head of lateral pterygoid.

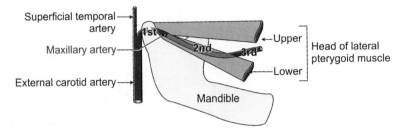

Fig. 10.1: Lateral pterygoid muscle showing three parts of maxillary artery

2. **Branches:** Branches of 1st and 2nd parts accompany the branches of maxillary nerve (Figs 10.2 and 10.3).

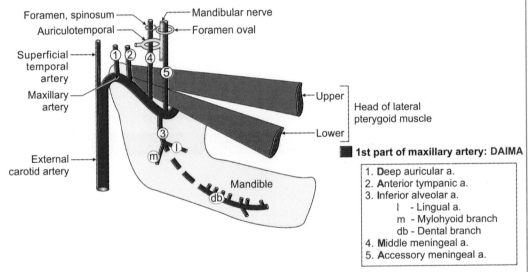

1st part of maxillary artery: DAIMA

1. **D**eep auricular a.
2. **A**nterior tympanic a.
3. **I**nferior alveolar a.
   - l - Lingual a.
   - m - Mylohyoid branch
   - db - Dental branch
4. **M**iddle meningeal a.
5. **A**ccessory meningeal a.

Fig. 10.2: Branches of 1st part of maxillary artery

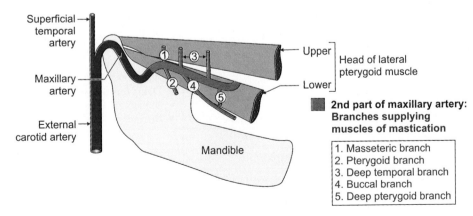

2nd part of maxillary artery: Branches supplying muscles of mastication

1. Masseteric branch
2. Pterygoid branch
3. Deep temporal branch
4. Buccal branch
5. Deep pterygoid branch

Fig. 10.3: Branches of 2nd part of maxillary artery

Head, Neck and Face

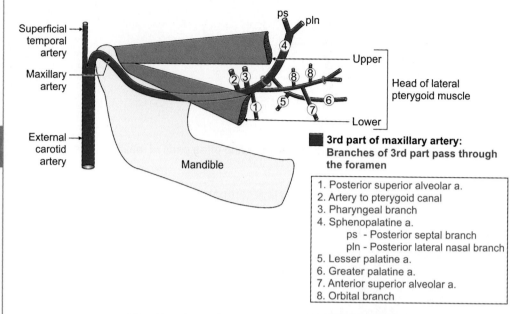

Fig. 10.4: Branches of 3rd part of maxillary artery

Table 10.1: Artery, foramina and distribution

Artery	Foramina	Distribution
• 1st part [🔑 DAIMA] **Bony branches**		
• **D**eep auricular artery		• External acoustic meatus
• **A**ccessory meningeal artery	• Foramina ovale	• Mainly to trigeminal ganglion.
• **I**nferior alveolar artery	• Mandibular canal	• Pulp of the mandibular teeth, body of the mandible, and • Lip and skin over the mandible
• **M**iddle meningeal artery	• Foramina spinosum	• Bones of the vault of skull
• **A**nterior tympanic artery	• Pterygopalatine fissure	• Inner surface of tympanic membrane
• 2nd part	—	• Muscular branches to muscles of mastication (1, 2 and 3) • Pterygoid (to pterygoids) • Deep temporal (to temporalis) • Masseteric (to masseter) • Buccal (to cheek)
• 3rd part		
• Sphenopalatine	• Sphenopalatine	• Main artery of nasal septum
• Posterior superior alveolar	• Posterior wall of maxilla	• Molar and premolar teeth and maxillary air sinus

Contd.

Table 10.1: Artery, foramina and distribution (Contd.)

Artery	Foramina	Distribution
• Greater palatine	• Greater palatine	• Soft and hard palate
• Lesser palatine	• Lesser palatine	• Soft palate and tonsil
• Pharyngeal branches	• Vomerovaginal and palatovaginal canal	• Pharynx

3. Applied anatomy

> Middle meningeal artery is the largest meningeal branch. Clinically, it is the most important branch of maxillary artery.
> It may be torn in fracture of the skull producing extradural haematoma that overlies the motor area of the cerebral cortex.

LAQ-20 Describe infratemporal fossa under the following heads:

1. Boundaries,

2. Contents, and

3. Applied anatomy

1. **Boundaries**
   A. **Location:** It is the space located deep to ramus of mandible.
   B. **Communication**
      a. Temporal fossa.
      b. Orbit.
      c. Middle cranial fossa
   C. **Openings**
      a. Foramen ovale,
      b. Foramen spinosum,
      c. Pterygomaxillary fissure, and
      d. Inferior orbital fissure.

Foramen rotundum—Tip

Box 10.1

Note: The foramen rotundum cannot be seen in the roof of infratemporal fossa.

   D. **Superiorly or roof:** It is formed by
      a. Inferior surface of greater wing of sphenoid bone.
      b. Mandibular surface and inferior surface of petrous part of temporal bone.
   E. **Anteriorly**
      a. Posterior surface of maxilla.
      b. Inferior orbital fissure.

F. **Medially**
   a. Lateral surface of lateral pterygoid plate.
   b. Tensor palatini.
   c. Superior constrictor.
   d. Pterygomaxillary fissure.

G. **Posteriorly**
   a. Anterior surface of styloid process of temporal bone.
   b. Carotid sheath.

H. **Laterally**
   a. Medial surface of ramus of mandible.
   b. Coronoid process.

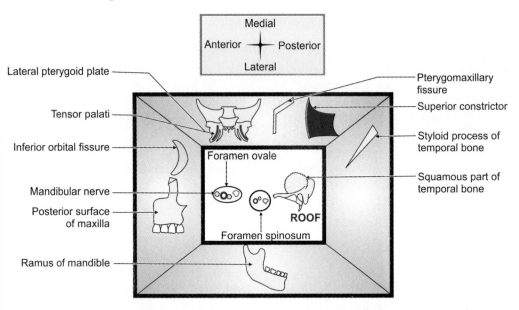

Fig. 10.5: Boundaries of infratemporal fossa

2. **Contents**
   A. Deep part of parotid gland
   B. **Muscles**
      a. Insertion of temporal is into the coronoid process,
      b. Medial pterygoid, and
      c. Lateral pterygoid.
   C. **Arteries:** Maxillary artery and its branches from 1st and 2nd parts are the contents of infratemporal fossa.
      a. Branches of 1st part. 🔑 **DAIMA**

      Deep auricular,
      Anterior tympanic,
      Inferior alveolar,

Middle meningeal, and

Accessory meningeal.

b. Branches of 2nd part (to muscles of mastication).

    I. Masseteric branch,

    II. Temporal branch,

    III. Pterygoid branch, and

    IV. Buccal branch.

D. **Pterygoid venous plexus.**

E. **Nerves**

a. Branches of mandibular division of trigeminal nerve.

    I. Branches from main trunk.

        i. Branch to medial pterygoid.

        ii. Meningeal branch.

    II. Branches from anterior trunk (mainly motor)

        i. Masseteric branch.

        ii. Branch to lateral pterygoid.

        iii. Deep temporal branch.

        iv. Buccal branch.

    III. Sensory branches are not the contents of infratemporal fossa.

b. Chorda tympani nerve

c. Posterior superior alveolar branches of maxillary nerve.

F. **Ganglion:** Otic ganglion.

3. | Applied anatomy |

➢ **LeFort and zygomatic fracture:** It is bilateral horizontal fracture of maxilla. It invariably involves infratemporal fossa. It damages the nerves, blood vessels and muscles in the region. The clinical manifestations are

- Injuries to the 2nd and 3rd divisions of trigeminal nerve and chorda tympani result into altered sensations in the oral cavity and face.
- Injuries involving otic ganglion interfere salivation.
- Damage to the motor nerve results in loss of chewing and swallowing movements.

➢ Fractures of the zygomatic bone involve infratemporal fossa and the maxillary air sinus. The infection of this region has grave consequences. It spreads in the middle cranial fossa through the various foramina present at the roof of the fossa.

➢ **Infection from**

- The impacted 3rd molar tooth also spreads to the infratemporal fossa. The main symptom of the infection is painful reflex muscle spasm.
- The infratemporal fossa may spread to orbit through inferior orbital fissure. It may result into cavernous sinus thrombosis.

➢ Infection also can spread to nose, palate and pharynx through pterygopalatine fissure.

Head, Neck and Face

LAQ-21	Describe temporomandibular joint under the following heads:

LAQ-21 **Describe temporomandibular joint under the following heads:**

1. Classification,
2. Ligaments,
3. Movements and muscles bringing movements,
4. Sets of movements
5. Axis of movement
6. Range of mandibular movements
7. Nerve supply, and
8. Applied anatomy

1. **Classification:** It is also called ginglymoarthrodial joint. It provides
   A. Hinge movement, and
   B. Gliding movement

   C. **Structurally:** Compound, complex, condylar, multiaxial, saddle shaped, atypical synovial joint.
      a. **Compound:** Two bones namely mandible and temporal bones and articular disc take part in the formation of TM joint.
         I. The inferior surface of the mandibular fossa of the squamous part of temporal bone,
         II. Superior surface of head of mandible, and
         III. Fibrocartilage articular disc.
      b. **Complex:** Joint cavity is separated by articular disc into upper menisco-temporal and lower menisco-mandibular compartments.
      c. **Condylar:** Left and right condyles of the head of mandible form a bicondylar articulation.
      d. **Multiaxial:** The movements are vertical, transverse and anteroposterior axis.
      e. **Saddle shaped:** The articular surface of head of mandible has convexo-concave surface which articulates with concavo-convex surface of mandibular fossa of temporal bone.
      f. **Atypical synovial:** The articular surfaces of the head of mandible and mandibular fossa of temporal bone are not covered by hyaline cartilage but are covered by fibrocartilage. Here collagen fibres predominate and cartilage cells are few. Because the concerned bones ossify in membrane.
   D. Functionally: Diarthrosis.
2. **Ligaments:** The ligaments can be divided into
   A. **Main ligaments**
      a. **Fibrous capsule**
         I. Attachments

Head, Neck and Face

i. Above
- Anteriorly: Anterior to articular tubercle.
- Posteriorly: Posterior to the squamotympanic fissure.
- Medially and laterally: To the margins of the mandibular fossa.

ii. Below: The capsule is attached at higher level near the articular margin of head of mandible. Posteriorly, it is attached to the neck lower down.

II. Nature of the capsule

Loose and lax above the disc ⬥▬➤ L and L

Tense and thick below the disc ⬥▬➤ T and T

III. Peculiarities
- i. It is spacious, lax and strong.
- ii. It gives attachment to lateral pterygoid muscle.

b. **Articular disc:** It is oval ⬬ in shape and fibrocartilage in nature (Fig. 10.6).

I. Morphologically, it represents lateral pterygoid muscle.

II. It is attached
- i. Anteriorly, medially and laterally near the head of mandible.
- ii. Peripherally to the inner side of the fibrous capsule.

III. Parts
- i. Anterior extension.
- ii. Posterior bilaminar extension.

IV. Variation in thickness: It is thick peripherally and thin in the centre.

V. Peculiarity: Gives attachment to lateral pterygoid muscle.

VI. Functionally, it divides the joint cavity into upper and lower compartments.
- i. The movement in the upper compartment is gliding.
- ii. The movement in the lower compartment is rotatory and gliding.

c. **Lateral ligament of TM joint**

I. It is a stout band of fibrous tissue.

II. It covers lateral aspect of capsule and strengthens it.

III. It extends from tubercle of root of zygoma to neck of the mandible.

IV. It tightens in retraction and protraction and relaxes in the rest position.

d. **Synovial membrane**

I. It lines the fibrous capsule above and below the disc but does not cover the disc.

II. It lines non-articular surface of articulating bones.

III. In newborn, even the articular surfaces are covered by synovial membrane.

B. **Accessory ligaments** (Fig. 10.6)

a. **Sphenomandibular ligament**

I. Introduction: It is an accessory ligament of temporomandibular joint, which lies on a deep plane away from fibrous capsule.

Head, Neck and Face

II. Attachments

    i. Above to the spine of sphenoid bone.

    ii. Below to the lingula of mandible.

b. **Stylomandibular ligament**

    I. It is a thickening of deep cervical fascia between angle of mandible and styloid process.

    II. It stretches

        i. From the

          • Apex, and

          • Adjacent anterior aspect of styloid process

        ii. To the

          • Angle of mandible, and

          • Posterior border.

    III. It is considered only accessory to the joint. The function is not exactly known.

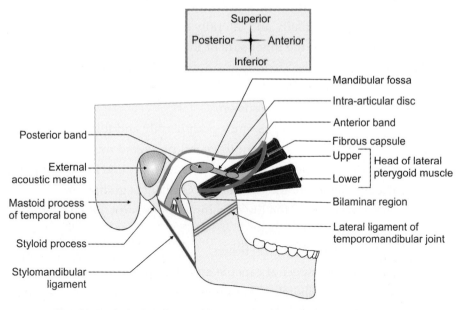

Fig. 10.6: Articular disc and ligaments of temporomandibular joint

3. **Movements and muscles bringing movements:** There are three sets of mandibular movements at the TM joint.

A. Movements and muscles bringing movements.

a. **Depression and elevation**

    I. *Depression is produced mainly by the lateral pterygoid.* The digastric, geniohyoid and mylohyoid muscles help when the mouth is opened wide or against resistance.

    II. Elevation is produced by the masseter, the temporalis and the medial pterygoid mucles of both sides.

b. **Side-to-side movement** (gliding movement): Lateral or side-to-side movements are produced by the medial and lateral pterygoids of each side acting alternately.

c. **Protraction and retraction**

 I. Protraction is done by the lateral pterygoid (principally its inferior head) and medial pterygoids.

 II. Retraction is produced by the posterior fibres of the temporalis. It may be resisted by the middle and deep fibres of the masseter, the digastric and geniohyoid muscles.

B. Position of articular disc and head of mandible in movements of TM joint

a. **When chin is depressed**

 I. In the upper compartment: Meniscofemoral compartment

 i. The articular disc and the head of mandible move forwards.

 ii. The movement is on the upper articular surface.

 iii. The movement continues till the head of mandible lies inferior to articular tubercle.

 II. In the lower compartment

 i. At the same time, the head of the mandible rotates on the lower surface of the disc.

 ii. The latter movement alone is capable of permitting simple chewing movements over a small range.

b. When small chewing movements are made without separating lips. The head of mandible moves in the mandibular fossa.

c. When the mouth is opened wide, the head of mandible swings forwards and downwards.

4. **Sets of movements:** There are three sets of mandibular movements at the TM joint. These are

A. **Depression and elevation**

a. In slight opening of the mouth or depression of the mandible, the head of mandible moves on the under surface of the disc like a hinge.

b. In *wide opening* of the mouth, the hinge-like movements is followed by gliding of the disc and the head of mandible, as in protraction. At the end of this movement, the head comes to lie under articular tubercle. These movements are reversed in closing the mouth or elevation of mandible.

c. *Active depression* is produced mainly by the lateral pterygoid. The digastric, geniohyoid and mylohyoid muscles help when the mouth is opened wide or against resistance.

d. Passive depression is produced by gravity.

e. Elevation is produced by the masseter, the temporalis and the medial pterygoid muscles of both sides.

B. **Side-to-side movement (gliding movement):** Lateral or side-to-side movements are produced by the medial and lateral pterygoid of each side acting alternately.

C. **Protraction and retraction**

a. In protraction, the articular disc glides forwards over the upper articular surface, the head of the mandible moving with it. Protrusion is done by the lateral (principally its inferior head) and medial pterygoids.

b. In retraction, the articular disc glides backwards over the upper articular surface, the head of mandible moving with it. It is produced by the posterior fibres of the temporalis. It may be resisted by the middle and deep fibres of the masseter, the digastric and geniohyoid muscles.

5. **Axis of movement**
   A. In small movement, the axis is through the head of mandible.
   B. In wider range of movements, the axis passes approximately through the mandibular foramen.

6. **Range of mandibular movements**
   A. Opening of the mouth
      a. Maximal opening of the jaw is about 50 mm.
      b. The functional range of opening is about 40 mm.
      c. Opening of jaw by rotation is about 25 mm.
      d. The last range of 15 mm is by anterior translateral (from side-to-side) gliding.
   B. In protrusion of the mouth: Maximal range of protrusion and lateral displacement are about 10 mm each.

7. **Nerve supply**
   A. Auriculotemporal nerve, a branch of posterior division of mandibular nerve.
   B. Masseteric nerve, a branch of anterior division of the mandibular nerve.

8. **Applied anatomy**

   ➢ **Lock jaw**
   • **Disc displacement:** The unique feature of articular disc is it is made up of elastic cartilage which is flexible. It serves as a cushion between two bony surfaces. The disc lacks arteries and nerves. Hence, it is pain insensitive.
      ▪ Anteriorly, it continues as lateral pterygoid muscle.
      ▪ Posteriorly, it continues as retrodiscal tissue. The retrodiscal tissue has rich nerve supply and blood supply.
   • Disc displacement is most common disorder. In most cases, disc is dislocated anteriorly. As the disc moves forwards, retrodiscal tissue is caught between two bones. This can be very painful as it has rich nerve supply.
   • The forward dislocated disc forms an obstacle for condylar movement. In order to open the jaw fully, the condyle has to jump over the backend with sense. This produces clicking sound. This condition is called *disc displacement with reduction.*
   • In later stages of disc dislocation, the condyles stay behind all the time unable to set back on the disc, the clicking sound disappears but mouth opening is limited. This is usually the most symptomatic stage.
   • The jaw is set to be locked as it is unable to open wide mouth. At this stage, the condition is called disc displacement without reduction. Fortunately, in majority of cases, the condition resolves by itself. This is called natural adaptation of retrodiscal tissue. This becomes a scar tissue and functionally replaces the disc. In fact, it becomes too similar to disc and is called pseudo-disc.

- *Forward dislocation is the commonest form of displacement.*
    - With the *mouth open*, the condyles are in the articular eminence and sudden violence, even muscular spasm (a convulsive yawn), may displace one or both temporomandibular joint.
- *Anterior dislocation readily occurs in the edentulous, i.e. person without teeth.* It is easily reduced; the joint is less stable because the increased elevation of the edentulous mandible permanently elongates lateral ligament.
- The reduction of the TM joint is easily achieved by pressing down on the molar teeth with thumbs placed in the mouth, and at the same time pushing the chin upward and backward. The downward pressure on the molar teeth overcomes the tension of the temporalis and masseter muscles which are in spasm. And the upward and backward pressure on the chin helps the head of mandible to put into original position.
- ➤ The lateral ligament of TM joint is very strong. It helps in following ways:
    - It prevents backward falling of head of mandible.
    - It prevents the fracturing of tympanic plate.
      This is very much true when a severe blow falls on the chin.
- ➤ The articular disc of the temporomandibular joint may become partially detached from the capsule. It results in noisy movements. It produces an audible click during movements at the joint.

SN-79   **Describe the factors responsible for the stability of temporomandibular joint**

Following factors maintain the stability of temporomandibular joint.
1. **Bones**
   A. Forward displacement is prevented by articular tubercles, and
   B. Backward displacement by post-glenoid tubercle.
2. **Ligament:** Lateral ligament of TMJ strengthens the capsule posterolaterally. It prevents the backward dislocation of mandible.
3. **Muscles**
   A. Protrusion is limited by the tension in temporalis.
   B. Retraction is limited by the tension in lateral pterygoid muscles.
4. **Position of mandible:** In occlusion, following factors play important role in stabilization of joint.
   A. Teeth themselves stabilize the mandible on maxilla. No strain is thrown on the joint when an upward blow is received by mandible.
   B. *Forward movement of the condyle is discouraged by the*
      a. Prominence of articular eminence, and
      b. Contraction of posterior fibres of temporalis.
   C. *Backward movement is prevented by the*
      a. Fibres of lateral ligament, and
      b. Contraction of the lateral pterygoid.

Head, Neck and Face

SN-80   Articular disc of TM joint (meniscus)

Introduction: It is the fibrocartilaginous structure separating the cavity of TM joint.

1. **Morphology**

  A. **Shape**—oval ⬬

  B. **Attachments**

    a. Anteriorly to the neck of mandible.

    b. Peripherally to the fibrous capsule.

    c. Medially and laterally to the neck of mandible.

  C. **Surfaces:** The superior surface of the disc is anteroposteriorly concavo-convex. The inferior surface of the disc is concave.

  D. **Extensions**

    a. Thick anterior band

    b. Thick posterior band

    c. Thin in the middle

  E. **Posterior band divides into two laminae with a venous plexus in between**

    a. Upper lamina: It is attached above to the mandibular fossa and is fibroelastic in nature.

    b. Lower lamina: It is attached to the mandible and is non-elastic.

  F. **Variation in thickness**

    a. Thick at periphery, and

    b. Thin in the centre.

2. **Peculiarities:** It gives attachment to lateral pterygoid muscle.

3. **Functions:** It divides the joint cavity into upper and lower compartments.

4. **Movements**

  A. Gliding movement in the upper compartment.

  B. Gliding and rotation movement in the lower compartment.

SN-81   Sphenomandibular ligament

Introduction: It is an accessory ligament of temporomandibular joint. It lies on a deep plane away from fibrous capsule.

1. **Attachment:** From spine of sphenoid bone to the lingula of mandible.

2. **Relations** (Fig. 10.7)

  A. **Laterally:** ⊶ MAIL

    a. <u>M</u>axillary artery.

    b. <u>A</u>uriculotemporal nerve.

    c. <u>I</u>nferior alveolar nerve.

    d. <u>L</u>ateral pterygoid muscle.

B. **Medially:** [🔑 MCP]

   a. **M**edial pterygoid muscle.

   b. **C**horda tympani nerve.

   c. Wall of the **p**harynx.

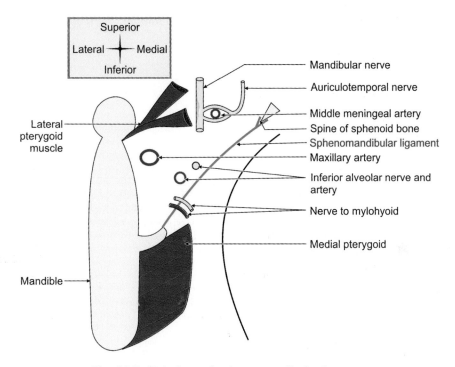

Fig. 10.7: Relations of sphenomandibular ligament

3. **Development:** It develops from the mesenchyme of the 1st pharyngeal arch. It is a remnant of dorsal part of Meckel's cartilage.

4. Applied anatomy

   • Sphenomandibular ligament is ruptured by
     – Fracture of neck of mandible, or
     – Dislocation of temporomandibular joint.
   • It leads to loss of taste sensations due to injury to chorda tympani nerve.

LAQ-22 **Describe muscles of mastication under the following headings:**

1. Proximal attachments,

2. Distal attachments,

3. Action, and

4. Nerve supply

Table10.2: Attachment and action of the muscles of mastication

Muscle	1. Proximal attachments	2. Distal attachments	3. Action
• Masseter: It has three parts. (Fig. 10.9)	• *Superficial part:* It arises from – Anterior 2/3rd of lower border of zygomatic arch – Zygomatic process of maxilla. • *Intermediate part* arises from middle 1/3rd of zygomatic arch. • *Deep part* arises from medial surface of zygomatic arch.	• All the fibres fuse and get attached into the lateral surface of ramus of mandible	• Elevates the mandible to close the mouth and clenches the teeth
• Temporalis (Fig. 10.8)	• Whole of the temporal fossa between inferior temporal line and infratemporal crest of the greater wing of sphenoid bone	• Main attachment is on the anterior and posterior borders of coronoid process	• Upper and anterior fibres elevate the mandible • Posterior fibres retract the mandible
• Lateral pterygoid: It has two heads	• *Superior head* arises from infratemporal surface and crest of the greater wing of sphenoid bone • *Inferior head* arises from lateral surface of lateral pterygoid plate	• Pterygoid fovea on the anterior surface of the neck of the mandible • Articular disc of TM joint • Capsule of TM joint	• It is indispensable for the active opening of the mouth • Both pterygoids acting together, protrude the mandible • Both the pterygoids contract alternately to produce side-to-side movements of the mandible
• Medial pterygoid: It has two heads	• *Superficial head:* It arises from tuberosity of maxilla – Pyramidal process of palatine bone • *Deep head* arises from medial surface of lateral pterygoid plate – Pterygoid fossa	• It is inserted into the rough area on the medial surface of angle of mandible • Adjoining part of the ramus of mandible • Area below and behind the mandibular foramen	• Moves the mandible upward, forward and medially and closes the mouth • It is a great chewing muscle • Both the pterygoids contract alternately to produce side-to-side movements of the mandible

4. Nerve supply : All the muscles of mastication are supplied by branches from anterior trunk of mandibular nerve except medial pterygoid which is supplied by branch from main trunk of mandibular nerve.

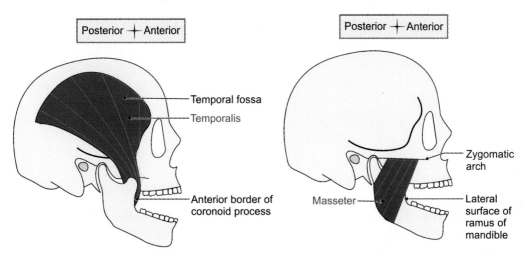

Fig. 10.8: Attachments of temporalis muscle

Fig. 10.9: Attachments of masseter muscle

| SN-82 | **Pterygoid venous plexus** |

Introduction: It is a plexus of veins present (Fig. 10.10)

A. Superficial to lateral pterygoid muscle.

B. Deep to lateral pterygoid muscle.

C. In the lateral pterygoid muscle.

D. Partly between temporalis and lateral pterygoid.

E. Partly between two pterygoid muscles.

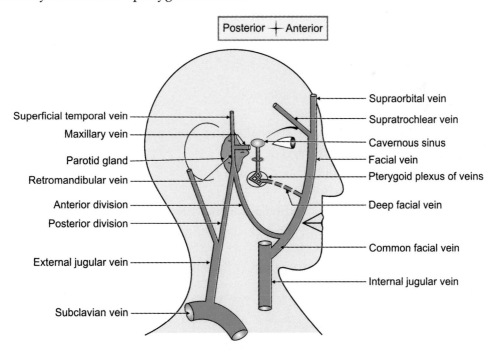

Fig. 10.10: Petrygoid plexus of veins

1. **Tributaries** of the plexus correspond to the branches of maxillary arteries. They are
   A. From muscles of mastication.
      a. Deep temporal
      b. Masseter
      c. Pterygoid
      d. Buccal
   B. Veins of palate
      a. Palatine
      b. Sphenopalatine
   C. Veins of cranium: Middle meningeal vein
2. **Termination:** It drains into maxillary vein which is formed at the lower border of lateral pterygoid muscle deep to the neck of mandible. They run back and join with the superficial temporal vein to form the retromandibular vein.
3. **Communications:** It has important communication with
   A. Inferior ophthalmic vein through veins of inferior orbital fissure.
   B. Cavernous sinus via emissary veins. These emissary veins pass through the foramen ovale and foramen of Vesalius (emissary sphenoidal foramen)
   C. Facial vein via deep facial veins.
4. **Role of pterygoid plexus:** (*Contraction of lateral pterygoid muscle facilitates venous return to heart. Hence, lateral pterygoid is called a peripheral heart.*) The veins of the plexus have valves and suck the blood from incompressible parts (face, bones and orbit) and pump it back into maxillary veins.
5. Applied anatomy : The infection from the face can spread to the cavernous sinus via the plexus.

SN-83 Lateral pterygoid muscle

Introduction: It is the muscle of mastication.
1. **Features:**
   A. **It acts as a peripheral heart.** It has plexus of veins present
      a. Superficial to lateral pterygoid
      b. In the lateral pterygoid
      c. Deep to lateral pterygoid
         These veins have valves and help in venous return.
   B. The emissary veins passing through the foramen ovale and foramen lacerum connect pterygoid venous plexus to cavernous venous sinus.
   C. It is a key muscle of the temporal and infratemporal regions.
2. **Origin:** It arises by two heads
   A. Upper head arises from
      a. Roof of infratemporal fossa.
      b. Infratemporal crests of greater wing of sphenoid bone.
   B. Lower head is larger and arises from lateral surface of lateral pterygoid plate.

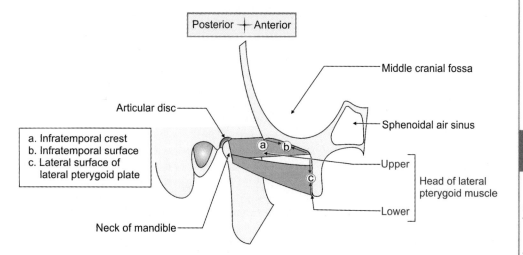

Posterior + Anterior

Middle cranial fossa

Articular disc

Sphenoidal air sinus

a. Infratemporal crest
b. Infratemporal surface
c. Lateral surface of
   lateral pterygoid plate

Upper

Head of lateral
pterygoid muscle

Lower

Neck of mandible

Fig. 10.11: Schematic diagram to show attachments of lateral pterygoid muscle

3. **Insertion:** The two heads lying edge-to-edge fuse and form a short tendon which is inserted into

A. Pterygoid fovea of the neck of mandible.

B. Capsule of temporomandibular joint.

C. Articular disc of temporomandibular joint.

4. **Relations**

A. **Superficial** (visualize mandible and structures attached and related to it.)

   a. Masseter,

   b. Ramus of mandible,

   c. Tendon of temporalis, and

   d. Maxillary artery.

B. **Deep**

   a. Mandibular nerve

   b. Middle meningeal artery

   c. Sphenomandibular ligament

   d. Deep head of medial pterygoid

C. **Structures emerging at the upper border**

   a. Deep temporal nerve

   b. Masseteric nerve

D. **Structures emerging at the lower border**

   a. Lingual nerve,

   b. Inferior alveolar nerve, and

   c. Middle meningeal artery.

E. **Between two heads of lateral pterygoid**

   a. 3rd part of maxillary artery.

   b. Buccal branch of mandibular nerve.

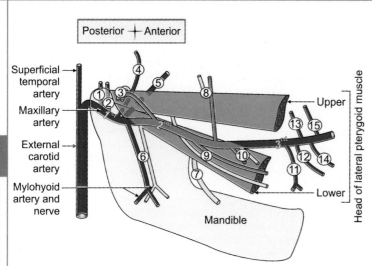

Fig. 10.12: Relations of lateral pterygoid muscle

Posterior + Anterior

Superficial temporal artery
Maxillary artery
External carotid artery
Mylohyoid artery and nerve
Mandible
Upper
Lower
Head of lateral pterygoid muscle

1. Deep auricular
2. Anterior tympanic
3. Masseteric nerve and artery
4. Middle meningeal
5. Accessory meningeal
6. Inferior alveolar artery and nerve
7. Lingual nerve
8. Deep temporal nerve and artery
9. Buccal artery and nerve
10. Pterygoid artery and nerve
11. Greater palatine
12. Posterior superior alveolar
13. Pharyngeal branch
14. Infraorbital
15. Artery to pterygoid canal

5. **Nerve supply**: It is supplied by a branch of anterior division of mandibular nerve.

6. **Action**

   A. It is indispensable muscle for the active opening of the mouth.[NEET]

   B. Protraction: It draws condyle and disc forward.

   C. Helps in side-to-side movements.

7. **Development**: It is developed from mesoderm of 1st pharyngeal arch.

LAQ-23 Describe mandibular nerve under the following headings:

1. Course and relations,

2. Development,

3. Branches, and

4. Applied anatomy

Introduction: It is 3rd division of trigeminal nerve. It is a mixed nerve supplying the muscles developed from 1st pharyngeal arch. It is also sensory to the skin and mucous membrane of mandible.

1. **Course and relations**

   A. It arises from trigeminal ganglion.

   B. It lies in the dura mater of middle cranial fossa lateral to the cavernous sinus.

   C. The sensory and motor roots pass through the foramen ovale.

   D. Both roots meet in the infratemporal fossa and a mixed nerve is formed.

   E. It begins as a trunk and divides into anterior and posterior divisions.

   F. The nerve lies deep to the upper head of lateral pterygoid and tensor palatini.

   G. Otic ganglion lies between mandibular nerve and lateral pterygoid.

2. **Development:** It is nerve of the 1st pharyngeal arch.

3. **Branches**

A. **From main trunk** (Fig. 10.13)

a. *Sensory:* Meningeal *(nervus spinosus):* It gives a cartilaginous branch to eustachian tube and enters the middle cranial fossa through foramen spinosum. It is accompanied by middle meningeal vessels. In the skull, it supplies
 I. Dura mater of middle cranial fossa,
 II. Mastoid antrum, and
 III. Mastoid air cells.

b. *Motor:* It gives motor branch to medial pterygoid and gives motor root to the otic ganglion. The root passes near or through the ganglion without synapse. Its fibres supply
 I. Tensor palatini, and
 II. Tensor tympani

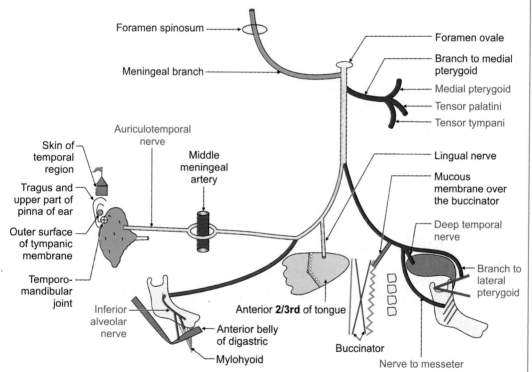

Fig. 10.13: Branches of mandibular nerve

B. **Branches from divisions:** After a distance of 4 to 5 mm, the nerve divides into a *'cat of nine tails'.* Six branches from anterior division and three branches from posterior division.

a. **Anterior division** (mainly motor): All the branches of anterior division are motor except buccal branch which is sensory.
 I. *Masseteric* nerve: It runs on upper border of lateral pterygoid and supplies
  i. Masseter muscle, and
  ii. Temporomandibular joint.

II. *Buccal* branch: It is purely sensory. It passes between two heads of lateral pterygoid. It runs in a fascial tunnel on the deep surface of temporal muscle and supplies

   i. External skin of cheek,

   ii. Internal mucous membrane,

   iii. Proprioceptive sensations of buccinator muscle, and

   iv. Gums of lower jaw opposite lower molar and premolar.

Along with parotid duct, buccal branch of mandibular nerve pierces buccinator.[NEET]

III. *Pterygoid* branches: They are two in number and supply

   i. Upper head of lateral pterygoid, and

   ii. Lower head of lateral pterygoid.

IV. *Temporal* branches: They are anterior and posterior and run on the upper border of lateral pterygoid. They supply the temporalis muscle.

  b. **Posterior division** (mainly sensory): All the branches of posterior division are sensory except nerve to mylohyoid which is motor.

> ### Exception proves the rule—Tip

Box 10.2

As a rule, anterior division is motor and posterior division is sensory. Every rule has an exception. On a lighter note: Exception proves the rule. If there are no exceptions, there are no rules.

All the branches of anterior division are motor except buccal branch which is sensory. All the branches of posterior division are sensory except nerve to mylohyoid which is motor.

I. *Auriculotemporal:* It arises by two roots.

> ### Last ritual of auriculotemporal nerve—Tip

Box 10.3

It hugs the middle meningeal artery since it is going to temple to have darshan.

It passes backwards between neck and ligament of mandible (sphenomandibular ligament). As the name suggests, it supplies structures surrounding the ear and temporal region.

   i. Skin of temporal region,

   ii. Temporomandibular joint,

   iii. Tragus,

   iv. Upper part of pinna of ear,

   v. Outer surface of tympanic membrane, and

   vi. Parotid gland (postganglionic secretomotor fibres from otic ganglion).

Great auricular nerve is great in following aspects
1. It is the largest ascending branch of cervical plexus.
2. It supplies skin over parotid gland and parotid fascia.
3. It supplies the area of skin of the ear which is pinched by a person who is great for the pinched person.

Box 10.4

Note: Skin over parotid gland and parotid fascia is supplied by great auricular nerve.

II. *Inferior alveolar* nerve
   i. It is a large branch of posterior division.
   ii. It emerges below the lower head of lateral pterygoid.
   iii. It lies anterior to its vessels and between sphenomandibular ligament and ramus of mandible.
   iv. It gives a branch called nerve to mylohyoid and enters the mandibular canal.
   v. *Nerve to mylohyoid* pierces sphenomandibular ligament. It supplies
     • Mylohyoid muscle, and
     • Anterior belly of digastric muscle.
   vi. Inferior alveolar nerve supplies
     • Three molar and two premolar teeth. It divides into
       * Mental nerve, and
       * Incisive nerve. It supplies pulps and periodontal membrane of the canine and incisors.
   vii. *Lingual nerve:* It appears below the lateral pterygoid muscle on the side of the pharynx. It joins with the chorda tympani at an acute angle. It emerges medial to mandible at third molar tooth. It carries
     • General and special sensations of anterior two-thirds of tongue (through chorda tympani)
     • Mucous membrane of floor of mouth.

4. **Applied anatomy**

➤ The sensory function of mandibular nerve is tested with a wisp of cotton on the skin of mandible.

➤ Motor function of mandibular nerve is tested by asking the patient to clench the teeth firmly. The contraction of the masseter can be felt by palpation when the teeth are clenched.

➤ Injury to trigeminal nerve causes paralysis of muscles of mastication. The chin is kept in the midline by the balanced tone of the muscles. In paralysis of the pterygoid muscles of one side, the chin is pushed to the paralyzed side by the muscles of opposite side.

Head, Neck and Face

➢ Pain arising from an area supplied by one branch of trigeminal nerve may be referred to another area of skin supplied by another branch of nerve. Thus, caries of the teeth of the lower jaw or ulcer of the tongue may cause pain in the ear because both are supplied by branches of mandibular nerve.

➢ A needle introduced to a depth of 4 cm in the coronal plane above the mandibular notch and in front of neck of mandible reaches the mandibular nerve. Usually, the needle is inserted until it strikes the lateral pterygoid plate. It is then passed posteriorly along the lateral pterygoid plate to reach the vicinity of foramen ovale.

➢ *Mandibular nerve block:* It is given for the extraction of the teeth of the lower jaw. The needle is inserted in the interval between pterygomandibular raphe and anterior margin of ramus of mandible. The tip of the needle is near the inferior alveolar nerve, just before it enters the mandibular canal. Anaesthetic injected here blocks the nerve.

➢ A lesion at the foramen ovale involves mandibular nerve and results in paraesthesia along the mandible, the lower (mandibular) teeth and the side of face. There is also paralysis of muscles of mastication and loss of jaw-jerk reflex as this nerve supplies both afferent and efferent fibres for the jaw-jerk reflex (Fig. 10.14).

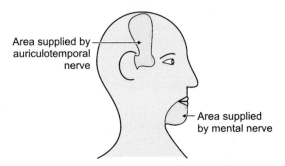

Area supplied by auriculotemporal nerve

Area supplied by mental nerve

Fig. 10.14: Loss of sensation in lesion of mandibular nerve

➢ *Mandibular neuralgia:* The pain along the distribution of mandibular division of trigeminal nerve is called mandibular neuralgia. It is often difficult to treat. This is treated by division of the sensory root of trigeminal nerve.

SN-84   Inferior alveolar (dental) nerve

Introduction: It is a branch of mandibular nerve. Its muscular part supplies mylohyoid and anterior belly of digastric. Its sensory part carries sensations of the teeth, pulp and periodontal membrane of lower jaw.

Ref. Figs 1.9 and 1.10

1. **Origin:** It arises from posterior division of mandible nerve, below the lower head of lateral pterygoid.

2. **Course and relations:** It lies anterior to its vessels between sphenomandibular ligament and ramus of mandible and enters the mandibular foramina. It runs along with vessels in the mandibular canal. It supplies three molars and two premolars.

3. **Branches**
   A. Mental nerve,
   B. Incisive nerve and
   C. **Nerve to mylohyoid:** It pierces the sphenomandibular ligament and supplies mylohyoid muscle.

4. Applied anatomy

   ➢ Inferior alveolar nerve block is used for the extraction of all teeth, except incisors.
   ➢ For inferior alveolar block, the needle is inserted orally through the buccinator above the 3rd molar tooth and in front of pterygomandibular raphe.

SN-85   Otic ganglion

It is a collection of cell bodies of postganglionic parasympathetic nerves. It is situated outside the central nervous system. The fibres supply parotid gland. Topographically (the description of anatomical region), it is related to the mandibular nerve and functionally it is related to glossopharyngeal nerve.

1. **Size:** 2–3 mm in size.
2. **Situation:** Infratemporal fossa at the base of foramen ovale.
3. **Synonym:** Arnold ganglion.
4. **Relations of otic ganglion**[NEET] (Fig. 10.15)
   A. **Superiorly:** Foramen ovale.
   B. **Anteriorly:** Medial pterygoid muscle.
   C. **Posteriorly:** Middle meningeal artery.
   D. **Medially:** Tensor veli palatini.
   E. **Laterally:** Mandibular nerve.

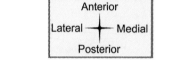

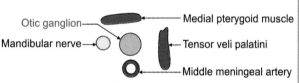

TS at the base of skull showing relations of otic ganglion

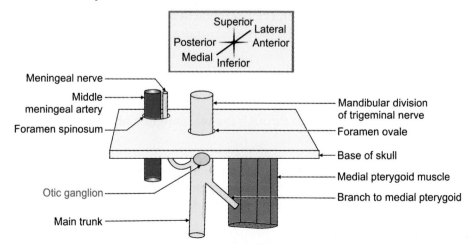

Fig. 10.15: Relations of otic ganglion

5. **Connections:**

A. **Parasympathetic or motor root**

   a. Preganglionic: Inferior salivatory nucleus—glossopharyngeal nerve—tympanic branch of glossopharyngeal nerve. It forms tympanic plexus along with caroticotympanic branch of internal carotid artery. A branch from plexus, a lesser petrosal branch is given that passes through foramen ovale—otic ganglion—relay.

   b. Postganglionic: Auriculotemporal nerve—parotid gland.

B. **Sensory:** Auriculotemporal nerve passes through otic ganglion without relay (Fig. 10.16).

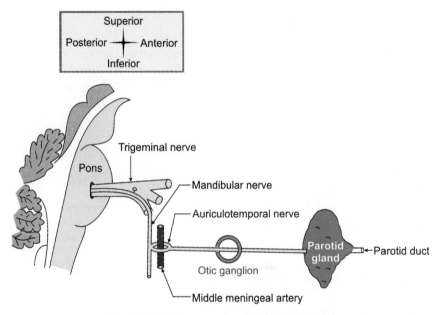

Fig. 10.16: Sensory fibres of otic ganglion

C. **Sympathetic**

   a. **Preganglionic:** Spinal nerve—superior cervical sympathetic ganglion.

   b. **Postganglionic:** Plexus around external carotid artery—maxillary artery—middle meningeal artery.

   Ref. Fig. 9.4

6. **Branches:**

A. Auriculotemporal nerve to parotid gland.

B. Nerve to medial pterygoid passes through the otic ganglion and supplies the

   a. Tensor palatini, and

   b. Tensor tympani.

C. The otic ganglion is connected to the chorda tympani nerve and the nerve of pterygoid canal. This communicating channel possibly forms an alternate route of the taste pathway from the anterior two-thirds of tongue to the geniculate ganglion of the facial nerve.

7. **Applied anatomy** : Injury to the auriculotemporal nerve manifests in the loss of salivation.

Submandibular Region

SN-86   Relations of hyoglossus muscle

1. **Superficial structures are grouped as**
   A. Nerves
      a. Hypoglossal nerve—12th cranial nerve, and
      b. Lingual nerve, a branch of posterior division of mandibular division of trigeminal nerve.
   B. Muscle: Styloglossus
   C. Structures related to word "submandibular"
      a. Submandibular ganglion,
      b. Deep part of the submandibular gland, and
      c. Submandibular duct.
   D. Veins accompanying it.

2. **Deep**
   A. Nerve: Glossopharyngeal nerve—9th cranial nerve.
   B. Artery: Lingual artery, a branch of external carotid artery.
   C. Muscles
      a. Muscle of tongue
         I. Inferior longitudinal muscle of the tongue.
         II. Genioglossus.
      b. Muscle of pharynx: Middle constrictor of the pharynx.
   D. Ligament: Stylohyoid.
      Ref: Fig. 11.9

3. **Structures passing deep to posterior border of hyoglossus, from above downwards are**
   A. Glossopharyngeal nerve.
   B. Stylohyoid ligament.
   C. Lingual artery.

SN-87   Mylohyoid muscle (oral diaphragm)

Introduction: It forms the diaphragm of the floor of the mouth.

1. **Proximal attachments:** It arises from the mylohyoid line present in the inner surface of body of mandible. It extends from 3rd molar tooth to mental spine (Fig. 11.1).

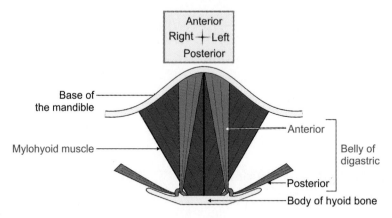

Fig. 11.1: Attachments of superficial relations of mylohyoid muscle

2. **Distal attachments**
   A. Anterior ¾ fibres interdigitate with each other in the midline. They extend between the symphysis menti and the hyoid bone and form mylohyoid raphe.
   B. It is only the posterior fibres which get inserted into the anterior surface of the body of hyoid bone.

3. **Nerve supply** : Nerve to mylohyoid, a branch of inferior alveolar nerve, branch of posterior division of mandibular nerve.

> **Box 11.1**
>
> **Note:** Nerve to mylohyoid pierces sphenomandibular ligament and supplies
> 1. Mylohyoid.
> 2. Anterior belly of digastric

4. **Action:** It elevates tongue and hyoid bone during swallowing.

5. **Relations:** The submandibular gland is the main relation to mylohyoid muscle. It has larger superficial and smaller deep part.

6. **Development:** It develops from mesenchyme of 1st pharyngeal arch.

SN-88   Carotid nerve

1. **Carotid nerve:** The internal carotid nerve arises from the upper end of the superior cervical sympathetic ganglion. It accompanies the internal carotid artery into the skull and forms the *internal carotid plexus.* The fibres from the plexus are distributed to
   A. All branches of the internal carotid artery,
   B. Pterygopalatine ganglion,

C. Eyeball, and

D. Dilator pupillae of the iris.

2. **Features**

A. It is composed mainly of postganglionic fibres arising from the superior cervical ganglion.

B. The nerve ascends along the internal carotid artery. It divides into branches that form a plexus over it.

C. This plexus has numerous connections.

3. **Connections:**

A. In the carotid canal, it forms *caroticotympanic nerves*. It enters the middle ear cavity and participates in the formation of tympanic plexus.

B. In the foramen lacerum, the plexus around internal carotid artery is called *deep petrosal nerve*. It joins the greater petrosal nerve and forms the nerve to the pterygoid canal (nerve of Vidian canal).[NEET]

a. The fibres reach the pterygopalatine ganglion.

b. They pass through the ganglion without relay and travel through the orbital branches. They supply the orbitalis muscle.

C. In the cavernous sinus, it communicates with the ophthalmic division of the trigeminal nerve. These fibres pass through nasociliary nerve. They travel through the long ciliary nerves and reach the eyeball. They supply the

a. Dilator pupillae muscle, and the

b. Blood vessels of the eyeball.

D. These fibres pass through ciliary ganglion without relay and then pass into the short ciliary nerves to supply the blood vessels of the eyeball.

E. It may be noted here that preganglionic sympathetic fibres for the eyeball begin in segment T1 of the spinal cord and ascend in the sympathetic trunk to the superior cervical ganglion in which the postganglionic neurons lie.

OLA-51 **What are the parts of submandibular gland?**

1. Superficial part of submandibular gland.
2. Deep part of submandibular gland.

OLA-52 **Where is the opening of submandibular duct?**

It opens in the floor of the mouth. It is on the summit of the sublingual papilla. It is demonstrated at the side of the frenulum of the tongue.

OLA-53 **Why the incision for removal of submandibular gland is placed more than 1" below the angle of mandible?**

The *marginal mandibular branch of the facial nerve* is situated at posteroinferior angle of jaw. To avoid the injury to the nerve, the incision is always taken 1" below the angle of mandible.

LAQ-24 **Describe submandibular gland under the following headings:**

1. Morphology

2. Relations

3. Blood supply

4. Lymphatic drainage

5. Nerve supply

6. Applied anatomy

1. **Morphology:** This is a large salivary gland situated in the anterior part of digastric triangle, in the submandibular region of mandible. It extends up to stylomandibular ligament.

   A. Division: The gland is divided by mylohyoid muscle into
      a. Large superficial part, and
      b. Small deep part.

   B. Ends: It has two ends:
      a. Anterior, and
      b. Posterior.

   C. Presents three surfaces
      a. Inferior,
      b. Lateral, and
      c. Medial.

2. **Relations:** Submandibular gland has larger superficial part and smaller deep part (Fig. 11.2).

   A. **Superficial part**
      a. Relations of inferior surface
         I. Skin,
         II. Superficial fascia,
         III. Platysma,
         IV. Deep fascia,
         V. Common facial vein,
         VI. Cervical branch of facial nerve,
         VII. Submandibular lymph node.
      b. Relations on lateral surface
         I. Submandibular fossa of mandible,
         II. Medial pterygoid muscle, and
         III. Facial artery.
      c. Medial surface is extensive and divided into three parts:
         I. Anterior
            i. Mylohyoid muscle,

ii. Mylohyoid vessels,

iii. Mylohyoid nerve, and

iv. Submental branch of facial artery.

II. Intermediate

i. Hyoglossus,

ii. Lingual nerve,

iii. Submandibular ganglion,

iv. Hypoglossal nerve, and

v. Intermediate tendon of digastric.

III. Posterior

i. Styloglossus,

ii. Stylopharyngeus,

iii. Digastric,

iv. Middle constrictor of pharynx,

v. Hypoglossal nerve, and

vi. Lingual artery.

Head, Neck and Face

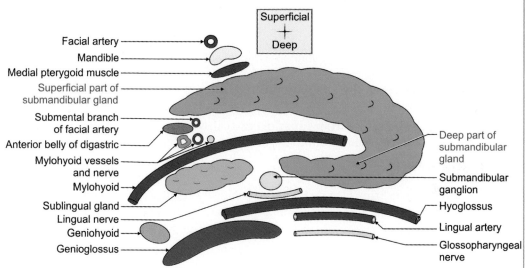

Fig. 11.2: Superficial and deep parts of submandibular gland

B. **Deep part:**

a. Laterally: Mylohyoid.

b. Medially: Hyoglossus and styloglossus.

3. **Blood supply**

A. **Arterial supply:** Glandular branch of facial artery.

B. **Venous drainage:** Common facial or lingual vein draining into internal jugular vein.

4. **Lymphatic drainage:** Submandibular lymph nodes.

5. **Nerve supply**

A. **Secretomotor fibres:** Arise from superior salivatory nucleus (Fig. 11.3).

a. Preganglionic fibres pass through facial nerve>chorda tympani> lingual nerve >submandibular ganglion.

b. Post-ganglionic fibres arise from ganglion and enter submandibular gland.

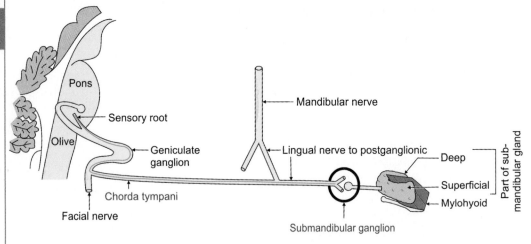

Fig. 11.3: Parasympathetic fibres of submandibular gland

B. Sensory fibres reach the ganglion through lingual nerve, branch of mandibular nerve.

C. Sympathetic fibres arise from superior cervical sympathetic ganglion. These fibres do not relay in the submandibular ganglion.

6. **Applied anatomy**

➢ The mandibular branch of facial nerve is closely related to the angle of jaw. The submandibular gland is excised by an incision 1" below the angle of jaw.

➢ The secretion of the submandibular gland is more viscous; hence, the incidence of *calculi* is more common in the *submandibular gland*.

➢ A stone in the submandibular duct (Wharton's duct) can be palpated bimanually in the floor of the mouth and can even be seen, if sufficiently large.

SN-89   Submandibular lymph nodes

1. **Situation:** They are situated in the digastric triangle beneath the deep cervical fascia. A few are embedded in the substance of submandibular salivary gland.

2. **Number:** They are usually three in number.

A. One in front of facial artery.

B. One behind the facial artery.

C. One on the anterior border of submandibular gland.

3. **Relation:** They are crossed by mandibular branch of facial nerve.

4. **Afferent**
   A. Centre of forehead,
   B. Medial angle of the eye,
   C. Side of nose,
   D. Cheek and angle of mouth,
   E. Whole of upper lip,
   F. Lateral part of lower lip,
   G. Anterior two-thirds of tongue,
   H. Upper gum through infraorbital foramen,
   I. Lower gum through the mental foramen, and
   J. Most of the air sinuses.

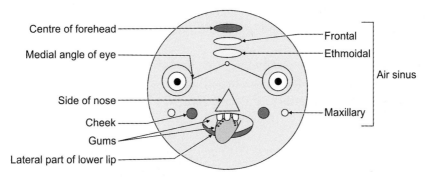

Fig. 11.4: Area drained by submandibular lymph nodes

5. **Efferent**
   A. Jugulo-omohyoid
   B. Jugulodigastric.

6. **Applied anatomy**: In malignancy of mandible, the submandibular gland along with submandibular lymph nodes is removed in the block dissection called hemi-mandibulectomy.

SN-90 **Histology of submandibular gland**

> The letters of the word signify the type of secretion they produce.
> Parotid- Pure serous.
> Sub-Mandibular: Serous More (predominantly serous)
> Sub-Lingual: Serous Less (predominantly mucous)

Box 11.2
- It is very simple to remember the types of salivary gland. There are mainly three salivary glands, namely parotid, submandibular and sublingual.
- Parotid is pure serous, submandibular and sublingual are mixed.
- Submandibular is predominant serous.

Contd.

Contd.

- Sublingual is predominantly mucous.
- Use the letter "P" for pure,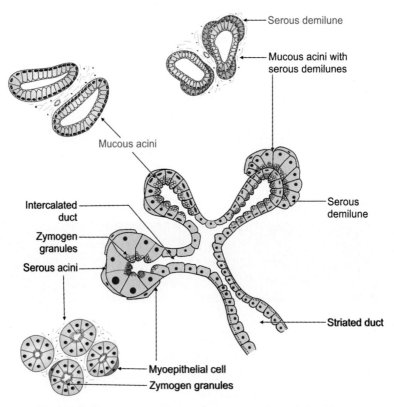
- Letter "M" for more, and the
- Letter "L" for less, things are easy to remember.
- Parotid gland: The word "Parotid" begins with the letter "P", hence remember parotid is pure serous.
- Sub-mandibular gland has letters "S" and the letter "M", hence serous more, i.e., predominant serous.
- Sub-lingual gland has the letters "S" and the letter "L" hence serous less, i.e., predominant mucous.

Features (Fig. 11.5)

1. Submandibular gland is mixed, predominantly serous salivary gland.
2. No lymphoid tissue.
3. Typical connective tissue—capsule, septa and stroma are present.
4. The parenchyma is divided by septa into lobules.
5. Most of the mucous secretory units are capped by serous demilunes (1/2 moon).

Fig. 11.5: Parenchyma and duct system of a salivary gland

6. Serous secretory units have a round nucleus which is located near the centre of the cell. This is in contrast with the mucous cells which have a flattened nucleus. It is pressed against the base of the cell.

7. Presence of myoepithelial cells in relation to acini.

8. Interlobular excretory ducts are located in the interlobar connective tissue septa. The septa divide the gland into lobules and lobes.

9. Intralobular ducts join to form the interlobular ducts and interlobar ducts. The terminal portion of these large ducts conveys saliva from salivary gland to the oral cavity. It constitutes the main ducts of each salivary gland. As these interlobular and interlobar excretory ducts get larger and larger, the lining epithelium goes on changing. The change is from stratified low cuboidal to stratified columnar cells.

SN-91 Submandibular ganglion

Introduction: It is a collection of cell bodies present in the course of parasympathetic nerve situated on the hyoglossus muscle, supplying the submandibular and sublingual glands.

A. It is topographically connected to lingual nerve, branch of mandibular nerve.

B. It is functionally connected to facial nerve.

1. **Gross anatomy**

   A. **Shape:** Fusiform .

   B. **Situation:** On hyoglossus muscle.

   C. **Relations**
      a. Superior: Lingual nerve.
      b. Inferiorly: Deep part of submandibular gland.

   D. **Connections**
      a. Parasympathetic.

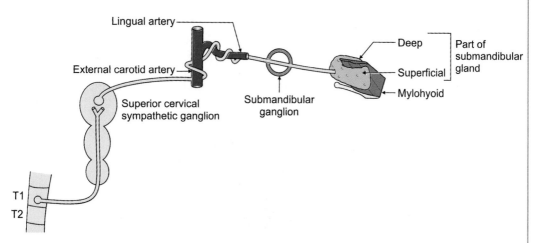

Fig. 11.6: Sympathetic root of submandibular ganglion

Head, Neck and Face

I. Preganglionic fibres: Superior salivatory nucleus>facial nerve>chorda tympani joins with lingual nerve>submandibular ganglion>relay.

II. Postganglionic fibres: Unnamed branches—to submandibular or sublingual gland.

b. Sympathetic fibres (Fig. 11.6):

I. Preganglionic fibres arise from spinal nerves>superior cervical sympathetic ganglion>fibres relay in the ganglion.

II. Postganglionic fibres form the plexus around external carotid artery>(lingual artery) the fibres do no relay (Fig. 11.6).

c. Sensory: Lingual nerve, a branch of mandibular division (V3) of trigeminal nerve.

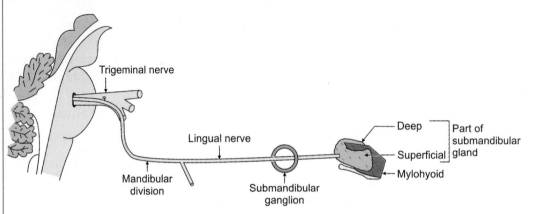

Fig. 11.7: Sensory root of the submandibular ganglion

2. **Branches:** 5 to 6 branches enter the submandibular, sublingual and anterior lingual glands.

SN-92   Hyoglossus muscle

1. **Origin:** It arises from
   A. The length of greater horn of hyoid bone.
   B. Lateral part of the body of hyoid bone.

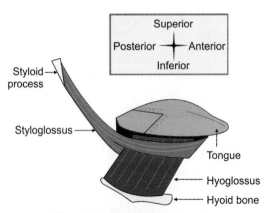

Fig. 11.8: Hyoglossus muscle

2. **Insertion:** Upper border interdigitates at right angles with the styloglossus and is attached to the side of tongue.

3. Nerve supply : Hypoglossal nerve—12th cranial nerve.

4. **Action:** It depresses the tongue.

5. **Relations**

   A. **Superficial from above downwards** "Yes" between 2 "No" ⚷

   a. Lingual branch of mandibular nerve

   b. Submandibular duct

   c. Hypoglossal nerve.

   B. **Deep relations from above downwards lying on middle constrictor of pharynx are** (Fig. 11.9)

   a. Glossopharyngeal nerve,

   b. Stylohyoid ligament, and

   c. Lingual artery.

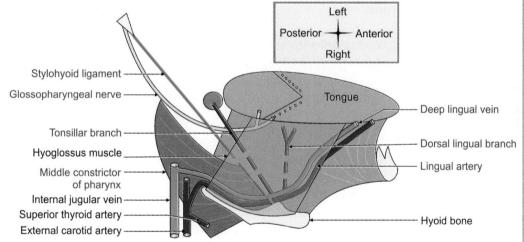

Fig. 11.9: Deep relations of hyoglossus muscle

Head, Neck and Face

Deep Structure in the Neck

OLA-54 **What forms right lymphatic duct?**

1. Right jugular trunk, and
2. Right subclavian trunk.

LAQ-25 **Describe scalenus anterior under the following headings:**
   1. Attachments,
   2. Nerve supply,
   3. Actions,
   4. Relations, and
   5. Applied anatomy

Scalenus (*scalene*—triangle with unequal sides) anterior is key muscle of neck extending from anterior tubercle of typical cervical vertebrae.

1. **Attachments:**
    A. **Proximal:** It arises from anterior tubercle of the typical cervical vertebrae, i.e. **C3, C4, C5** and **C6.**
    B. **Distal:** It is inserted by a narrow tendon to the
        a. Scalene tubercle on the inner border of 1st rib,
        b. To a ridge on the upper surface of the rib between the grooves for subclavian artery and vein.

2. **Nerve supply** : Ventral rami of 4th, 5th and 6th cervical nerves.

3. **Actions:** Acting from above, it elevates 1st rib and acts as accessory muscle for inspiration.

4. **Relations**
    A. **Anterior (from before backwards)** (Fig. 12.1)

a. Skin,
b. Superficial fascia,
c. Platysma, and
d. Investing layer of deep cervical fascia.
e. Clavicle and muscles attached to clavicle, i.e.
    I. Subclavius, and
    II. Sternocleidomastoid.
f. Carotid sheath and its contents
    I. Common carotid artery,
    II. Internal jugular vein, and
    III. Vagus nerve.
g. Termination of thoracic duct on the left side.

h. Thyrocervical trunk and three branches. 🔑 SIT on it.
    Suprascapular artery,
    Inferior thyroid artery, and
    Transverse cervical artery
i. Prevertebral fascia,
j. Phrenic nerve. It runs vertically downward.

Head, Neck and Face

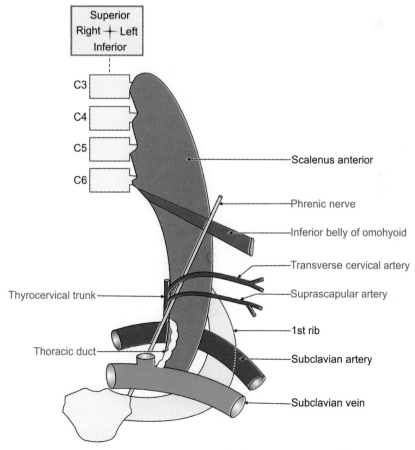

Fig. 12.1: Anterior relations of scalenus anterior muscle

B. **Posterior**
 a. 2nd part of subclavian artery,
 b. Roots of brachial plexus,
 c. Scalenus medius, and
 d. Suprapleural membrane.
C. **Superior:** Longus capitis
D. **Medial** (Fig. 12.2)
 a. Scalenovertebral triangle containing
  I. 1st part of vertebral artery, and
  II. Vertebral vein.
 b. Sympathetic trunk
E. **Lateral:** Brachial plexus.

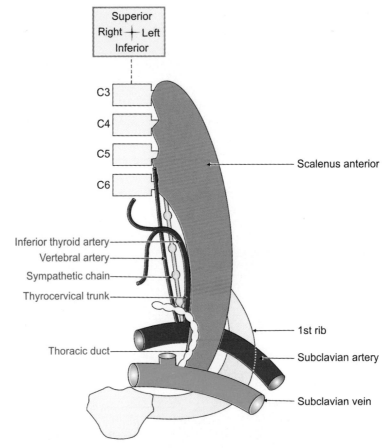

Fig. 12.2: Medial relations of scalenus anterior muscle

5. Applied anatomy

> **Cervical rib:** Additional rib from 7th cervical vertebra. It passes between scalenus anterior and medius. Clinical manifestations are

- Wasting of hypothenar muscles
- Sensory loss of medial 1½ finger of the hand and part of the forearm due to compression of lower trunk of brachial plexus.

SN-93   Anastomotic sites of carotid and subclavian arteries

Table 12.1: Anastomosis between carotid and subclavian arteries

Site	Carotid artery	Subclavian artery
• Circle of Willis	• Posterior communicating artery—branch of internal carotid artery	• Posterior cerebral artery—branch of basilar artery
	• Ascending pharyngeal artery—branch of external carotid artery	• Ascending cervical branch of inferior thyroid artery
	• Deep branch of the descending branch of the occipital artery	• Deep cervical artery—branch of costocervical trunk
• Posterior border of thyroid gland	• Superior thyroid artery—branch of external carotid artery	• Inferior thyroid artery—branch of thyrocervical trunk
• Larynx	• Superior laryngeal artery—branch of superior thyroid artery	• Inferior laryngeal artery—branch of inferior thyroid artery
• Pharynx	• Superior thyroid artery—branch of external carotid artery	• Pharyngeal branch—branch of inferior thyroid artery
	• Descending branch of occipital artery—branch of external carotid artery	• Superficial cervical artery—branch of thyrocervical trunk
	• Descending branch of occipital artery—branch of external carotid artery	• Deep cervical branch of costocervical trunk
	• Ascending pharyngeal artery—branch of external carotid artery	• Ascending cervical branch of vertebral artery

Head, Neck and Face

OLA-55   Why superior thyroid artery is ligated close to superior pole and inferior thyroid artery away from the inferior pole in thyroidectomy?

1. Superior thyroid artery and external laryngeal nerve are away from each other at superior pole. Hence, it is safe to ligate superior thyroid artery at superior pole, to avoid injury to the external laryngeal nerve.
2. Inferior thyroid artery and the recurrent laryngeal nerve are intimately related at inferior pole. It is not safe to ligate the inferior thyroid artery at inferior pole. Hence, one is advised to ligate inferior thyroid artery away from inferior pole to avoid injury to recurrent laryngeal nerve.

OLA-56   What are the lining epithelial cells of thyroid gland?

1. Follicular cells
2. Parafollicular cells

OLA-57 | What are parafollicular cells? What do they secrete?

1. Parafollicular cells occur as single cells or in clumps on the periphery of the follicles.
2. They stain somewhat lighter than the follicular cells
3. They are readily visible in the canine (dog) thyroid.
4. They synthesize and secrete the hormone *calcitonin*.

OLA-58 | What is the colloid in thyroid follicles made up of?

1. The colloid is formed by the follicular cells.
2. Its main component is thyroglobulin.
3. Thyroglobulin is the inactive storage form of thyroid hormone.

OLA-59 | State the two types of cells in parathyroid gland. What does the para-thyroid gland secrete?

Parathyroid glands contain two types of cells (Fig. 12.3)
1. **Principal or chief cells**
    A. These are the most numerous cells.

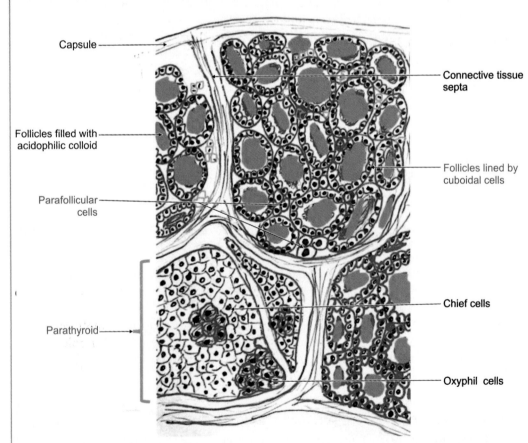

Fig. 12.3: Histology of thyroid and parathyroid glands

B. They are polygonal 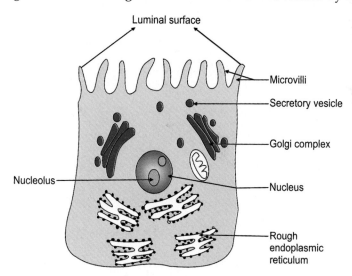 in shape.

C. They are arranged in clumps or irregular cords.

D. The cytoplasm of the cells shows numerous secretory granules.

E. Each cell has a centrally located spherical nucleus.

F. Large capillaries are present in between the cords and clumps.

G. They secrete parathyroid hormone (PTH or parathormone).

2. **Oxyphil cells**

A. They are larger in size but fewer in number than chief cells.

B. They are arranged in clumps.

C. Their function is not clear.

OLA-60 **Describe production of thyroid hormones from follicular cells to its release into the capillary.**

1. **Synthesis and storage**

A. Thyroglobulin is synthesised by rough endoplasmic reticulum.

B. It is carried to Golgi complex.

C. It is packed into vesicles.

D. These vesicles are transported to the apical surface of the cell.

E. The thyroglobulin is discharged into the lumen of the follicle by exocytosis.

Fig. 12.4: Follicular cell

2. **Iodide uptake**

A. Under the influence of TSH, follicular cells take up iodine from the blood.

B. Iodide is oxidised to iodine by enzyme thyroid peroxidase.

3. **Iodination of thyroglobulin**

A. Iodination of thyroglobulin occurs at the luminal surface of the follicular cells.

B. Triiodothyronine (T_3) and tetraiodothyronine (T_4, also known as thyroxine) are formed.

Head, Neck and Face

4. Release of thyroid hormones

A. Stimulation of follicular cells by TSH causes endocytosis of thyroglobulin.

B. Numerous colloid resorption droplets containing iodinated thyroglobulin are formed.

C. Lysosomes fuse with the colloid resorption droplets.

D. These droplets release T_4 and T_3 hormones.

E. They enter blood circulation.

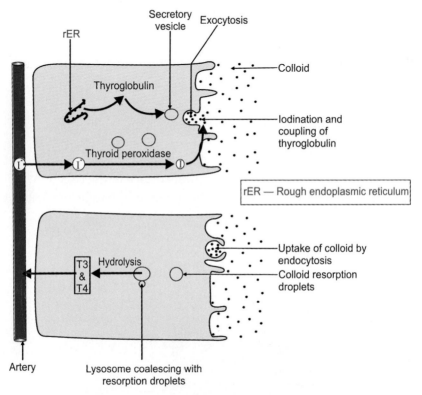

Fig. 12.5: Steps of thyroid hormone synthesis

LAQ-26 Describe thyroid gland under the following heads:

1. Gross anatomy,

2. Histology,

3. Development, and

4. Applied anatomy.

(*Thyreos*—shield, *cides*—form)

1. Gross anatomy

A. **Situation**

a. It is situated in front of **C5, C6, C7** and **T1** vertebrae.

Association memory—Tip

> **Box 12.1**
>
> Relations of number of cervical vertebrae of thyroid gland are remembered by associating with the number of cervical vertebrae related to ventral rami of brachial plexus.

    b. Each lobe extends from oblique line of thyroid cartilage to the 6th tracheal ring.

    c. The isthmus extends from the 2nd to the 3rd tracheal ring.

B. Dimensions and weight

    a. Each lobe measures 2″ × 1″ × 1″.

    b. The isthmus measures ½″ × ½″

    c. Weight: About 25 g

C. Capsules

    a. True capsule: It is condensation of peripheral part of connective tissue of gland.

    b. False capsule: It is condensation of pretracheal layer of deep cervical fascia (Fig. 12.6).

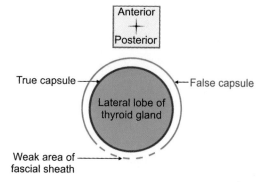

Fig. 12.6: False capsule

D. Surfaces of

    a. Lateral lobes 🔑 **(Preventive and social medicine)**

      <u>P</u>osterior

      <u>S</u>uperficial

      <u>M</u>edial

    b. Isthmus

      I. Anterior, and

      II. Posterior.

E. Borders of

    a. Lateral lobe

      I. Anterior, and

      II. Posterior.

    b. Isthmus

      I. Upper, and

      II. Lower.

F. **Relations of lateral lobe of thyroid gland** (Fig. 12.7)

a. Relations to surface

I. Superficial 4S

S̲ternohyoid,

S̲ternothyroid,

S̲uperior belly of omohyoid, and

S̲ternomastoid.

II. Medial ◐━ MTN

M̲uscles:
- Inferior constrictor, and
- Cricothyroid.

T̲ubes:
- Trachea, and
- Oesophagus.

N̲erves:
- External laryngeal nerve, and
- Recurrent laryngeal nerve.

III. Posterolateral: Carotid sheath.

b. Relations to border

I. Anterior: Superior thyroid artery (anterior descending branch).

II. Posterior: Parathyroid gland is important structure. Other structures are

◐━ ITA

I̲nferior thyroid artery.

T̲horacic duct (only on left side).

A̲nastomosis between superior and inferior thyroid arteries.

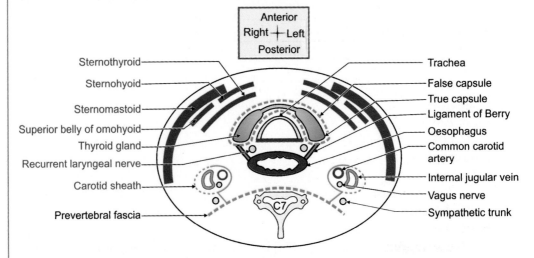

Fig. 12.7: Relations of thyroid gland at the level of the isthmus

G. **Blood supply**

a. **Arterial** (Fig. 12.8): [🔑━━ ITA]

I. Inferior thyroid artery:

i. It is a branch of thyrocervical trunk.

ii. It is chief artery of thyroid gland.

iii. It supplies
- Lower 2/3rd of lobe of the gland, and
- Lower half of isthmus.

iv. It penetrates deep surface of gland and anastomoses with descending branch of superior thyroid artery.

v. The anastomosis takes place at the junction of upper 1/3rd with lower 2/3rd of the posterior border.

vi. It has intimate relation with the recurrent laryngeal nerve near the gland.

II. *Superior thyroid artery*

i. It is a branch of external carotid artery.

ii. It supplies
- Upper 1/3rd of the gland, and
- Upper half of isthmus.

iii. It descends up to apex of thyroid gland and divides into anterior and posterior branches. The branches descend on the respective borders.
- The anterior branch anastomoses with artery of opposite side at superior border of isthmus.
- Posterior branch anastomoses with inferior thyroid artery on posterior border.

iv. It is closely related to external laryngeal nerve.

III. Thyroid ima: It either arises from brachiocephalic trunk or arch of aorta. It supplies isthmus of thyroid gland.

IV. Numerous accessory thyroid arteries, branches of oesophageal and tracheal arteries. These branches supply the gland from the medial or deep surface.

b. **Venous drainage:** The veins of the thyroid gland form a plexus which is situated deep to the capsule. They do not accompany arteries. They drain as follows (Fig. 12.9)

I. Superior thyroid vein ⎫

II. Middle thyroid vein ⎬ Drain into internal jugular vein

III. Kocher's vein ⎭

IV. Left and right inferior thyroid veins drain into brachiocephalic vein.[NEET]

Note: Kocher's vein is the 4th vein of thyroid gland. It drains lower pole of thyroid gland when present. It is occasionally present between middle and inferior thyroid veins.

Superior thyroid vein is related to lateral border of superior belly of omohyoid muscle.

The middle thyroid vein is related to medial border of superior belly of omohyoid muscle.

Head, Neck and Face

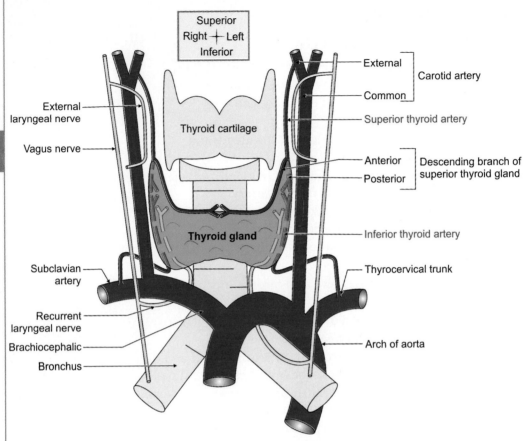

Fig. 12.8: Arterial supply of thyroid gland

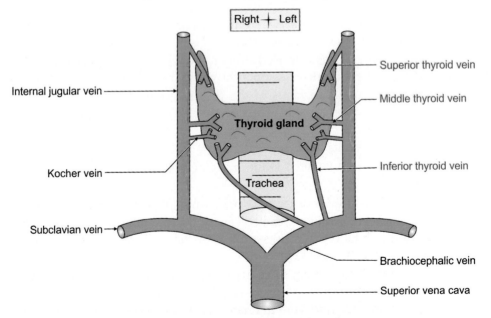

Fig. 12.9: Venous drainage of thyroid gland

H. **Lymphatic drainage** (Fig. 12.10): They are arranged into

    a. Upper group: Prelaryngeal and jugulodigastric group of lymph nodes.

    b. Lower group: Pretracheal group of lymph nodes along recurrent laryngeal nerve.

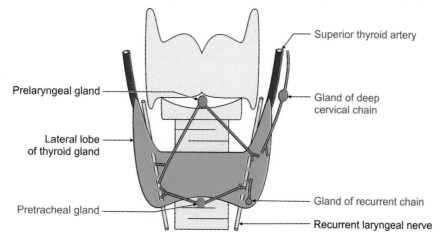

Fig. 12.10: Lymphatic drainage of thyroid gland

I. **Nerve supply**: They are derived

    a. Mainly from middle cervical sympathetic ganglion.

    b. Partly by superior and inferior sympathetic ganglion.

    c. Function: Vasoconstriction.

2. **Histology** (Fig. 12.11):

    A. Lumen of follicles shows colloid material.

    B. Follicles are lined by cuboidal epithelium.

    C. There are clear or light cells called parafollicular cells which produce *calcitonin*.

    D. They are polyhedral with oval, eccentric nuclei.

    E. They are present between follicular cells and lie on basement membrane.

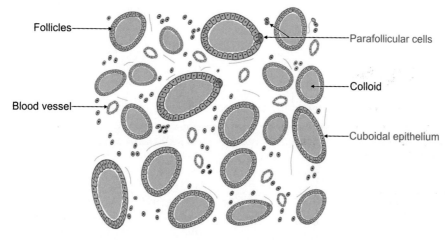

Fig. 12.11: Histology of thyroid gland

3. Development
   A. **Chronological age**
      a. It develops in the 4th week of intrauterine life.
      b. The descent of thyroid gland is completed at 7th cervical vertebra. (Number is equal to the number of alphabets of "thyroid".)
      c. The secretion of thyroid commences from the 4th month of IUL.
   B. **Germ layer:** It develops from endoderm of
      a. 2nd pharyngeal arch.
      b. 4th pharyngeal pouch.
   C. **Site:** Floor of the primitive pharynx behind the tuberculum impar (unpaired) of the developing tongue.
   D. **Sources**
      a. It develops as a **median thyroid diverticulum** extending from foramen caecum to thyroid cartilage.
      b. The distal part becomes bifid.
      c. The duct divides into a series of double cellular plates.
      d. The colloid accumulates within the bilaminar plates.
      e. The bilaminar plate is converted into primary thyroid follicle.
      f. The buds arise from the primary thyroid follicle and differentiate into secondary or definite follicles.
      g. The caudal pharyngeal complex (ultimobranchial body) joins each side of the lower end of thyroglossal duct to give origin to parafollicular cells.
      h. The duct disappears, its cephalic end persists as a foramen caecum and its caudal end occasionally forms the pyramidal lobe.
   E. **Anomalies:**
       ITA

      Incomplete descent of thyroid gland.
      Thyroglossal duct.
      Thyroglossal cyst.
      Agenesis of thyroid gland.
      Lingual thyroid

4. Applied anatomy

Table.12.2: Arteries of thyroid gland and details of relations of nerves

Artery	Nerve related	Site of intimate relation	Safe site of ligation
• Superior thyroid	• External laryngeal	• Away from lateral lobe of thyroid gland	• Tied near the gland during thyroid-ectomy
• Inferior thyroid	• Recurrent laryngeal	• Close to the gland	• Tied away from the gland during thyroidectomy

➢ ◆━ ITA During thyroid operation, inferior thyroid artery should be tied away from the gland to avoid injury to recurrent laryngeal nerve.

➢ The superior thyroid artery should be tied near the gland to avoid the injury to the external laryngeal nerve.

➢ **Thyroid Swelling moves with Swallowing but does not Swift (move) on protrusion of tongue**.

➢ Kocher vein, if present, may bleed profusely during thyroid operation. Therefore, an attempt should be made to search and ligate.

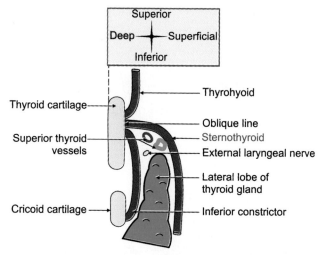

Fig. 12.12: Applied anatomy of thyroid gland

Note: 1. Sternothyroid muscle attached to oblique line prevents upward enlargement of the gland

2. The thyroid gland always enlarges downward

Attachment of sternothyroid muscle to oblique line prevents upward enlargement of thyroid gland.

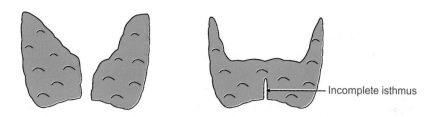

Fig. 12.13: Absence of isthmus   **Fig. 12.14:** Incomplete isthmus

OLA-61 Name the arteries supplying thyroid gland.

1. Inferior thyroid artery
   A. Chief artery of thyroid gland
   B. Branch of thyrocervical trunk

C. Supplies
    a. Lower 2/3rd of lateral lobe of thyroid gland, and
    b. Lower half of the isthmus of thyroid gland.
2. **Superior thyroid artery**
    A. 1st ventral branch of external carotid artery
    B. Supplies
        a. Upper 1/3rd of lateral lobe of thyroid gland.
        b. Upper half of the isthmus of thyroid gland.
3. **Thyroid ima (lowest) artery**
    A. Branch of arch of aorta
    B. Rarely present.

SN-94　Isthmus of thyroid gland

Introduction: It is median quadrilateral part of gland.
1. **Morphology** (Fig. 12.15)
    A. **Dimension:** 1.25 cm in length and breadth
    B. **Surfaces:** Anterior and posterior
    C. **Borders:** Upper and lower.
    D. **Extent:** From 2nd to 3rd tracheal ring.

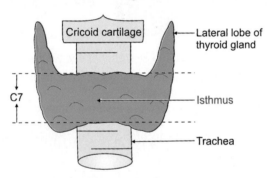

Fig. 12.15: Level of isthmus of thyroid gland

2. **Relations** (Fig. 12.16)
    A. **Upper border**
        a. Site of anastomosis of anterior descending branch of right and left superior thyroid arteries.
        b. Pyramidal lobe: A small conical mass of thyroid tissue.
        c. **Levator glandulae thyroideae:** A fibromuscular band connecting upper border of isthmus to pyramidal lobe of thyroid gland.

Levator glandulae thyroideae—Tip

Box 12.2
Note: It is supplied by external laryngeal nerve. It is remnant of median thyroid diverticulum. It never represents remnant of the thyroglossal duct.

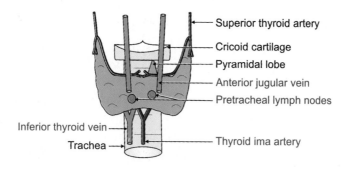

Fig. 12.16: Relations of structures at the isthmus of thyroid gland

B. **Lower border** is related to
   a. Inferior thyroid vein: It emerges from lower border of isthmus of thyroid gland.
   b. Arteria **thyroidea ima (lowest):** It enters lower border of isthmus of thyroid gland.
C. **Anterior surface:** It is related to
   a. Skin
   b. Superficial fascia containing anterior jugular vein
   c. Deep fascia of neck
   d. Sternohyoid
   e. Sternothyroid
D. **Posterior surface:** Posterior surface of the isthmus firmly adhere to 2nd, 3rd and 4th tracheal cartilages. The pretracheal fascia is fixed between them.

3. **Applied anatomy**: In tracheostomy, the isthmus of thyroid gland is cut and an opening is made through the 2nd and 3rd tracheal rings (Fig. 12.17).

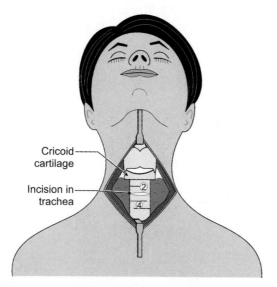

Fig. 12.17: Incision of isthmus during tracheostomy

SN-95 Thyroglossal duct

Introduction: A duct extending from the foramen caecum of tongue to thyroid primordium. It is present in embryonic life. It is formed by endoderm of 3rd and 4th pharyngeal arches (Fig. 12.18).

1. **Fate:** Distal part usually differentiates to form pyramidal lobe of thyroid gland and the remainder part obliterates.

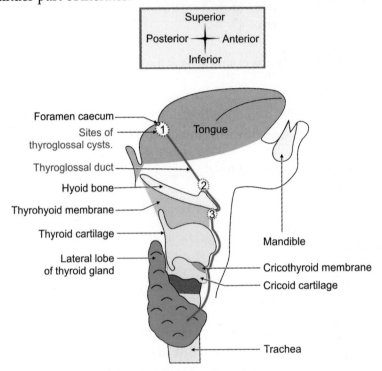

Fig. 12.18: Thyroglossal duct
Note: Dotted outlined structure indicates sites of thyroglossal cyst

2. **Chronological age:** At 7th week of intrauterine life.

3. **Applied anatomy:** Persistence of fragment of thyroglossal duct results into thyroglossal cysts or fistula.

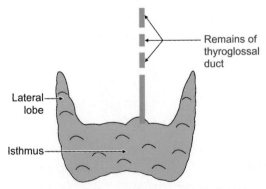

Fig. 12.19: Remains of thyroglossal duct

SN-96 Thyroglossal cyst

1. **Aetiology:** It results from persistence of a portion of a thyroglossal duct.
2. **Incidence:** It is the commonest congenital anomaly.
3. **Site:** Below the level of hyoid bone.
4. **Age:** It is evident in the late teens presumably because the lining of the thyroglossal duct becomes secretory.
5. **Clinical manifestations**
   A. It presents as a swelling along the course of duct.
   B. The swelling moves with swallowing and when the tongue is protruded out.
   C. There is recurrence of thyroglossal cyst, if the whole of the thyroglossal duct is not removed.
   Ref. Fig. 12.18

SN-97 Parathyroid glands

These are two pairs (superior and inferior) of small endocrine glands.
1. **Site:** On posterior border of lateral lobe of thyroid gland. They are present within the capsule of thyroid gland.
2. **Gross**
   A. **Weight:** 50 mg each.
   B. **Dimensions:** 6 × 4 × 2 mm.
   C. **Position** (Fig. 12.20)
      a. Superior parathyroid gland
         I. It is more constant in position.
         II. It lies at the middle of posterior border of lateral lobe of thyroid gland.
         III. It lies inside the true capsule and dorsal to recurrent laryngeal nerve.

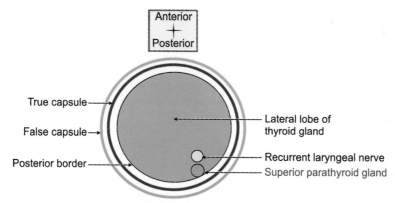

Fig. 12.20: Position of superior parathyroid gland in relation to recurrent laryngeal nerve

      b. The inferior parathyroid gland (Fig. 12.21)
         I. It is ventral to the recurrent laryngeal ner+ve.
         II. The position of inferior parathyroid gland is variable.
         III. The relations of the structures with various positions are shown in Table 12.3.

Head, Neck and Face

Table 12.3: Location of parathyroid gland and relation with artery and nerve

Type	Position of inferior parathyroid gland	Relation to	
		Inferior thriroid artery	Recurrent laryngeal nerve
1.	Outside thyroid capsule	Above	
2.	At lower pole within thyroid capsule	Below	
3.	Within the substance of lateral lobe, near posterior border.	—	Ventral to recurrent laryngeal nerve

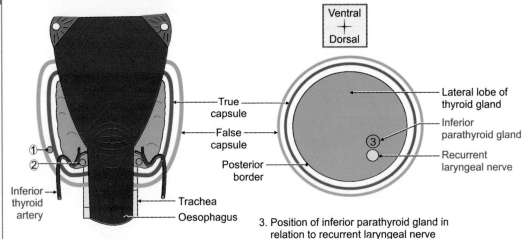

1. Position of inferior parathyroid gland out side the capsule and above inferior thyroid artery
2. Position of inferior parathyroid gland at lower pole within thyroid capsule below inferior thyroid artery
3. Position of inferior parathyroid gland in relation to recurrent laryngeal nerve

Fig. 12.21: Variations of positions of inferior parathyroid gland

3. **Blood supply:** It has rich blood supply.

A. Arterial supply :

   a. Ascending branch of inferior thyroid artery, branch of thyrocervical trunk. This branch anastomoses with posterior branch of superior thyroid artery.

   b. It also receives blood from anastomotic channel between superior and inferior thyroid arteries.

B. Venous drainage

   a. Superior thyroid vein
   b. Middle thyroid vein } drain into internal jugular vein.
   c. Inferior thyroid vein drains into left brachiocephalic vein.

4. Applied anatomy

  ➤ Tumours of the parathyroid gland enlarge downwards. The descent depends upon the relation of false capsule.

    • If tumour is outside the false capsule, it descends in the posterior mediastinum of thorax.

• If tumour is within the false capsule, it descends in the superior mediastinum of thorax.

SN-98   Subclavian artery

Introduction: It is the main artery of upper limb and supplies considerable part of posterior triangle of neck and brain.

1. **Origin**
   A. Right subclavian artery arises from brachiocephalic trunk.
   B. Left subclavian artery arises from arch of aorta.
2. **Extent:** It extends from sternoclavicular joint to outer border of 1st rib. At outer border of 1st rib, it continues as axillary artery.
3. **Course and relations:** The artery is divided into three parts by scalenus anterior muscle (Fig. 12.22).
   A. 1st part of subclavian artery is medial to scalenus anterior.
   B. 2nd part is posterior to scalenus anterior.
   C. 3rd part is lateral to scalenus anterior muscle.

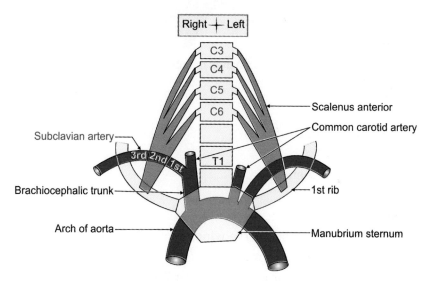

Fig. 12.22: Origin, course and termination of subclavian artery

4. **Branches:** **VIT, C, D**

   This mnemonic is right for the right side, i.e VIT for 1st part, C for 2nd part and D for 3rd part. However, on the left side, the branch "C" denoting "Costocervical"arise from 1st part. In that case, there is no branch from 2nd part (Fig. 12.23).

   A. **1st part**
      <u>V</u>ertebral artery.
      <u>I</u>nternal thoracic artery.
      <u>T</u>hyrocervical trunk which divides into **SIT**

Suprascapular.

Inferior thyroid.

Transverse cervical.

Costocervical trunk (on left side).

B. **2nd part:** Costocervical trunk (on right side).

C. **3rd part:** Dorsal scapular artery.

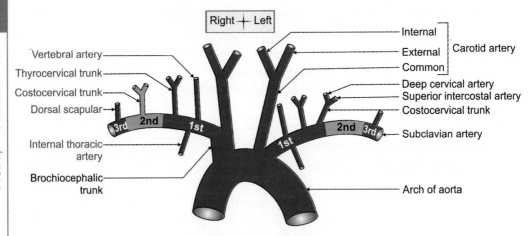

Fig. 12.23: Branches of subclavian artery

5. **Relations (Fig. 12.24)**

A. **1st part**

a. **Anterior:** Ansa subclavia

b. **Posterior**

I. Suprapleural membrane,

II. Apex of lung, and

III. Sympathetic trunk.

c. Right recurrent laryngeal nerve winds around the right subclavian artery.

d. **Lateral:** Scalenus anterior muscle.

B. **2nd part:** Scalenus anterior is present anteriorly.

C. **3rd part:** Scalenus anterior is present medially.

6. **Development**

A. Sources:

a. Right subclavian artery is derived from

I. Proximal part from the right 4th arch artery.

II. Right dorsal aorta cranial to

III. Distal part from the right 7th cervical intersegmental artery.

b. Left subclavian artery is developed entirely from the left 7th cervical inter-segmental artery.

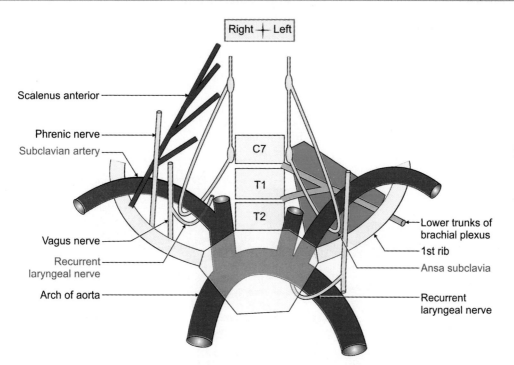

Fig. 12.24: Relations of subclavian artery

B. Abnormal right subclavian artery is[NEET 2016]
   a. Derived by
       I. Right 7th cervical intersegmental artery
       II. Right dorsal aorta caudal to right 7th cervical intersegmental artery.
   b. The sources which are disappearing are
       I. Proximal part from the right 4th arch artery.
       II. Right dorsal aorta cranial right 7th cervical intersegmental artery
C. Clinical manifestation: The abnormal right subclavian artery goes posteriorly, winds oesophagus and causes dysphagia lusoria.

7. **Applied anatomy**: *Subclavian steal syndrome* takes place in obstruction of the subclavian artery proximal to the origin of vertebral artery. Some amount of blood is stolen from the brain through the opposite vertebral artery. This is to provide collateral circulation to the affected arm. This may result in ischaemic neurological symptoms.

SN-99 Internal jugular vein

It is direct continuation of sigmoid venous sinus.
1. **Extent:** It extends from jugular foramen to sternal end of clavicle. It joins the subclavian vein to form brachiocephalic vein.
2. **Tributaries** (Fig. 12.25)
   A. Inferior petrosal sinus,
   B. Pharyngeal vein,

Head, Neck and Face

C. Common facial vein,

D. Lingual vein,

E. Superior thyroid vein, and

F. Middle thyroid vein,

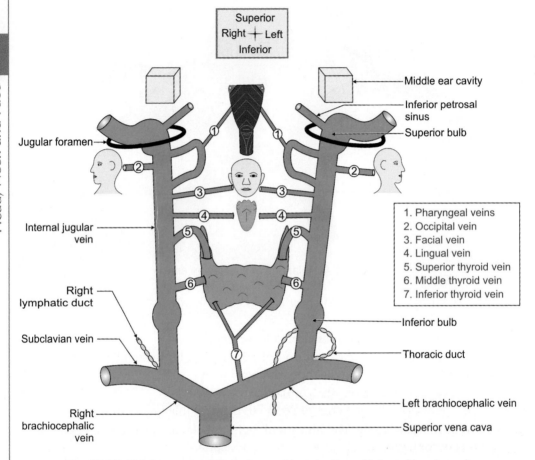

Fig. 12.25: Origin, course, tributaries and termination of internal jugular vein

3. **Relations** (Figs 12.26 and 12.27)

A. **Posteriorly:** The relations from above downwards are

   a. Rectus capitis lateralis,

   b. Transverse process of atlas,

   c. Levator scapulae,

   d. Scalenus medius and cervical plexus of nerves,

   e. Scalenus anterior and phrenic nerve,

   f. Thyrocervical trunk,

   g. 1st part of vertebral artery, and

   h. 1st part of subclavian artery.

B. **Anterolaterally**
   a. It is crossed by superior belly of omohyoid and posterior belly of digastric.
   b. Below the omohyoid: Sternohyoid and sternothyroid.
C. **Medially**
   a. Common carotid artery.
   b. Vagus nerve.

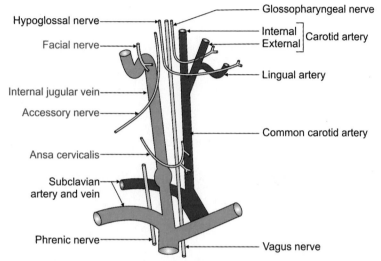

Fig. 12.26: Relations of nerves to right internal jugular vein

4. **Applied anatomy**

➢ The internal jugular vein is accessible deep to the supraclavicular fossa. The vein is used for recording venous pulse pressure (Fig. 12.28).
➢ In the congestive cardiac failure, the internal jugular vein is most dilated vein.
➢ The deep cervical lymph nodes lie along the internal jugular vein.

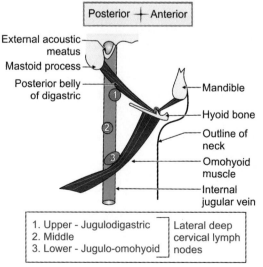

Fig. 12.27: Relations of lymph nodes to internal jugular vein

Head, Neck and Face

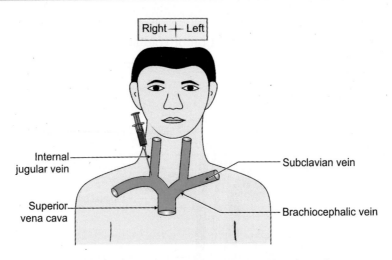

Fig. 12.28: Applied anatomy of internal jugular vein

LAQ-27	Describe glossopharyngeal nerve under the following heads:

1. Functional components,

2. Nuclei,

3. Course and relations,

4. Extracranial course,

5. Branches, and

6. Applied anatomy

Glossopharyngeal nerve: Nerve of 3rd pharyngeal arch

1. Functional components

Table 12.4: Functional components and the functions of the glossopharyngeal nerve

Functional components	Functions
• General somatic afferent	• Pain, touch and temperature from posterior one-third of tongue, tonsil, soft palate and oral part of pharynx.
• Special Visceral afferent SVAd	• Taste sensations from the circumvallate papillae and posterior one-third part of tongue.
• General visceral afferent sensation	• From baroreceptor and chemoreceptor of the carotid body and carotid sinus

Contd.

Table 12.4: Functional components and the functions of the glossopharyngeal nerve (Contd.)

Functional components	Functions
• Branchial efferent (Special Visceral efferent). Sa VE	• Motor to stylopharyngeus
• General Visceral efferent (GiVE) glands	• Secretomotor fibres to parotid gland

2. **Nuclei:** The three nuclei in the upper part of medulla are (Fig. 12.29)
   a. Nucleus ambiguus (brachiomotor)
   b. Inferior salivatory nucleus (parasympathetic)
   c. Nucleus of tractus solitarius (gustatory)

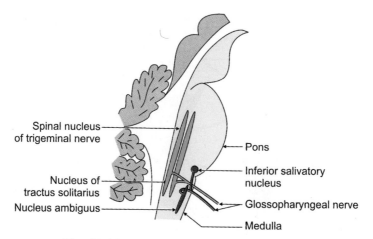

Fig. 12.29: Nuclei of glossopharyngeal nerve

3. **Course and relations** (Fig. 12.30)

    A. The nerve arises by 3 to 4 rootlets from posterolateral sulcus of medulla oblongata.

    B. It passes through jugular foramen in a separate dural sheath.

    C. In the foramen, it has two vessels in front and two behind and two nerves accompanying it.

        a. The vessels in front are

            I. Inferior petrosal sinus, and

            II. Meningeal branch of ascending pharyngeal artery.

        b. The vessels behind are

            I. Sigmoid sinus, and

            II. Meningeal branch of occipital artery.

        c. The accompanying nerves are

            I. Vagus, the 10th cranial nerve, and

            II. Accessory, the 11th cranial nerve.

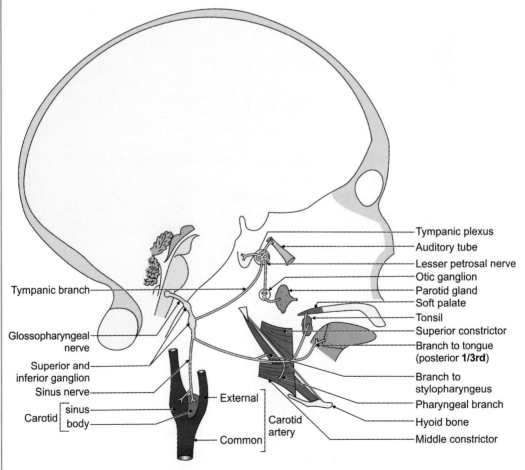

Fig. 12.30: Course and distribution of glossopharyngeal nerve

4. **Extracranial course**
   A. The nerve descends between internal jugular vein and internal carotid artery.
   B. It lies deep to styloid process (i.e. styloid process and the muscles attached to styloid process).
   C. It passes between external and internal carotid arteries.
   D. It passes in the gap present between superior constrictor and middle constrictor. It is accompanied by stylopharyngeus muscle.
   E. It lies on muscles of pharynx.
      a. Here it gives a pharyngeal branch.
      b. It enters the submandibular region passes deep to hyoglossus muscle where it breaks up into
         I. Tonsillar, and
         II. Lingual branch.
5. **Branches**

> ### Glossopharyngeal/Carotico Parotico Tonsili Tympani—Tip

Box 12.3

The word glossopharyngeal indicates glosso = tongue, pharyngeal = pharynx.
It is sensory nerve of pharynx and tongue.
It is motor nerve to muscle of pharynx, i.e. stylopharyngeus.
In addition to this the nerve is renamed as
Carotico Parotico Tonsili Tympani
   Meaning thereby supplies
   Carotico—Carotid body, and carotid sinus,
   Parotico—Parotid gland,
   Tonsili—Tonsils, and
   Tympani—Middle ear cavity.

A. **Tympanic branch**
   a. It arises from inferior ganglion and enters the tympanic canaliculus in front of the jugular fossa.
   b. It reaches the middle ear cavity.
   c. It joins with caroticotympanic nerve (a branch of plexus around internal carotid artery), and form tympanic plexus.[NEET] The branches from the plexus are
      I. Lesser petrosal nerve: It carries preganglionic parasympathetic fibres to the otic ganglion. It supplies parotid gland.
      II. Branch to middle ear cavity: It supplies
         i. Bony part of eustachian tube,
         ii. Mastoid antrum,
         iii. Mastoid air cells, and
         iv. Tympanic membrane.

B. **Muscular branch:** Stylopharyngeus muscle.

C. **Sinus branch:** It arises just below the jugular foramen. It descends along the internal carotid artery up to the carotid bifurcation and supplies

   a. Carotid sinus, and

   b. Carotid body. This branch mediates 'carotid reflex'.

D. **Parotid branch:** The lesser petrosal nerve, a branch of tympanic plexus, carries the parasympathetic fibres. It ends in the otic ganglion where the fibres relay. Post-ganglionic fibres from the otic ganglion are distributed to the parotid gland through the auriculotemporal nerve.

E. **Pharyngeal branch** supplies

   a. Fossae,

   b. Palatine tonsil, and

   c. Soft palate.

F. **Lingual branch** carries general and taste sensations from posterior one-third of tongue. It also carries taste sensations from the circumvallate papillae.

6. Applied anatomy

➢ The glossopharyngeal nerve is tested clinically by

- Tickling the posterior wall of pharynx. There is loss of reflex contraction of throat muscle in the lesion of glossopharyngeal nerve.
- Taste sensations from posterior one-third of tongue.

➢ Isolated lesion of glossopharyngeal nerve is almost unknown.

➢ Following are the features of glossopharyngeal nerve

- Loss of taste sensations in posterior one-third of tongue.
- Patient will have difficulty in swallowing.
- Patient will have decreased secretion from parotid gland.
- Patient will have paralysis of stylopharyngeus muscle.
- Gag reflex will be lost.

➢ Whenever an adult complains of constant pain in the middle ear and has no evidence of middle ear disease, a cancer of the pharynx is suspected.

➢ Involvement of carotid branch following surgery leads to transient or sustained hypertension.

LAQ-28 Describe hypoglossal nerve under the following heads:

   1. Course and relations,

   2. Extracranial course,

   3. Branches and distribution, and

   4. Applied anatomy

---

1. **Course and relations:** The rootlets arise from anterolateral sulcus of medulla oblongata. The nerve leaves the skull through hypoglossal canal (Figs 12.31 and 12.32).

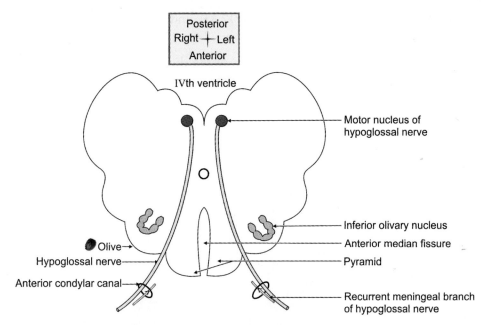

Fig. 12.31: TS of medulla oblongata showing the nucleus and exit of hypoglossal nerve

2. **Extracranial course**
   A. The nerve 1st lies deep to the internal jugular vein and descends between internal jugular vein and the internal carotid artery.

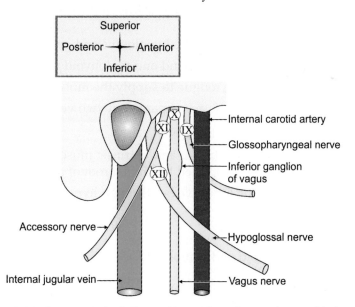

Fig. 12.32: Course and relations of hypoglossal nerve in carotid sheath

   B. It is present deep to the
      a. Parotid gland,
      b. Styloid process and muscles attached to process, i.e. stylohyoid.

c. Posterior belly of the digastric (Fig. 12.33), and

d. Stylohyoid muscle.

C. At the lower border of posterior belly of the digastric, it curves forwards and crosses the internal carotid artery and then external carotid artery. It crosses the loop of lingual artery anteriorly.

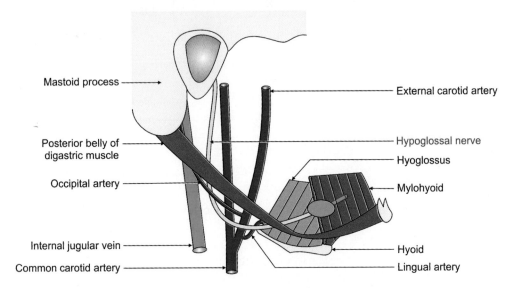

Fig. 12.33: Course and relations of hypoglossal nerve in digastric triangle

D. The nerve then runs forwards on the hyoglossus and genioglossus muscles.

E. It passes deep to submandibular gland and mylohyoid muscle.

F. It enters the substance of the tongue to supply the muscles of tongue.

G. On the hyoglossus muscle, it is accompanied by two venae comitantes.

3. **Branches and distribution** (Fig. 12.34)

A. Muscular branches supply intrinsic and extrinsic muscles of the tongue except the palatoglossus, which is supplied by cranial root of accessory nerve.

B. Other branches containing C1 nerve but through hypoglossal nerve (Fig. 12.35).

a. Meningeal branch.

b. Superior root of ansa cervicalis.

c. Branches to thyrohyoid and geniohyoid.

4. Applied anatomy

➤ Hypoglossal nerve is tested clinically by asking the patient to protrude the tongue.

➤ Lesion of the hypoglossal nerve produces protrusion of the tongue to the side of lesion. The position of the tongue indicates side of the lesion.

➤ If the lesion is infranuclear, there is gradual atrophy on the side of lesion.

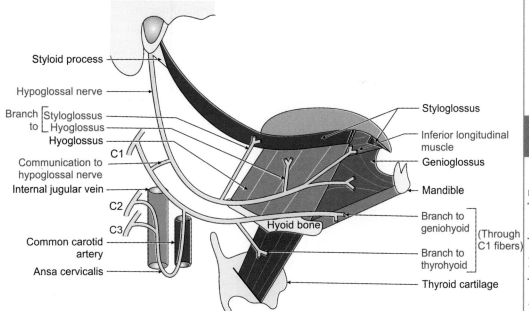

Fig. 12.34: Branches of hypoglossal nerve

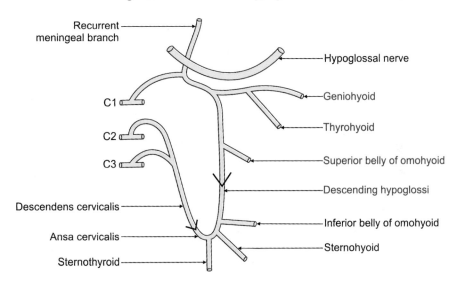

Fig. 12.35: Distribution of C1 fibres via hypoglossal nerve

Head, Neck and Face

SN-100   Anterior condylar canal (hypoglossal canal)

1. **Site:** It lies in the posterior cranial fossa.
2. **Situation:** It lies medial to and below the lower border of jugular foramen. It is at the junction of basilar and condylar part of occipital bone.
3. **Transmits**
   A. Hypoglossal nerve (XII).

B. Recurrent branch of hypoglossal nerve, 12th cranial nerve.

C. Meningeal branch of ascending pharyngeal artery (external carotid artery).

D. Emissary vein from the basilar venous plexus.

SN-101 Development of thymus

1. **Chronological age:** 6th week of intrauterine life.

    A. It is larger at birth.

    B. It continuously increases till puberty.

    C. After puberty, it undergoes atrophy.

2. **Germ layer**

    A. **Hassall's corpuscle:** It is developed from the **ventral part of endoderm of the 3rd pharyngeal pouch**.

    B. Lymphoid tissue is developed from mesoderm of the 3rd pharyngeal arch.

3. **Site:** Primitive pharynx.

4. **Sources:** It is very closely associated with the inferior parathyroid gland. It gets separated from the inferior parathyroid gland as the thymic rudiment. This is divided into

    A. Thinner portion which forms the cervical part of the thymus.

    B. Broader portion is divided into two parts, which enters into thorax and forms thoracic part.

       These two parts unite with each other by means of connective tissue and the thymus is formed.

5. **Anomalies**

    A. **DiGeorge syndrome:** It is failure of differentiation of 3rd pouch into thymus and parathyroid. It is associated with hypoplasia or aplasia of thymus and parathyroid glands. It manifests as

       a. Immunodeficiency resulting to low grade susceptibility to opportunistic pathogens, and

       b. Low calcium level resulting in tetany.

    B. Abnormal site is the commonest anomaly of thymus. It may remain along the course of development.

    C. Cervical part of the thymus may get fragmented and give rise to accessory thymic tissue.

LAQ-29 Describe lymphatic drainage of head, face and neck.

Lymphatics of head, face and neck are classified as (Fig. 12.36)

1. Anatomical classification

2. Clinical classification

1. **Anatomical classification**

    A. **Peripheral group—outer circle**

       a. Site: Present at the junction of head and neck.

I. Groups
- i. Submental
  - Site: Deep to mylohyoid
  - Afferent
    * Tip of tongue,
    * Incisor teeth, and
    * Floor of mouth.
  - Efferent: Jugulo-omohyoid
- ii. Submandibular
  - Site: Superficial submandibular gland
  - Afferent
    * Anterior 2/3rd of tongue,
    * Floor of mouth,
    * Anterior part of nasal cavity, and
    * Teeth.
  - Efferent: Jugulo-omohyoid
- iii. Preauricular (parotid)
  - Afferent:
    * Forehead,
    * Eyelid,
    * Temple,
    * External ear, and
    * Eyelid.
- iv. Postauricular (mastoid)—middle ear
- v. Occipital:
  - Afferent: Posterior part of scalp,
  - Efferent: Deep cervical

B. **Deep circle—inner circle**
  a. Site: Deep to investing layer of deep cervical fascia
  b. Groups
     I. Pretracheal/prelaryngeal
     II. Retropharyngeal

C. **Inner to inner circle:** Mucosa associated lymphoid tissue (Waldeyer's ring)
  a. Site: Submucosal aggregation of lymphoid tissue.
  b. Groups:
     I. Lingual tonsil,
     II. Palatine tonsil,
     III. Tubal tonsil, and
     IV. Adenoids (pharyngeal tonsil).

Head, Neck and Face

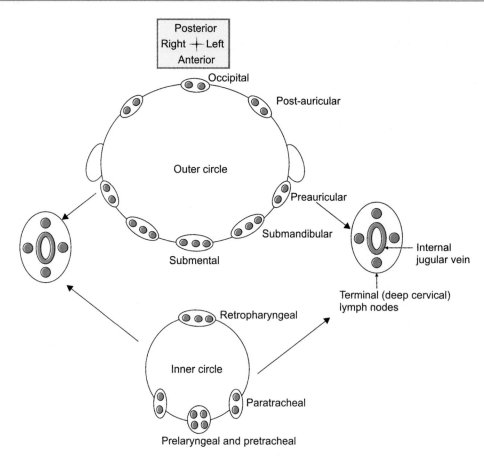

Fig. 12.36: Lymphatic drainage of head and neck

D. **Deep cervical lymph nodes**
  a. Jugulodigastric nodes: The node of **tonsil**
     I. Site: Triangular area present between
        i. Internal jugular vein
        ii. Common facial vein
        iii. Posterior belly of digastric muscle
     II. Area: Tonsil
  b. Jugulo-Omo Hyoid Node—JOHN—means—Tongue.
     I. Site: Area above the intermediate tendon of omohyoid on internal jugular vein
     II. Area: Tongue
  c. Efferents: Deep cervical lymph nodes.
     I. Right deep cervical node drain to right lymphatic duct.
     II. Left deep cervical node drain to thoracic duct.
2. Clinical classification of lymph nodes is based on involvement of lymph nodes at various levels (Fig. 12.37).

A. Level I lymph
   a. Ia: Submental
   b. Ib: Submandibular
B. Level II: Upper jugular—upper part of internal jugular vein
C. Level III: Midjugular—middle part of internal jugular vein
D. Level IV: Lower jugular—lower part of internal jugular vein
E. Level V: Lymph nodes are present in posterior triangle. They are associated with spinal accessory nerve.
   a. Va
   b. Vb
F. Level VI: Lymph nodes are situated between hyoid bone to sternum. They are present in anterior triangle.
G. Level VII: Supramediastinal lymph nodes.

All these lymph nodes ultimately drain in deep cervical lymph nodes: Jugulodigastric and jugulo-omohyoid lymph nodes.

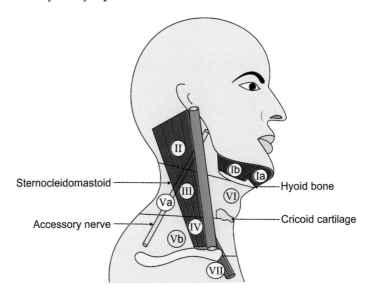

Fig. 12.37: Levels of lymph nodes in neck

3. Applied anatomy

   ➤ In radical neck dissection, the surgeons remove following structures
      • All lymph nodes,
      • Sternocleidomastoid,
      • Internal jugular vein, and
      • Spinal root of accessory nerve.
   ➤ In modified radical neck dissection, surgeons remove all lymph nodes sparing
      • Sternocleidomastoid
      • Internal jugular vein
      • Spinal root of accessory nerve

Head, Neck and Face

Prevertebral and Paravertebral Regions

OLA-62 **Where does trachea commence and terminate?**

It begins at 6th cervical vertebra and ends at the plane which passes from angle of Louis to lower border of 4th thoracic vertebra.

OLA-63 **What is tracheostomy and when is it done? What are the structures prone to injury?**

1. A transverse incision made through the skin of the neck and anterior wall of the trachea is called tracheostomy.
2. Indications of tracheostomy
   A. Patients with extensive laryngeal damage,
   B. Infants with severe airway obstruction,
   C. For evacuation of excessive secretions,
   D. For long continued artificial respiration.
3. Structures prone to injury
   A. Isthmus of thyroid gland,
   B. Inferior thyroid vein, and
   C. Arteria thyroidea ima.

LAQ-30 **Describe vertebral artery under the following heads:**
   1. Origin,
   2. Branches and distribution,
   3. Relations, and
   4. Applied anatomy

1. **Origin:** It is the 1st branch of 1st part of subclavian artery. It is the *largest* branch of subclavian artery. It is one of the two principal sets of arteries of the brain. In addition, it also supplies spinal cord, meninges, surrounding muscles and bones.

2. **Branches and distribution:** It is divided into four parts (Figs 13.1 and 13.2).

A. 1st part is cervical and is horizontal. It extends from the origin to entry into foramen transversarium.

B. 2nd part is vertebral and is vertical. It extends from 6th cervical vertebra to 1st cervical vertebra through foramen transversarium. It gives

a. Spinal, and

b. Muscular branches.

C. 3rd part is suboccipital and is horizontal, arching over the atlas vertebra behind the superior articular facet. It is present in the suboccipital triangle. It gives only muscular branches.

D. 4th part is cranial and is vertical. It extends from posterior atlanto-occipital membrane to the lower border of pons. It gives

a. Meningeal branches, which supply meninges of posterior cranial fossa.

b. Branches to brain and spinal cord.

    I. Posterior spinal artery (branch of vertebral artery) gives two branches which run anterior and posterior to dorsal root of spinal nerve.

    II. Anterior spinal artery (branch of vertebral artery): It arises from terminal part of vertebral artery and unites as it descends with the fellow of the opposite side to form anterior median trunk. It supplies medial part of medulla oblongata including pyramid and hypoglossal nuclei.

    III. Posterior inferior cerebellar artery: It is the most tortuous artery in the body. It is the largest branch of vertebral artery. It supplies

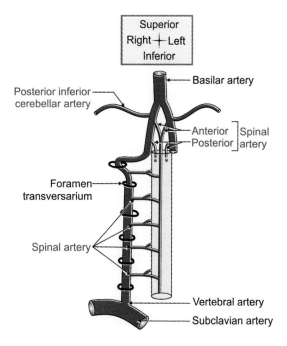

Fig. 13.1: Branches of vertebral artery

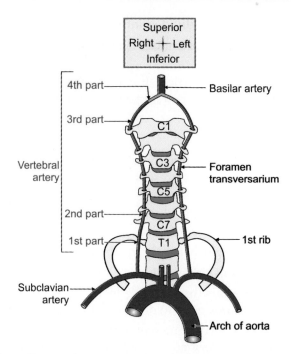

Fig. 13.2: Extent of 1st, 2nd, 3rd, and 4th parts of vertebral artery

    i. Lateral part of medulla,
    ii. 4th ventricle by forming choroid plexus,
    iii. Inferior vermis and inferolateral surface of cerebellar hemisphere,
    iv. Meningeal branch, and
    v. Medullary branches.

3. **Relations**

    A. The sympathetic plexus of the vertebral artery runs around the artery.
    B. Middle cervical ganglion lies anteromedially to vertebral artery.
    C. Inferior cervical ganglion lies posteromedially to vertebral artery.

4. **Applied anatomy**

  ➤ **Medial medullary syndrome:** The lesion of the anterior spinal artery is manifested by
    • Impairment of volitional (desired) movement on the contralateral side due to involvement of corticospinal tract, and
    • Ipsilateral loss of movements of tongue, wasting of muscles of tongue. It is due to involvement of hypoglossal nerve nucleus situated in the medulla.
  ➤ **Lateral medullary syndrome (Wallenberg's syndrome):** It is due to the lesion of posterior inferior cerebellar artery. This is manifested by
    • Loss of pain and thermal sensation of the same side of the face and opposite 1/2 of the body.
    • Paralysis of the vocal cords, soft palate and pharyngeal muscles of the same side.
  ➤ **Subclavian steal syndrome:** It takes place in obstruction of the subclavian artery proximal to the origin of vertebral artery. Some amount of blood is diverted

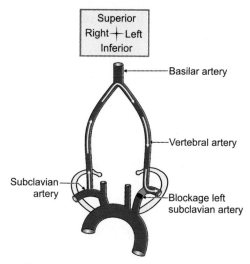

Fig. 13.3: Subclavian steal syndrome

from the brain through the vertebral artery of the opposite side to maintain collateral circulation (Fig. 13.3).

SN-102 Phrenic nerve

1. **Origin:** It is mainly formed from **C4**, with unimportant contribution from **C3** and **C5**. It is one of the most important nerves in the body, the principal motor supply to its own ½ of diaphragm.[NEET] It also supplies peritoneum, pleura and pericardium.
2. **Course and relations** (Fig. 13.4)
   A. The nerve is formed at the lateral border of scalenus anterior, at the level of upper border of thyroid cartilage.
   B. It runs vertically downwards on the anterior surface of scalenus anterior.[NEET]

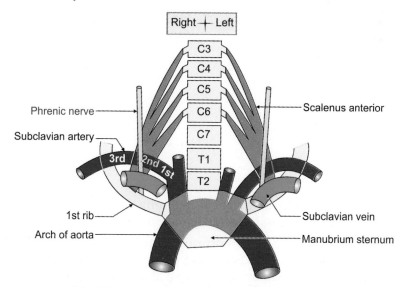

Fig. 13.4: Course and relations of phrenic nerve

C. It lies behind subclavian vein and in front of subclavian artery.

D. The nerve lies deep to

　a. Prevertebral fascia,

　b. Inferior belly of omohyoid,

　c. Transverse cervical artery,

　d. Suprascapular artery, and

　e. Internal jugular vein.

E. The nerve runs downward on the cervical pleura behind the commencement of brachio-cephalic vein. It crosses the internal thoracic artery and enters the thorax.

F. In thorax, phrenic nerve descends in front of hilum of lungs.[NEET]

G. Right phrenic nerve is shorter and more vertical.[NEET]

H. Note:

　a. Vagus nerve descends behind the hilum of lung.

　b. Right vagus nerve is shorter in length.

3. **Branches** (Fig. 13.5)

A. **Motor branches to diaphragm:** Phrenic nerve is main motor nerve to the diaphragm.

B. **Sensory branches**

　a. Central part of diaphragm.

　b. Pleura,

　c. Pericardium, and

　d. Peritoneum.

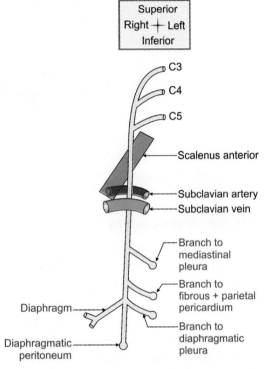

Fig. 13.5: Root value, branches of phrenic nerve

4. Applied anatomy

➢ The phrenic nerve may be injured by penetrating wounds of the neck or damaged. The damage is due to pressure of malignant tumours in the mediastinum.

➢ If phrenic nerve is damaged, the corresponding 1/2 dome of the diaphragm will be paralyzed. **The paralyzed 1/2 dome of the diaphragm will be relaxed and pushed up into the thorax by the positive abdominal pressure.** As a result, the lower lobe of the lung on that side may collapse.

➤ Phrenic avulsion is done to give rest to diaphragm. While dissecting phrenic nerve, one must keep in mind the possibility of accessory phrenic nerve in mind. If present, it might tear the subclavian vein with alarming symptoms. This is because the main trunk loops around the vessel. The accessory phrenic nerve, *branch of nerve to subclavius, is an important nerve of unimportant muscle*.

LAQ-31	Describe atlantoaxial joints under the following heads:

1. Articulating surface,

2. Classification,

3. Ligaments,

4. Movements and muscles bringing movements, and

5. Applied anatomy

Table 13.1: (1) Articulating surface, (2) Classification, (3) Ligaments

	Median atlantoaxial joint	Lateral atlantoaxial joint
1. Articulating surface	• Dens or odontoid process of the axis • Anterior arch of atlas	• Inferior articular facet of the lateral mass of atlast • Superior articular facet of the axis
2. Classification of the joints	• Pivot joint	• Plane synovial joint

3. Ligaments of the joints	• **Transverse ligament of atlas:** It extends between the two tubercles on the medial side of lateral masses of atlas
	• **Apical ligament:** It connects the tip of the dens to the dorsal surface of basilar part of occipital bone.
	• **Alar ligaments:**
	  – It extends from upper part of lateral surface of the dens to the medial surface of condyles.
	  – These are strong ligaments
	  – They are stretched during flexion and relaxed during extension.
	  – They check excessive rotation.
		• **Capsular ligament:**
		  – Loose: The laxity of the fibrous capsule permits forward or backward gliding movements during rotation of the atlas
		  – Attached to the peripheral margin of articular surface
		  – Excessive stretching of the fibrous capsule is prevented by curvatures of articular surfaces

4. **Movements and muscles producing movements:** Movements at all three joints are rotatory movements and take place around a vertical axis. The dens form a pivot around which the atlas rotates (carrying the skull with it). It is called "NO" movement.

Head, Neck and Face

A. **Ipsilateral:** The muscles bring flexion of the neck on the same side. They are
   a. Obliquus capitis inferior,
   b. Rectus capitis posterior major and minor,
   c. Longissimus capitis,
   d. Spleniu capitis, and
   e. Sternocleidomastoid of opposite side.
B. **Contralateral:** Sternocleidomastoid brings rotation of the neck on the opposite side.

5. Applied anatomy : Death by hanging may be due to
   ➤ Rupture of the transverse ligament of atlas, or
   ➤ Fracture of the dens of axis.
   As a result, the atlas is dislocated from the axis. The dens compresses the spinal cord and results in death.

LAQ-32 Describe atlanto-occipital joints under the following heads:

1. Classification,

2. Ligaments,

3. Movements and muscle bringing movements, and

4. Applied anatomy

1. **Classification**
   A. **Structural:** Biaxial, simple, ellipsoid variety of synovial joint. **AB'S** ◆━
      a. Axis: Biaxial
      b. Depending upon number of bones simple since there are 2 articulating bones
         I. Occipital condyle
         II. Superior articular facet of atlas.
      c. Shape: Ellipsoid
2. **Ligaments** (Fig. 13.6)
   A. **Fibrous capsule**
      a. Attached to peripheral margin of articular surface.
      b. It is thick posterolaterally, thin and loose anteromedially.
   B. **Synovial membrane:** Internally, lines the fibrous capsule.
   C. **Anterior atlanto-occipital membrane**
      a. It connects the anterior arch of atlas with the anterior margin of foramen magnum.
      b. Laterally, it continues with the anterior part of capsular ligament.
      c. Anteriorly, it is strengthened by the anterior longitudinal ligament.
      d. It prevents excessive movements.
   D. **Posterior atlanto-occipital membrane**
      a. It extends from posterior margin of foramen magnum to the posterior arch of atlas.
      b. Laterally, it continues as the posterior part of capsular ligament.

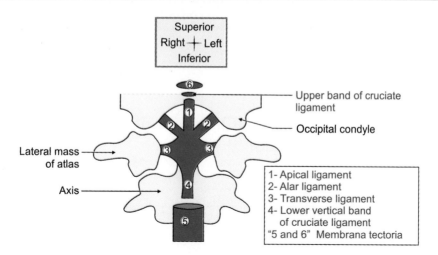

Fig. 13.6: Ligaments of atlanto-occipital and atlantoaxial joints

3. **Movements and muscles bringing movements:** Flexion and extension collectively called "YES" movement.

A. **Flexion**

    a. Longus capitis

    b. Rectus capitis anterior

    c. Sternocleidomastoid

B. **Extension**

    a. Rectus capitis posterior major

    b. Rectus capitis posterior minor

    c. Obliquus capitis

    d. Semispinalis capitis

    e. Splenius capitis

    f. Longissimus capitis

    g. Trapezius.

C. **Lateral flexion**

    a. Sternomastoid (acting unilaterally).

    b. Obliquus capitis.

4. **Applied anatomy**

➤ The atlantoaxial region of the cervical spine can be visualized in transoral anteroposterior radiographs.

➤ The transoral route is also utilized in surgical approaches to this region, with upward retraction of the soft palate and division of the posterior wall of the pharynx.

Mouth and Pharynx

SN-103 Ludwig's angina

Introduction: It is cellulitis (inflammation of the fascia) of the floor of the mouth.

1. **Site:** A swelling appears below the chin and inside the mouth. It is deep to mylohyoid.
2. **Boundaries:** It is limited
   A. Laterally by two halves of mandible, and
   B. Posteriorly by hyoid bone. This is because of the attachments of investing layer of deep cervical fascia to the base of mandible and hyoid bone.
3. **Cause:** It is usually secondary to caries of molar teeth.
4. **Complications:** If infection spreads backwards, it causes oedema of glottis. It may result into asphyxia.
5. **Applied anatomy:** The abscess is drained by a deep incision below the mandible by dividing the mylohyoid muscle.

SN-104 Buccinator

Introduction: It is an accessory muscle of mastication. It is indispensable for the return of bolus from the vestibule to the oral cavity (Fig. 14.1).

1. **Action** (Fig. 14.2)
   A. Accessory muscle of mastication.
   B. It is useful in blowing.

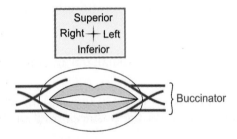

Fig. 14.1: Buccinator

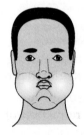

Fig. 14.2: Action of buccinator

2. **Development:** It is developed from the mesenchyme of 2nd branchial arch.
3. **Proximal attachments:**
   A. It has bony origin from the bone above and below the oral cavity, i.e. maxilla and mandible.
   B. Fibrous band from pterygomaxillary ligament.
   C. Raphe part from pterygomandibular raphe.
4. **Distal attachments:**
   A. Upper and lower fibres to the respective lip.
   B. Middle fibres decussate and push to the lips.
5. **Peculiarities:** It is pierced by parotid duct opposite the crown of upper 2nd molar tooth. It has double nerve supply.

6. Nerve supply
   A. Proprioceptive by buccal branch of mandibular division of trigeminal nerve (Vth cranial nerve).
   B. Motor by buccal branch of facial nerve (VIIth cranial nerve).

SN-105   Uvula (small grape)

1. **Definition:** It is conical projection hanging from inferior surface of soft palate.
2. **Folds:** Two curved folds of mucous membrane extend laterally and downwards.
   A. **Anterior fold:** Palatoglossal arch or anterior pillar of fauces. It contains palatoglossus.
   B. **Posterior fold:** Palatopharyngeal arch or posterior pillar of fauces. It contains palatopharyngeus.

SN-106   Passavant's ridge

1. **Definition:** Palatopharyngeus is a longitudinal muscle of pharynx. The upper fibres of both sides encircle and form a circular bundle. They act as a sphincter. They give an elevated appearance called Passavant's ridge.
2. **Relations:** Internal to the superior constrictor.
3. **Site:** Posterior wall of nasopharynx.
4. **Function:** Prevents entry of food in nasopharynx.

5. Applied anatomy
   ➢ It is hypertrophied in cases of complete cleft palate.
   ➢ In case of paralysis of the ridge, the food regurgitates into nasopharynx.

LAQ-33   Describe muscles of soft palate under the following heads:
   1. Muscles,
   2. Attachments,
   3. Insertion,
   4. Action,
   5. Nerve supply, and
   6. Blood supply

Head, Neck and Face

Head, Neck and Face

Table 14.1: Origin, insertion and actions of muscles of soft palate

1. Muscles	2. Attachments	3. Insertion	4. Action
Tensor palati	• Lateral side of auditory tube • Adjoining part of the base of the skull (greater wing and scaphoid fossa of sphenoid bone)	Muscle descends, converges to form a delicate tendon which winds round the pterygoid hamulus, passes through the origin of the buccinator, and flattens out to form the palatine aponeurosis. Aponeurosis is attached to: • Posterior border of hard palate • Inferior surface of palate behind the palatine crest	• Tightens the soft palate chiefly the anterior part • It dilates the auditory tube hence, it is known as **dilator tubae**
Levator palati	• Inferior aspect of auditory tube • Adjoining part of inferior surface of petrous part of temporal bone	Muscle enters the pharynx bypassing over the upper concave margin of the superior constrictor, runs downwards and medially and spreads out in the soft palate. It is inserted into the upper surface of the palatine aponeurosis	• Elevates soft palate and closes the pharyngeal isthmus • Opens the auditory tube, like the tensor palatini
Musculus uvulae	• Posterior nasal spine • Palatine apo-neurosis	Mucous membrane of uvula	• Pulls up the uvula
Palatoglossus	• Oral surface of palatine apo-neurosis	Descends in the palato-glossal arch, to the side of the tongue at the junction of its oral and pharyngeal parts	• Elevates the base of the tongue and closes the oropharyngeal isthmus
Palato-pharyngeus	• Anterior fasciculus: From posterior border of hard palate • Posterior fasciculus: From palatine-aponeurosis	• Descends in the palato-pharyngeal arch and spreads out to form the greater part of long-itudinal muscle coat of pharynx. It is inserted into: • Posterior border of the lamina of the thyroid cartilage • Wall of the pharynx and its median raphe	• Pulls up the wall of the pharynx and shortens it during swallowing

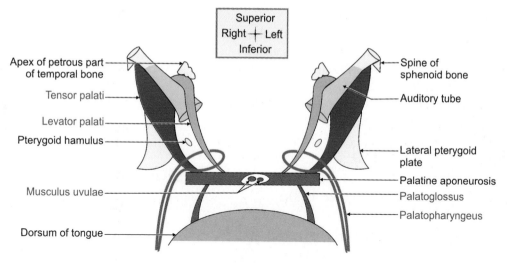

Fig. 14.3: Muscles of soft palate

5. Nerve supply

   A. **Motor nerves:** All muscles of the soft palate are supplied by pharyngeal plexus except tensor palatini, which is supplied by the mandibular nerve. The fibres of this plexus are derived from the cranial part of the accessory nerve (through vagus).

   B. **General sensory nerves are derived from**

     a. Lesser palatine nerves, which are branches of the maxillary nerve (through the pterygopalatine ganglion) and from the

     b. Glossopharyngeal nerve.

   C. **Special sensory (gustatory) nerve:** The fibres travel through the greater petrosal nerve—geniculate ganglion of the facial nerve—nucleus of the solitary tract.

   D. **Secretomotor nerves:** Lesser palatine nerves. They are derived from the superior salivatory nucleus and travel through the greater petrosal nerve.

6. Blood supply of soft palate

   A. Arterial supply :

     a. Greater palatine, branch of maxillary artery.

     b. Ascending palatine, branch of facial artery.

     c. Palatine artery, branch of ascending pharyngeal artery.

     All these arteries anastomose freely in the soft palate.

   B. Venous drainage : Most of the venous blood is drained laterally through wall of pharynx. The veins are paratonsillar veins which open into pharyngeal venous plexus and the pterygoid plexus.

SN-107   Palatine aponeurosis

Introduction: It is expanded tendon of insertion of tensor veli palatini muscle.

1. **Features**
    A. **Attachments:** Anteriorly, posterior border of hard palate.
    B. **Structure:** It is thin, firm fibrous sheet.
    C. Encloses musculus uvulae.
2. **Functions**
    A. It supports the muscles of soft palate.
    B. It gives strength to soft palate.

SN-108   Waldeyer's ring

It is a ring of submucosal lymphoid tissue which surrounds the beginning of respiratory and gastrointestinal tracts (Fig. 14.4).

1. **Formation**
    A. **In front and below:** Lingual tonsil.
    B. **On each side:** Palatine tonsil.
    C. **Above and on each side:** Tubal tonsil.
    D. **Above and behind:** Nasopharyngeal tonsil. The internal ring of Waldeyer drains into precervical chain of lymph node and deep cervical lymph node which together constitute the "external ring of Waldeyer".

2. **Functions**
    A. It filters tissue fluid coming from inner surface of oral cavity.
    B. It prevents the entry of organisms from outside and thereby acting as a guard.
    C. It serves as the first line of defense and protects the body against ingested and inspired bacteria by producing antibodies against such invading organisms. When the tonsil itself becomes infected, it becomes a source for the spread of infection.

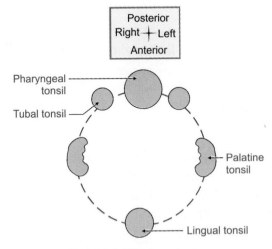

Fig. 14.4: Waldeyer's ring

3. Applied anatomy

  ➤ Waldeyer's ring forms a strong defense system to prevent the spread of infection from the oral and nasal cavities into the lower respiratory tract consisting of larynx, trachea, bronchi and lungs.

➤ The lymphatic ring helps in defensive mechanism of the respiratory and alimentary systems by destroying the entry of microorganisms from the external environment.

➤ In pre-antibiotic era: Enlargement of the lymphoid follicle in the Waldeyer's ring was blocking the respiratory tract.

SN-109 Palatine tonsil

1. **Gross:** Tonsils are collection of lymphoid tissue situated bilaterally in the lateral wall of oropharynx.

A. **Situation:** Tonsillar sinus between palatoglossal and palatopharyngeal folds.

B. **Dimension:** 2 cm.

C. **Capsule:** Capsule is condensed connective tissue present on the lateral side. It can easily be separated from the pharyngeal muscular wall except at its anteroinferior part.

D. **Morphology**

    a. Two surfaces: Medial and lateral.

    b. Two borders: Anterior and posterior.

    c. Two ends: Upper and lower.

2. **Relations** (Fig. 14.5)

A. **Surface**

    a. **Medial:** Presence of 8–12 crypts.

    b. **Lateral: Bed of tonsil**[NEET]

        I. Capsule of tonsil

        II. Peritonsillar space which contains paratonsillar vein.

        III. Superior constrictor which is lined by pharyngobasilar fascia inside and buccopharyngeal fascia outside.

        IV. **Artery**

            i. Facial artery and its branches

                • Ascending palatine and

                • Tonsillar

            ii. Ascending pharyngeal artery.

        V. **Muscle**

            i. Styloglossus muscle,

            ii. Medial pterygoid muscle, and

            iii. Posterior belly of digastric.

        VI. Glosspharyngeal nerve

        VII. **Gland:** Submandibular and parotid gland.

B. **Border**

    a. **Anterior:** Palatoglossus.

    b. **Posterior:** Palatopharyngeus.

Head, Neck and Face

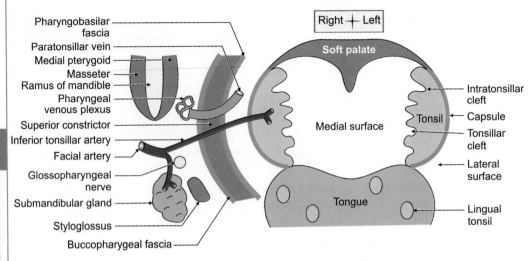

Fig. 14.5: Relations of palatine tonsil

3. **Blood supply**

A. Arterial supply

a. Main source: Inferior tonsillar branch of facial artery. It enters the tonsil from its lateral surface (Fig. 14.6A).

b. Additional sources (Fig. 14.6B):

I. Anterior tonsillar, a branch of lingual artery.

II. Posterior tonsillar, a branch of
   i. Ascending palatine branch of facial artery
   ii. Ascending pharyngeal artery

III. Superior tonsillar, a branch of descending palatine.

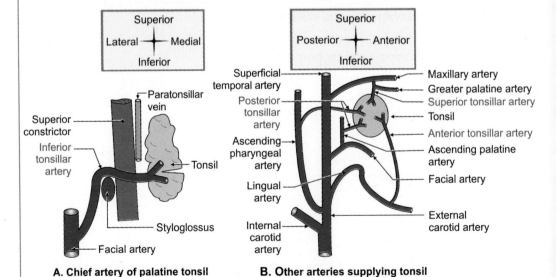

A. Chief artery of palatine tonsil   **B. Other arteries supplying tonsil**

Fig. 14.6: Arterial supply of palatine tonsil

B. **Venous drainage**

a. Into the pharyngeal venous plexus.

b. Principal drainage is by the paratonsillar vein, which opens into pharyngeal venous plexus (Fig. 14.7).

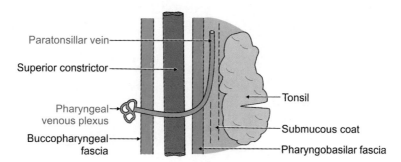

Fig. 14.7: Venous drainage of tonsil

4. **Nerve supply** : Glossopharyngeal nerve.

5. Development

A. **Chronological age:** It develops in the 4th week of intrauterine life.

B. **Germ layer:** The epithelium develops from the endoderm of the 2nd pharyngeal pouch and remaining structures from the local mesenchymal tissue.

C. **Source:**

a. Tonsillar fossa develops from ventral part of the 2nd pharyngeal pouch. The endodermal cells proliferate outwards as solid buds which are subsequently canalized to form tonsillar pits and crypts. Lymphocytes either develop from mesoderm of adjoining arches or from circulating lymphocytes.

b. Tonsil is aggregation of lymphocytes. It belongs to lymphatic system which develops from secondary mesoderm. It is called neural crest cells.[NEET]

D. **Site:** On the lateral side of oral cavity.

6. **Histology** : It is lymphoid organ consisting of (Fig. 14.8)

A. Stratified squamous non-keratinized epithelium covering the free surface.

B. With crypts

C. Fibrous capsule on the outer side, and

D. Lymphoid tissue (diffuse and lymph nodule)

7. **Applied anatomy**

➤ Referred pain from the infected tonsil extends to the middle ear, because both are supplied by the glossopharyngeal nerve.

➤ The capsule of the tonsil is removed during tonsillectomy because it is attached to deep surface of the tonsil and extends to form septa which conduct nerves and vessels.

Head, Neck and Face

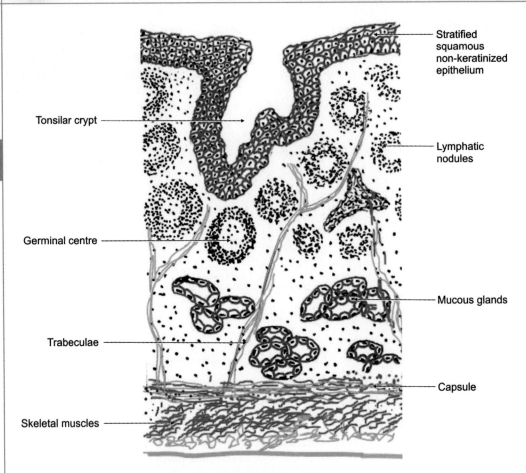

Fig. 14.8: Histology of palatine tonsil

➢ After tonsillectomy, all clots in the tonsillar fossa are removed. It prevents the interference of retraction of blood vessels.

➢ Quinsy is infection of peritonsillar space (peritonsillar abscess.)

➢ Rupture of paratonsillar vein is most common cause of tonsillar haemorrhage in tonsillectomy procedure.

After tonsillectomy and after postpartum haemorrhage are the areas where clot formation is prevented.

Box 14.1

Such removal of clots is also done in uterus after delivery to prevent postpartum haemorrhage.

8. **Lymphatic drainage**: Tonsil is not fully covered by a capsule. There is no subcapsular sinus or afferent lymphatics. Dense plexuses of the fine lymphatic vessel surround

each follicle and form efferent lymphatics. They drain into jugulodigastric lymph nodes.

9. **Site:** It is present below and behind angle of mandible. It is ▲ lar interval between the junction of internal jugular vein, facial vein and posterior belly of digastric. This is considered principal lymph node of tonsil since it is primarily enlarged in tonsil.

OLA-64 Pharyngeal tonsil

1. **Features**

   A. It is also called 'the *adenoids*'.

   B. It consists of a collection of lymphoid tissue beneath the epithelium of the roof and posterior wall of the pharynx.

   C. It is one of the important members of *Waldeyer's ring*.

   D. It is unpaired organ.

   E. It is prominent in children.

   F. It usually undergoes atrophy after puberty.

2. **Applied anatomy**

   ➤ Marked hypertrophy of adenoids blocks the posterior nasal openings. It makes the patient to snore loudly at night and to breathe through the open mouth.

   ➤ In chronic inflammation, it may

   - Block the nasopharynx and cause mouth breathing.
   - Block the auditory tube and cause deafness and middle ear infection.
   - Inflammation of the pharyngeal tonsils (adenoids) is called *adenoiditis*.
   - Sometimes the palatine and pharyngeal tonsils are removed during the tonsillectomy and adenoidectomy operation.

LAQ-34 Describe pharynx under the following heads:

1. Parts,
2. Structure of pharynx,
3. Muscles of pharynx,
4. Blood supply,
5. Nerve supply, and
6. Applied anatomy

1. **Parts:** It is a wide, muscular tube situated behind the nose, mouth and larynx. It is divided into three parts:

   A. Nasopharynx,

   B. Oropharynx, and

   C. Laryngopharynx.

Table 14.2: Subdivisions of pharynx and their details

Particulars	Nasopharynx	Oropharynx	Laryngopharynx
• Situation	• Behind nose	• Behind oral cavity	• Behind larynx.
• Extent	• Base of skull (body of sphenoid) to soft palate	• Soft palate to upper border of epiglottis	• Upper border of epiglottis to lower border of cricoid cartilage
• Communications	• Anteriorly with nose	• Anteriorly with oral cavity • Above with naso-pharynx • Below with laryn-gopharynx	• Inferiorly with oesophagus
• Nerve supply	• Pharyngeal branches of pterygopalatine ganglion	• Ninth and tenth nerves	
• Relations: Anterior	• Posterior nasal aperture	• Oral cavity	• Inlet of larynx • Posterior surface of cricoid • Arytenoid cartil-age
• Posterior	• Body of sphenoid bone	• Body of 2nd and 3rd cervical vertebrae	• 4th and 5th cervical vertebrae
• Lateral	• Opening of auditory tube	• Palatoglossal and palatopharyngeal fold containing palatine tonsil	• Pyriform fossa present between thyroid membrane and aryepiglottic fold
• Lateral wall	• Opening of auditory tube	• Tonsillar fossa con-taining palatine tonsils	• Pyriform fossa
• Lining epithelium	• Ciliated columnar epithelium	• Stratified squamous non-keratinised epith-elium	• Stratified squamous non-keratinised epithelium
• Function	• Passage for air (respiratory function)	• Passage for air and food	• Passage for food

2. **Structures of pharynx**

   A. Mucosa.

   B. Submucosa.

   C. **Pharyngobasilar fascia:** Fibrous sheet filling the gap extending from base of skull to upper margin of superior constrictor muscle.

D. **Muscular coat**

    a. Outer circular muscle consists of

        I. Superior constrictor,

        II. Middle constrictor, and

        III. Inferior constrictor.

    b. Inner longitudinal layer consists of

        I. Stylopharyngeus.

        II. Salpingopharyngeus.

        III. Palatopharyngeus.

3. **Muscles of pharynx** are described as inner longitudinal and outer circular.

    A. **The circular muscles of pharynx are described as follows** (Fig. 14.9)

        a. **Proximal attachments**

            I. **Superior constrictor:** It has four parts

                i. **Pterygopharyngeus** arises from

                    • Posterior border of medial pterygoid plate, and

                    • Pterygoid hamulus.

                ii. **Buccopharyngeus** arises from pterygomandibular raphe.

                iii. **Mylopharyngeus** arises from posterior end of mylohyoid line of mandible.

                iv. **Glossopharyngeus** arises from side of tongue.

            II. **Middle constrictor**

                i. **Chondropharyngeus**arises from

                    • Lower part of stylohyoid ligament, and

                    • Lesser cornu of hyoid bone.

                ii. **Ceratopharyngeus** arises from upper border of greater cornu of hyoid bone.

            III. **Inferior constrictor** arises from

                i. Thyropharyngeus (propulsive part):

                    • From oblique line of thyroid cartilage, and

                    • The tendinous band across the cricothyroid muscle.

                ii. Cricopharyngeus (sphincter part: From side of the cricoid)

        b. **Distal attachments**

            I. Pharyngeal tubercle, and

            II. Median pharyngeal raphe.

    B. **Longitudinal muscles of pharynx are described in Table 14.3.**

Head, Neck and Face

Table 14.3: Origin and insertion of longitudinal muscles of pharynx

Muscles	Origin	Features	Insertion
• Stylopharyn-geus	• Arises from the medial surface of the base of styloid process	• Muscle descends, converges to form a delicate tendon which winds wound the pterygoid hamulus, passes through the origin of the buccinator, and flattens out to form the palatine aponeurosis	• Posterior border of lamina of thyroid cartilage
• Palatophary-ngeus	• Anterior fasciculus: From posterior bor-der of hard palate. • Posterior fasciculus: From palatine aponeurosis		• Posterior border of lamina of thyroid cartilage • Wall of pharynx and its median raphe
• Salpingo-pharyngeus	• Anterior end of the cartilage of audi-tory tube		• Blends with palato-pharyngeus

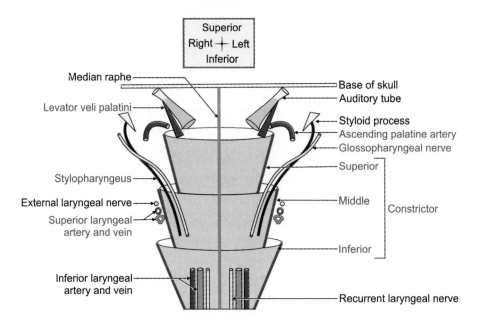

Fig. 14.9: Constrictor muscles of pharynx and structures passing between them

4. **Blood supply**

A. Arterial supply

    a. Ascending pharyngeal, branch of external carotid artery.

    b. Ascending palatine (branch of facial artery)

    c. Tonsillar artery

d. Dorsal lingual branch of lingual artery

e. Greater palatine branch of maxillary artery.

B. **Venous drainage:** Form a plexus which drains into internal jugular and facial veins.

C. **Lymphatic drainage**

a. Retropharyngeal, and

b. Deep cervical group of lymph nodes.

5. **Nerve supply**: Pharyngeal plexus which is formed by

A. **Sensory**

a. **General:** Pharyngeal branch of glossopharyngeal nerve.

b. **Special:** Taste fibres through internal laryngeal nerve, a branch of superior laryngeal nerve, branch of vagus nerve.

B. **Motor**

a. **Somatomotor:** Pharyngeal branch of vagus—chiefly motor.

b. **Secretomotor:** Fibres from greater petrosal nerve.

c. **Vasomotor:** Pharyngeal branch of superior cervical sympathetic ganglion.

Table 14.4: Nerve supply of inferior constrictor

No.	Nerve	Function
1.	• Accessory nerve	• Motor
2.	• Pharyngeal branch of glossopharyngeal	• Sensory
3.	• Pharyngeal branch of superior cervical sympathetic ganglion	• Vasomotor
4.	• External and recurrent laryngeal nerves	• Motor

6. **Applied anatomy**

➤ **Dysphagia:** Difficulty in swallowing.

➤ Killian's dehiscence.

LAQ-35 **Describe inferior constrictor muscles under**

1. Gross anatomy

2. Applied anatomy

1. **Gross anatomy**

A. **Inferior constrictor:** It is the thickest of the three constrictor muscles and is usually described in two parts.

a. **Thyropharyngeus**

I. **Proximal attachment:** It arises from oblique line of the lamina of thyroid cartilage.

II. **Distal attachment:** Pharyngeal raphe

III. **Arrangement of fibres:** The upper muscle fibres of inferior constrictor overlap middle constrictor.

Head, Neck and Face

IV. **Nerve supply** : Cranial root of accessory nerve (pharyngeal plexus).

V. **Action:** It constricts lower part of pharynx.

b. **Cricopharyngeus:** It is rounded and thicker than the flat sheets of other constrictors. It extends from one side of cricoid arch to other side of cricoid arch.

I. **Proximal attachment:** It arises from the side of the arch of the cricoid cartilage.

II. **Distal attachment:** It blends with circular oesophageal fibres around the narrowest part of pharynx.

III. **Nerve supply**

Table 14.5: Nerve supply of inferior constrictor

No.	Nerve	Function
1.	• Cranial part of accessory nerve	• Motor
2.	• Pharyngeal branch of glossopharyngeal	• Sensory
3.	• Pharyngeal branch of superior cervical sympathetic ganglion	• Vasomotor
4.	• External and recurrent laryngeal nerves	• Motor

c. **Action:** It acts as a sphincter at the junction of the laryngopharynx and the oesophagus.

2. **Applied anatomy**

➢ On the posterior surface of pharynx, there is a gap between two components of inferior constrictor, called "pharyngeal dimple" or "Killian's dehiscence". The mucosa and submucosa of pharynx may bulge through the weak area to form the pharyngeal diverticulum.

➢ In spasm of cricopharyngeus, there is failure of the relaxation of cricopharyngeus. The bolus of food fails to move downward. Hence, it is pushed in the region of Killian's dehiscence producing a pharyngeal diverticulum. It is also called pharyngeal pouch.

➢ Patient presents dysphagia (difficulty in swallowing), if pharyngeal pouch is filled with food.

➢ Third stage of swallowing is brought by inferior constrictor of pharynx. In this stage, the food passes from lower part of the pharynx to the oesophagus.

SN-110 Pharyngobasilar fascia (pharyngeal aponeurosis)

Introduction: Between the base of skull and upper border of superior constrictor, there is a gap called "sinus of Morgagni". It is closed internally by a rigid membrane called pharyngobasilar fascia (Fig. 14.10).

1. **Extent:** It extends from the upper border of superior constrictor muscle of pharynx to the base of the skull.

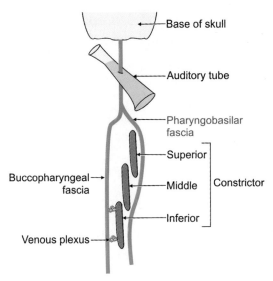

Fig. 14.10: Pharyngobasilar fascia (pharyngeal aponeurosis)

2. **Attachments**
   A. **Above**
      a. Basilar part of occipital bone.
      b. Petrous part of temporal bone.
      c. Posterior border of medial pterygoid plate.
      d. Pterygomandibular raphe.
   B. **Below:** It gradually becomes areolar and merges in pharyngeal muscles and **never extends below superior constrictor muscle.**
   C. **Features**
      a. It is non-expansible sheet of fascia.
      b. It is strengthened by pharyngeal ligament, a midline thickening.
   D. **Structures piercing:** Auditory tube.
   E. **Function:** It keeps the wall of nasopharynx permanently open for breathing.
      Ref. LAQ-34, Fig. 14.9

SN-111 Pterygomandibular raphe

Introduction: It is a thin band of tendinous fibres between buccinator anteriorly and superior constrictor posteriorly (Fig. 14.11).
1. **Extent:** It extends
   A. From hamulus of medial pterygoid plate
   B. To the posterior end of mylohyoid line of the mandible.
2. **Relations**
   A. **Medially:** Mucous membrane of the mouth.
   B. **Laterally:** Adipose tissue and ramus of mandible.
3. **Attachments**
   A. Anteriorly to the central part of buccinator, and
   B. Posteriorly to the superior constrictor of pharynx.

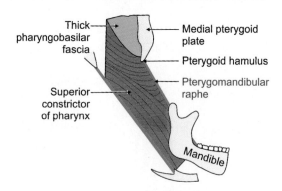

Fig. 14.11: Pterygomandibular raphe

4. **Surface anatomy** : In wide opened mouth, the raphe raises a fold of mucosa that marks internally the posterior boundary of cheek. It is important landmark for the inferior alveolar nerve block.

5. **Applied anatomy** : The pterygomandibular space lies lateral to the pterygomandibular raphe. It contains lingual and inferior alveolar nerves. This is the site for the injection for inferior alveolar nerve block.

SN-112 Auditory tube

Introduction: It is a funnel ▽ shaped tube which connects middle ear cavity to nasopharynx (Fig. 14.12).

1. **Gross**

    A. **Length:** 36 mm.

2. **Parts:** Two parts (Table 14.6).

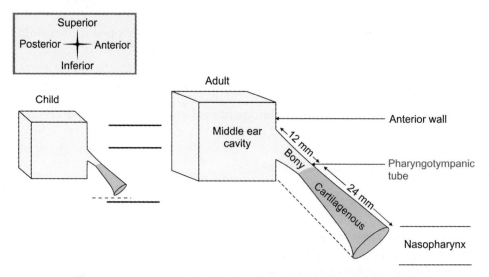

Fig. 14.12: Right pharyngotympanic tube in child and then adult

Table 14.6: Bony and cartilaginous parts of auditory tube

Particulars	Bony	Cartilaginous
• Site	• Petrous parts of temporal bone.	• Sulcus tubae
• Length (in mm)	• 12 (1/3rd)	• 24 (2/3rd)
• Formation	• Bony	• Cartilaginous
• Opening	• Middle ear	• Pharynx
• Relations	• Below: Tympanic plate of temporal bone • Medially: Carotid canal	Anterolaterally: • Spine of sphenoid • Middle meningeal artery • Mandibular nerve • Otic ganglion • Tensor veli palati • Chorda tympani

3. **Age difference**

Table 14.7: Auditory tube in child and adult

Particulars	Child	Adult
• Length (in mm)	• 18 (½)	• 36
• Position	• Straight	• Oblique
• Bony part	• Two-thirds	• One-third
• Tubal elevation	• Absent	• Present

4. **Blood supply:**
    A. Middle meningeal artery (maxillary artery).
    B. Ascending pharyngeal artery (external carotid artery).

5. **Venous drainage**: Pterygoid venous plexus.

6. **Nerve supply**: There are three nerves supplying various parts of auditory tube (Fig. 14.13).
    A. Bony part of auditory tube is supplied by a branch from tympanic plexus.
    B. Cartilaginous part is supplied by meningeal branch of mandibular nerve.
    C. Ostium of the auditory tube is supplied by pharyngeal branch of pterygopalatine ganglion.

7. **Functions**
    A. Maintains equilibrium of air pressure on either side of tympanic membrane.
    B. Increased pressure in middle ear forces the auditory tube to open with a click.

8. **Applied anatomy**
    ➤ In children, infection of oral cavity, nasal cavity or pharynx usually spreads to the middle ear because auditory tube is short in length and horizontal in position.
    ➤ Sometimes tube is blocked due to inflammation of tubal tonsil.
    ➤ The tube can dysfunction due to
        • Blockage of tube due to cold,

Head, Neck and Face

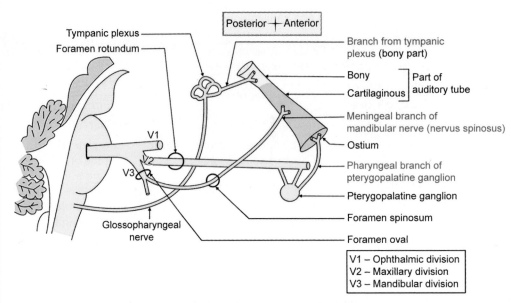

Posterior — Anterior

Tympanic plexus

Foramen rotundum

Branch from tympanic plexus (bony part)

Bony
Cartilaginous — Part of auditory tube

Meningeal branch of mandibular nerve (nervus spinosus)

V1

V3

Ostium

Pharyngeal branch of pterygopalatine ganglion

Pterygopalatine ganglion

Foramen spinosum

Glossopharyngeal nerve

Foramen oval

V1 – Ophthalmic division
V2 – Maxillary division
V3 – Mandibular division

Fig. 14.13: Nerve supply of auditory tube

- Congestion of nasal mucosa or tube
- Pressure variation
➤ **Glue ear** (otitis media with effusion): Absorption of air in the middle ear. Air is replaced by fluid. It leads to conductive deafness and sometimes pain in air. In children, it leads to learning disability.
➤ Barotrauma: Due to significant difference of pressure on both sides of tympanic membrane, there can be damage to middle ear. This situation occurs in
  - Rapid ascent as in mountaineering
  - Scuba (**S**elf-**c**ontained **u**nderwater **b**reathing **a**pparatus) diving
  - Pilots who travel the air craft without using air pressure cabin.
  - In landing or taking off
  - From hill you are rapidly coming down
➤ The tympanic membrane may pull inward or outward depending upon pressure ingredients. This separates tympanic membrane and develops severe pain in the ear.
➤ Conductive deafness is defined as a type of deafness which is due to impaired function of those components of ear which are involved in the conduction of sound energy.
➤ Following are the causes for conductive deafness
  - Causes in external auditory meatus
  - Large wax in the external ear
  - Foreign body in external ear
  - Infection in external ear
  - Tympanic membrane is dysfunctional or perforated or because of barotauma
  - Problems in the middle ear
    - Problems in ossicles
    - Air is replaced by fluid
    - Cholestatoma in the middle ear

SN-113 Tensor palatini (dilator tubae)

1. **Proximal attachments:** It arises from
   A. Lateral side of cartilaginous part of auditory tube. It is outside pharynx.
   B. Sulcus tubae,
   C. Spine of the sphenoid bone, and
   D. Scaphoid fossa of medial pterygoid plate of sphenoid bone.
2. **Distal attachments:** It is inserted in the form of aponeurosis which is attached to
   A. Posterior border of hard palate.
   B. Inferior surface of hard palate behind palatine crest.
3. **Peculiarities**
   A. It is more active in blowing and less active in sleeping.
   B. Its tendon hooks round the pterygoid hamulus and passes medially to expand to form the palatine aponeurosis of its lower half.
4. **Relations**
   A. It lies anterior to levator palatini muscle.
   B. Laterally, it is related to
      a. Mandibular nerve
      b. Auriculotemporal nerve
      c. Chorda tympani nerve
      d. Otic ganglion, and
      e. Middle meningeal artery.
5. **Blood supply**
   A. Ascending palatine branch of facial artery.
   B. Greater palatine branch of maxillary artery.
6. **Actions**
   A. Its primary role is to open the pharyngotympanic tube, e.g. during deglutition and yawning. Thus, it equalizes the pressure between the middle ear and nasopharynx, and
   B. Tightens the soft palate, chiefly the anterior part.
   C. It dilates the auditory tube; hence, it is known as dilator tubae.
7. **Development:** It develops from mesoderm of 1st pharyngeal arch.
8. **Nerve supply**: It is supplied by the mandibular nerve, nerve of 1st pharyngeal arch.

SN-114 Development of palate (Fig. 14.14)

1. **Chronological age:**
   A. Eighth week of intrauterine life.
   B. Palatogenesis begins at the end of 5th week. However, it is not completed until 12th week.
   C. Critical period of development: End of 6th week to the beginning of 9th week.

Head, Neck and Face

2. **Germ layer:** Mesoderm of pharyngeal arches.
3. **Site:** At the primitive oral cavity.
4. **Sources:** It consists of two parts
   A. **Primary palate:** It is an area in front of incisive fossa. It is developed by fusion of
      a. Medial nasal process, and
      b. Maxillary process.
   B. **Secondary palate:** Permanent palate lies behind primitive palate. It is developed from fusion of
      a. Left and right palatine process of both maxillae in midline.
      b. The fusion between the primitive and permanent palates takes place in a 'Y' shaped manner. The fusion extends from before backwards.
   C. **Anterior 3/4th of permanent palate:** Ossifies and fuses with nasal septum.
      a. Posterior 1/4th of the permanent palate does not fuse with lower edge of nasal septum and hangs as soft palate.

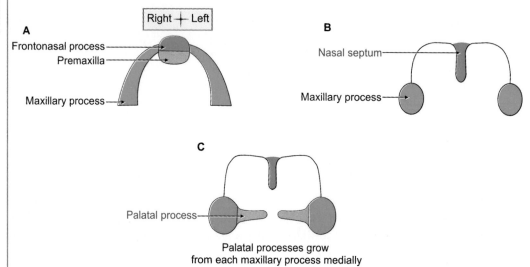

Fig. 14.14: Development of palate

5. **Anomalies**
   A. Cleft palate
   B. Cleft lip

SN-115 Cleft palate

Introduction: It is failure of fusion of primitive and permanent palates. It varies in degree of severity (Fig. 14.15).

1. **1st degree:** Bifid uvula.
2. **2nd degree:** Ununited palatal process.
3. **3rd degree:** Ununited palatal process and a cleft of one side of premaxilla.

4. **4th degree:** It is rare. Ununited palatal process and cleft on both sides of premaxilla.

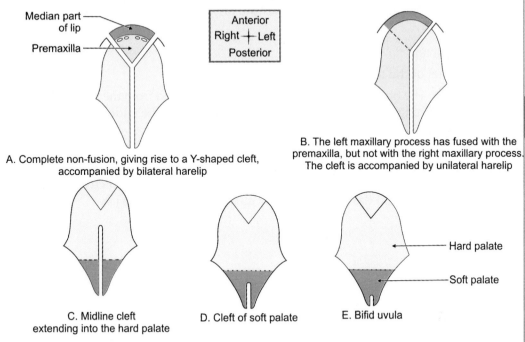

A. Complete non-fusion, giving rise to a Y-shaped cleft, accompanied by bilateral harelip

B. The left maxillary process has fused with the premaxilla, but not with the right maxillary process. The cleft is accompanied by unilateral harelip

C. Midline cleft extending into the hard palate

D. Cleft of soft palate

E. Bifid uvula

Fig. 14.15: Types of the cleft palate

SN-116   Cleft lip

1. **Incidence:** It is most common abnormality. The incidence is 1:750 births.
2. **Cleft lip:** Due to failure or union of the
   A. Medial nasal process with the
   B. Maxillary process of the mandibular arch.
3. **Situation:** It may be unilateral or bilateral. It is more frequently unilateral. It runs down from the nostril.

SN-117   Development of oral mucosa

1. **Parts:** The mouth cavity consists of two parts
   A. The primitive mouth is derived from ectodermal stomodeum.
   B. The definitive mouth is developed from endoderm of the cephalic part of foregut.
2. **Division of stomodeum:** The stomodeum is divided by the development of the primitive and permanent palate into
   A. **Nasal:** The nasal component of the stomodeum forms the
      a. Mucous membrane of the nasal cavity,
      b. Nasal septum, and
      c. Palate.

B. **Oral cavities:** The oral component of the stomodeum forms the

   a. Mucous linings of the cheek (vestibule of the mouth),

   b. Lips,

   c. Gums, and

   d. Enamel of the teeth.

3. **Germ layers:** The floor of the definitive mouth is developed from the foregut because the mucous lining of the tongue is entirely derived from the endodermal elements of the branchial arches.

4. **Process of development:** The epithelial cells lining the margins of the primitive oral fissure proliferate outward into the surrounding mesenchyme. Eventually the epithelial cells breakdown, and the endodermal alveolus-labial sulcus thus formed separates the lips and the cheek from the gums and teeth of the jaw.

Nose and Paranasal Sinuses

| OLA-65 | Why are the boils of nose and ear painful? |

Nose and ear are firmly attached to cartilages. There is no space for expansion of infection or pus. Hence, the cutaneous nerves are irritated and cause pain.

| OLA-66 | What is epiphora? |

It is an abnormal overflow of tears down the cheek. It is mainly due to stricture of the passage. It is also called ill lacrimation.

LAQ-36	Describe nasal septum under the following heads:
	1. Formation,
	2. Blood supply,
	3. Nerve supply, and
	4. Applied anatomy

It is usually deviated to one side and each nasal cavity somewhat asymmetrical.

1. **Formation:** Partly by bones and partly by cartilage.[NEET]
   A. **Bony part** (Fig. 15.1)
      a. Major part is formed by
         I. **Vomer:** Below and behind.
         II. Perpendicular plate of ethmoid.
      b. Small bones taking part are
         I. Nasal spine of frontal bone,
         II. Anterior nasal spine of maxilla, and
         III. Rostrum of sphenoid
      c. Crests of
         I. Nasal bone,
         II. Maxilla, and
         III. Palatine bone.

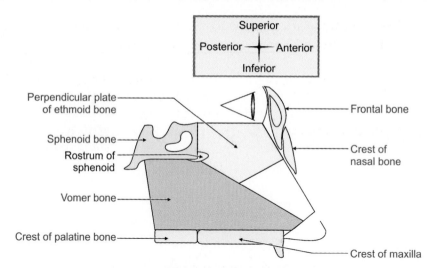

Fig. 15.1: Bones forming nasal septum

B. **Cartilaginous part is formed by** (Fig. 15.2)
   a. Septal cartilage.
   b. Septal process of inferior nasal cartilage.

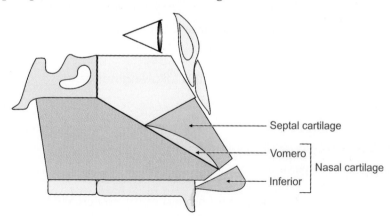

Fig. 15.2: Cartilages forming nasal septum

C. Cuticular part is formed by fibrofatty tissue.

2. **Blood supply**

   A. Arterial supply :
      a. The main arteries of the nasal septum are (Fig. 15.3)
         I. Anterior ethmoidal artery, branch of ophthalmic artery, supplies anterior superior part.
         II. Sphenopalatine artery, branch of maxillary artery, supplies posterior inferior part.
      b. Less important arteries are (Fig. 15.4)
         I. Superior labial, a branch of facial artery,

II. Greater palatine artery, branch of maxillary artery, and

III. Posterior ethmoidal artery, branch of ophthalmic artery.

Note:

    i. All the arteries supplying the nasal septum are branches of external carotid artery except anterior and posterior ethmoidal arteries which are branches of ophthalmic artery which is a branch of internal carotid artery.[NEET]

    ii. All the arteries give septal branches which form important anastomosis at anteroinferior quadrant of nasal septum. It is called Kiesselbach plexus.

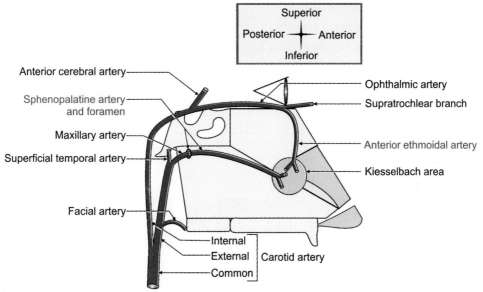

Fig. 15.3: Most important arteries of nasal septum

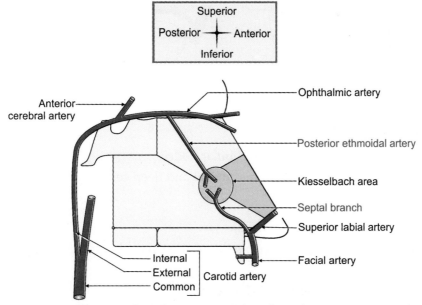

Fig. 15.4: Less important arteries of nasal septum

B. **Venous drainage** (Fig. 15.5)

a. Anterosuperior part is drained by superior ophthalmic vein, which opens into cavernous sinus.

b. Posteroinferior part is drained into pterygoid venous plexus.

c. Upper part of the septum is drained into inferior cerebral vein.

d. Lower mobile part of septum drains into facial vein which drains into internal jugular vein. An infection from this part may extend into cavernous sinus via

   I. Deep facial vein, and

   II. Pterygoid venous plexus.

   This belongs to dangerous area of face.

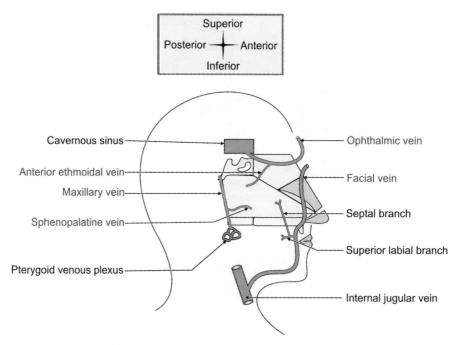

Fig. 15.5: Venous drainage of nasal septum

C. **Lymphatic drainage**

a. Anterior half: To the submandibular nodes.

b. Posterior half: To the retropharyngeal and deep cervical nodes.

3. **Nerve supply**

A. General sensory nerves (Fig. 15.6).

a. **Anterosuperior part:** Anterior ethmoidal nerve, a branch of ophthalmic nerve **(V1)**.

b. **Posteroinferior part:** Nasopalatine branch of pterygopalatine ganglion.

B. Special sensory nerves are olfactory nerves (Fig. 15.7).

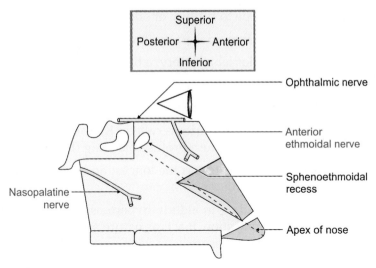

Fig. 15.6: General sensations of nasal septum

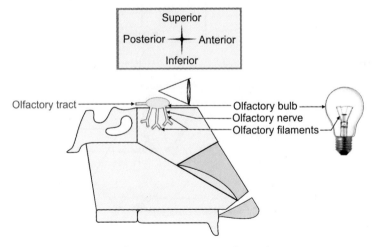

Fig. 15.7: Special sensations of nasal septum

4. **Applied anatomy**

> Deviation of nasal septum may be due to cartilage or bone. It may be due to
> • Birth injury (most common cause).
> • Congenital malformation.
>   – Excessive nasal deviation produces unilateral nasal obstruction and is treated by submucous resection of the septum (SMR)—septoplasty
> Little's area or Kiesselbach's area for epistaxis.

SN-118 Little's area or Kiesselbach's area

Introduction: It is an area on anteroinferior part of nasal septum. The nose bleeding is relatively common because nasal mucosa is highly vascular. The mild epistaxis results from nose pricking which tears the veins in the vestibule.

Head, Neck and Face

1. The profuse bleeding occurs due to rupture of one of the following arteries:

   A. Septal branch of anterior ethmoidal artery (branch of ophthalmic artery).

   B. Septal branch of the superior labial artery, a branch of facial artery.

   C. Septal branch of sphenopalatine artery

   D. Septal branch of greater palatine artery } (maxillary artery).

2. The anastomosis formed by these arteries is called **"Kiesselbach's plexus"**. Even a small ulcer affecting this area can cause profuse bleeding (Fig. 15.8).

3. Septal branch of sphenopalatine artery is the longest and tortuous. It is also called **"artery of nose bleeding"** or *"rhinologist's artery"*.

4. Sudden and severe nasal bleeding in elderly hypertensive patient may be due to rupture of the venous communication. It acts as nature's safety procedure to reduce increased intracranial vascular pressure.

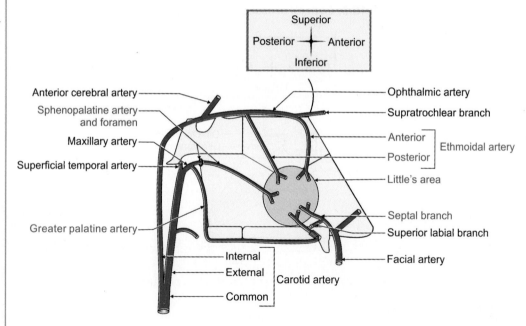

Fig. 15.8: Little's area

LAQ-37	Describe lateral wall of nose under the following heads:

1. Formation,

2. Features,

3. Blood supply,

4. Nerve supply, and

5. Applied anatomy

1. **Formation** (Fig. 15.9)[NEET]
   A. **Bony part is formed by**
      a. Conchae of
         I. Superior }
         II. Middle } concha of ethmoid bone
         III. Inferior nasal concha
      b. Lacrimal
      c. Maxilla
      d. Nasal
      e. Perpendicular plate of palatine bone.
      f. Medial pterygoid plate of sphenoid bone.
   B. **Cartilaginous part is formed by**
      a. Upper nasal cartilage,
      b. Lower nasal cartilage, and
      c. Alar cartilage.
   C. Cuticular part is formed by fibrofatty tissue.

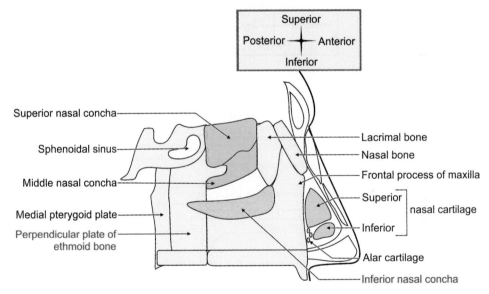

Fig. 15.9: Bones and cartilage forming the lateral wall of nose

2. **Features** (Table 15.1)
   A. **The epithelium of lateral wall is as follows:**
      a. Above superior concha: Olfactory epithelium.
      b. Below superior concha: Respiratory mucosa.
      c. Below inferior concha: Erectile tissue.
   B. **Lateral wall shows bony projections called nasal conchae. These are:**
      a. **Superior concha:** A projection of ethmoid bone. This is the smallest concha, situated above the middle concha. It encloses a space called superior meatus.
      b. **Middle concha:** A projection of ethmoid bone. It encloses middle meatus.
      c. **Inferior concha:** It is independent bone. It encloses inferior meatus.

Head, Neck and Face

Table 15.1: Features present in the lateral wall of nose

Site	Opening (Fig. 15.10)
• Sphenoethmoidal recess	• Sphenoidal air sinus
• Superior meatus	• Posterior ethmoidal air sinus
• Middle meatus	• Middle ethmoidal air sinus
• Ethmoidal bulla: Rounded elevation produced by upper margin of ethmoidal bulla. • Hiatus semilunaris deep semicircular sulcus below the bulla	
• At anterior end	• Frontal air sinus
• Middle part	• Anterior ethmoidal air sinus
• Posterior end	• Maxillary air sinus
• Inferior meatus	• Nasolacrimal duct

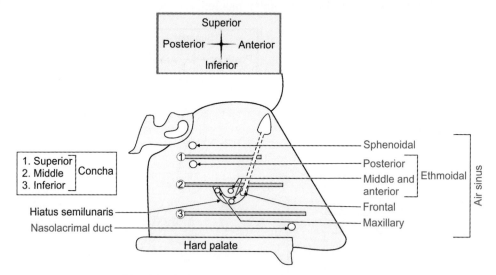

Fig. 15.10: Openings in the lateral wall of nose

3. Blood supply

A. Arterial supply

Table 15.2: Arterial supply of lateral wall of nose (Figs 15.11 and 15.12)

Quadrant	Anterior	Posterior
• Superior	• Anterior ethmoidal artery (ophthalmic artery)	• Sphenopalatine artery (maxillary artery)
• Inferior	• Alar branch of facial artery • Greater palatine artery (maxillary artery)	• Greater palatine artery (maxillary artery)

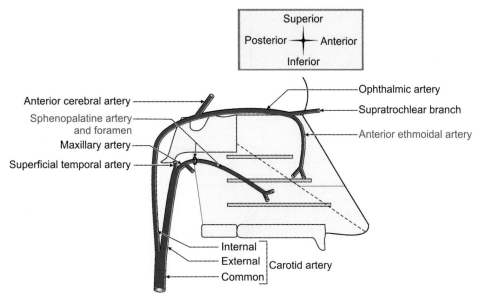

Fig. 15.11: Most important arteries of lateral wall of nose on right side

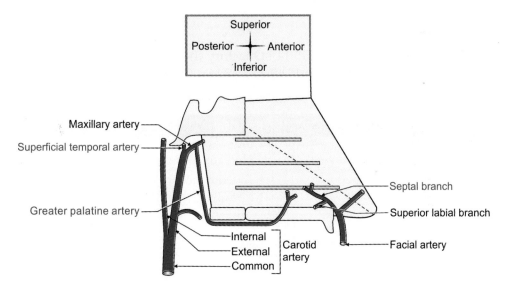

Fig. 15.12: Less important arteries of lateral wall of nose on right side

B. **Venous drainage** (Fig. 15.13)

   a. Anterior veins form a plexus and drain into facial vein.

   b. Posterior veins drain into pharyngeal plexus of veins.

   c. Middle part drains into pterygoid plexus of veins.

C. **Lymphatic drainage**

   a. Anterior ½ drains into submandibular lymph nodes.

   b. Posterior ½ drains into retropharyngeal and deep cervical lymph nodes.

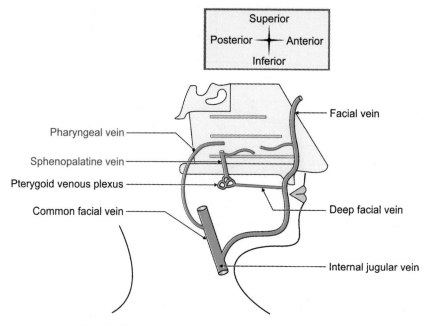

Fig. 15.13: Venous drainage of lateral wall of nose

4. **Nerve supply**

A. **Special sensory nerve** (Fig. 15.14): Olfactory (I)—upper part.
B. **General sensory nerve** (Figs 15.15 and 15.16): Trigeminal (V).

Table 15.3: Sensory nerves supply the lateral wall of the nose

Quadrant	Anterior	Posterior
• Superior	• Anterior ethmoidal nerve (ophthalmic nerve) (V1)	• Posterior superior lateral nasal branches from pterygopalatine ganglion (maxillary nerve) V2.
• Inferior	• Anterior superior alveolar nerve	• Anterior palatine branch from pterygopalatine ganglion

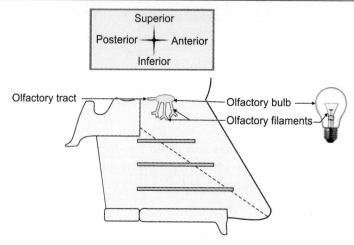

Fig. 15.14: Special sensations of lateral wall of nose (right side)

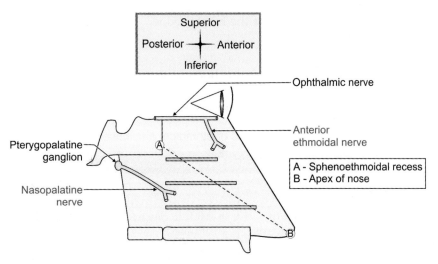

Fig. 15.15: Nerves carrying general sensations of lateral wall of nose on right side

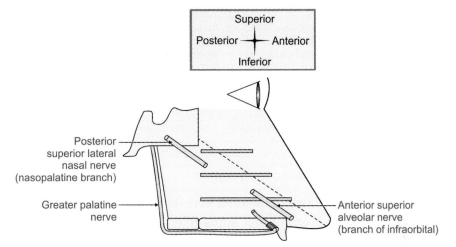

Fig. 15.16: Less important nerves carrying general sensations of lateral wall of nose

5. **Applied anatomy**

   ➢ Common cold is the commonest viral infection of nose.
   ➢ Paranasal air sinus may get infected from the infection of nose.
   ➢ Hypertrophy of mucosa over the inferior nasal concha is a common feature of allergic rhinitis presenting as sneezing, nasal blockage and excessive watery discharge.

OLA-67 Ethmoidal air sinuses

Introduction: They are small numerous spaces present in the labyrinth of the ethmoid bone.

1. **Features:**
   A. They are completed from

a. Above by the orbital plate of the frontal bone,

b. Behind by the

    I. Sphenoidal conchae and

    II. Orbital process of the palatine bone, and

c. Anteriorly by the lacrimal bone.

2. The sinuses are divided as given in Table 15.4.

Table 15.4: Details of ethmoidal air sinuses

Features	Anterior	Middle	Posterior
• Number of cells	• 1 to 11	• 1 to 7	• 1 to 7
• Opened into	• Anterior part of hiatus semilunaris present in middle meatus of nose	• Middle meatus of nose	• Superior meatus of nose
• Blood supply	• Anterior ethmoidal artery branch of ophthalmic artery		• Posterior ethmoidal vessels
• Nerve supply	• Anterior ethmoidal nerve, branch of ophthalmic nerve (V1)	• Anterior ethmoidal nerve, branch of ophthalmic nerve (V1) • Orbital branches of pterygopalatine ganglion	• Posterior ethmoidal nerve (V1) • Orbital branches of pterygopalatine ganglion
• Lymphatic drainage	• Submandibular lymph nodes		• Retropharyngeal lymph nodes

3. **Applied anatomy**

➤ Fracture of the medial wall of the orbit may damage ethmoidal air sinus.

➤ Malignant tumour of ethmoidal sinus may erode the orbit and results in exophthalmos.

➤ If nasal drainage is blocked, infections of the ethmoidal cells may break through the fragile medial wall of the orbit.

➤ Severe infections from ethmoidal air sinus may cause blindness. It is because of close proximity with optic canal, which gives passage to the optic nerve and ophthalmic artery.

➤ Spread of infection from ethmoidal cells can also affect the dural nerve sheath of the optic nerve. It results in *optic neuritis*.

SN-119 Frontal sinus

1. **Morphology**

    A. **Number:** There are two frontal air sinuses. Each is situated between the inner and outer tables of frontal bone.

    B. **Situation:** It is deep to supraorbital margin of fontal bone.

    C. **Shape:** ▲ lar.

D. **Symmetry:** There is an oblique septum separating the right and left sinuses. Hence, they are asymmetrical.

E. **Dimensions**
  a. **Vertical:** 3 cm
  b. **Transverse:** 2.5 cm
  c. **Anteroposterior:** 1.8 cm.

F. **Age changes:** It is rudimentary at birth.

G. **Communications:** It opens into anterior part of hiatus semilunaris. This is ½ moon (shaped depression present in middle meatus part of lateral wall of nose.

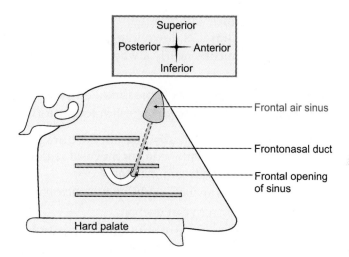

Fig. 15.17: Frontal air sinus

2. **Features and relations**
  A. Anterior wall of the sinus is thick and is related to the skin of the forehead.
  B. The posterior wall is thin and related to the meninges and frontal lobe of brain.
  C. Its inferior wall forms the roof of the orbit.
  D. The frontonasal duct begins in the opening of the sinus, which is located in the floor of the sinus.

3. **Blood supply**
  A. Arterial supply :
    a. Supraorbital artery, branch of ophthalmic artery.
    b. Anterior ethmoidal artery, a branch of ophthalmic artery arising from main trunk.

  B. Venous drainage : Supraorbital vein drains into angular vein—facial vein—internal jugular vein.

4. Lymphatic drainage : Submandibular nodes.

5. Nerve supply : Supraorbital nerve, branch of ophthalmic division of trigeminal nerve.

Head, Neck and Face

6. **Development:** Frontal air sinuses are the only sinuses not present at birth, they appear during the 2nd year.

7. Surface anatomy : Join following three points
   A. Point at nasion
   B. Point 3 cm above the nasion
   C. Point at the supraorbital margin at the junction of its medial one-third and lateral two-thirds.

8. Applied anatomy
   ➤ Pain of frontal sinusitis may be referred to the skin of the forehead and adjacent skin since they have same nerve supply.
   ➤ Frontal air sinus communicates with maxillary air sinus through infundibulum. It is located at higher level. It tracks down into the maxillary air sinus.
   ➤ The patients with frontal sinusitis nearly always have a maxillary sinusitis.

OLA-68 Why is headache the commonest presentation in involvement of nose, paranasal sinuses, teeth, gums, eyes (refractory error) and meninges?

1. The dura is sensitive to stretching. Pain arising from the dura is generally referred, perceived as a headache. It arises in cutaneous or mucosal regions. It is supplied by the cervical nerve or division of the trigeminal nerve.
2. The trigeminal nerve has three branches—ophthalmic, maxillary and mandibular.
3. The ophthalmic nerve is sensory nerve of eyeball.
4. The maxillary nerve is the sensory nerve of nose (common cold, boils), paranasal air sinuses (sinusitis), gums and teeth of upper jaw.
5. The mandibular nerve is the sensory nerve of gums and teeth of the lower jaw.
6. Hence, headache is a uniformly common symptom in
   A. Refractive errors of the eyes,
   B. Nose (common cold, boils) and the paranasal air sinuses (sinusitis),
   C. Infections and inflammations of teeth and gums, and
   D. Infection of the meninges as in meningitis.

OLA-69 What are the junctions of paranasal sinuses?

Frontal air sinus and maxillary air sinus in the middle meatus in the lateral part of nose.

SN-120 Paranasal sinuses

Introduction: These are air-filled spaces within the bones present around air passage (Fig. 15.18).

1. **Functions**
   A. They add resonance to the voice.
   B. They improve the timbre of the voice.
   C. They condition the inhaled air by adding humidity.

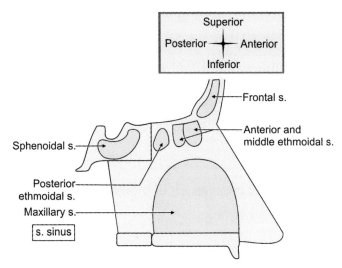

Fig. 15.18: Paranasal sinuses

2. Applied anatomy

> Infection of the sinus is known as sinusitis. It causes headache and persistent, thick, purulent discharge from the nose. Diagnosis is done by X-ray. A diseased sinus is opaque.
> Frontal sinusitis and ethmoidal sinusitis can produce a brain abscess in the frontal lobe.
> Carcinoma of the maxillary sinus produces symptoms depending upon the growth.

Table 15.5: Gross anatomy of air sinuses

Particulars	Frontal	Maxillary	Sphenoid	Ethmoid
• Number	• 1 on each side	• 1 on each side	• 1 on each side	• 3 on each side
• Opening	• Middle meatus	• Middle meatus	• Sphenoeth-moidal recess	• Anterior and middle opens into middle meatus and posterior opens into superior meatus.
• Arterial supply	• Supraorbital artery (ophth-almic artery)	• Facial artery • Infraorbital artery • Greater pala-tine artery	• Posterior ethmoidal • Internal carotid	• Anterior, middle and posterior ethmoidal arteries
• Venous drainage	• Anastomosing vein between supraorbital and superior ophth-almic veins	• Facial vein • Pterygoid plexus of vein	• Pterygoid plexus of vein • Cavernous sinus	• Anterior, middle and posterior ethmoidal veins

Contd.

Head, Neck and Face

Table 15.5: Gross anatomy of air sinuses (Contd.)

Particulars	Frontal	Maxillary	Sphenoid	Ethmoid
• Nerve supply	• Supraorbital nerve	• Infraorbital • Anterior, middle and posterior superior alveolar nerves	• Posterior ethmoidal nerve • Orbital branches of pterygopalatine ganglion	• Posterior ethmoidal nerve
• Lymphatic drainage	• Submandibular nodes		• Retropharyngeal nodes	

OLA-70 What is the clinical importance of maxillary sinus?

1. It may become infected either from the
   A. Nasal cavity, or
   B. Caries of the upper molar teeth.
2. Antral puncture is carried out using a trocar and cannula. It is passed through the nasal cavity in an outward and backward direction. The trocar passes below the inferior concha.
3. *Caldwell-Luc operation:* It is removing a portion of the medial wall of the sinus below the inferior concha. It is done to facilitate the drainage.
4. The carcinoma of the maxillary sinus produces.
   A. Obstruction of the nares and epistaxis by medial invasion.
   B. Blockage of the nasolacrimal duct by invasion of duct.
   C. Diplopia by invasion of the orbit.
   D. Facial pain by the invasion of infraorbital nerve.
   E. Ulceration in the palatal roof by invasion of sinus.
   F. Swelling of the face by spreading laterally.
   G. Posterior spread may involve the palatine nerves and produce severe pain referred to the teeth of the upper jaw.

SN-121 Maxillary air sinus (antrum of Highmore)

Introduction: The largest and important paranasal air sinus present in maxilla, lined by ciliated columnar epithelium (Fig. 15.19).

1. **Importance**
   A. Helps in conditioning of the air by adding humidity.
   B. Acts as resonating chamber for production of sounds.
   C. Increases the quality of voice (timbre).
   D. Reduces the weight of the skull.

2. **Gross anatomy:** Shape is pyramidal .
   A. Base is formed by nasal surface of body of maxilla and forms lateral wall of nose.
   B. **Apex:** Towards the zygomatic bone.

3. **Boundaries**

A. **Superior wall or roof:** Orbital surface of maxilla.

B. **Inferior wall or floor:** Alveolar surface of maxilla.

C. **Anterior wall:** Anterior surface of maxilla.

D. **Posterior wall:** Posterior surface of maxilla.

4. **Dimension**

A. **Vertical:** 3.5 cm.

B. **Transverse:** 2.5 cm

C. **Anteroposterior:** 3.25 cm.

5. **Opening:** Maxillary air sinus opens in the middle meatus by two openings.

A. Upper opening is present in lower part of hiatus semilunaris. The opening is at higher level and is called antrum of Highmore (dental surgeon). The dimensions of opening are reduced

a. Superiorly by

I. Uncinate process of ethmoid bone

II. Descending part of lacrimal bone

b. Inferiorly by: Inferior nasal concha.

c. Posteriorly by: Perpendicular plate of palatine bone.

d. Internally by: Thick mucosa.

B. Lower opening is present at posterior end of hiatus.

6. **Relations of maxillary air sinus**

A. **Anterolaterally related to**

a. Infraorbital nerves

b. Infraorbital vessels

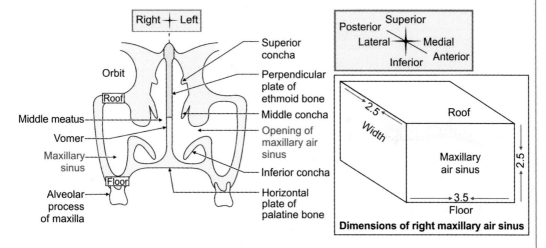

Fig. 15.19: Maxillary air sinus

c. Origin of muscles of upper lip

d. Anterior superior alveolar vessels and nerves.

B. **Posteriorly**

a. Infratemporal fossa,

b. Pterygopalatine fossa,

c. Posterior superior alveolar vessels and nerves.

C. Floor is related to roots of teeth especially 2nd premolar and 1st molar.

D. Roof is related to the floor of the orbit and eyeball.

E. Medially, it is related to lateral wall of nose.

F. Laterally, it is related to cheek.

7. **Development:** Developed from splitting of maxilla. It is the 1st paranasal air sinus to develop. It develops in the 4th month of intrauterine life. It grows rapidly during 6–7 years and reaches full size after the eruption of all permanent teeth.

8. **Blood supply**

A. **Arterial supply** (Fig. 15. 20)

a. Infraorbital artery

b. Greater palatine artery

c. Posterior superior alveolar artery

} Branches of maxillary artery.

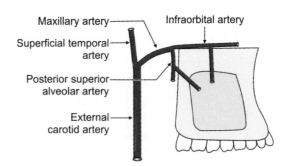

Fig. 15.20: Arterial supply of maxillary air sinus

B. **Venous drainage**

a. Infraorbital vein drains into angular vein.

b. Greater palatine vein drains into pterygoid venous plexus.

9. **Nerve supply** (Fig. 15.21)

A. Infraorbital nerve (continuation of maxillary nerve).

B. Greater palatine nerve (pterygopalatine ganglion).

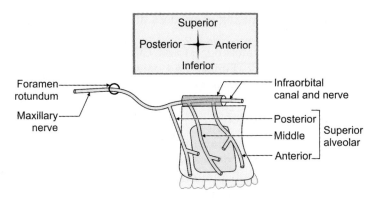

Fig. 15.21: Nerve supply of maxillary air sinus

10. **Lymphatic drainage** : By submandibular lymph node.

11. **Applied anatomy**

➤ **Sinusitis:** Inflammation of maxillary air sinus presents headache, which is maximum at 12:00 noon. At 12:00 noon, there is maximum expansion of the air which is not accommodated in the maxillary air sinus. Hence, it passes to the frontal air sinus.

➤ It can be visualised by taking X-rays of paranasal sinus.

➤ Abscess of maxillary air sinus is drained by antral puncture.

➤ The opening of maxillary air sinus is located much higher than the floor. There is poor natural drainage. Hence, the maxillary sinus is most commonly infected.

➤ Maxillary sinus becomes infected either from the
  • Nasal cavity or from
  • Caries of the upper molar teeth.

➤ The maxillary sinus is sometimes called the *'secondary reservoir'* of the frontal air sinus. The frontal sinus drains into the hiatus semilunaris in the middle meatus, via infundibulum. It is close to the opening of maxillary sinus.

➤ The mucus or pus from maxillary sinus cannot be drained into the nasal cavity when the head is erect, until it is filled up to the top.

➤ In severe cases, drainage of maxillary sinus may require a surgical intervention. The **'antral puncture'** is done by passing a trocar and cannula through the nasal cavity. It is directed in an outward and backward direction below the inferior nasal concha. It produces a hole in the lower part of the lateral wall of the nasal cavity.

➤ For more adequate drainage, a portion of anterior wall of the sinus below the inferior nasal concha is removed. Or, the sinus is fenestrated in the region of gingivolabial fold (Caldwell-Luc operation).

12. **Applied anatomy of relations of maxillary air sinus**

➤ **A tumour in the sinus may push**
  • Orbital floor and displace the eyeball.
  • Project into the nasal cavity causing nasal obstruction and bleeding.

Head, Neck and Face

- Protrude into cheek causing numbness and swelling when the infraorbital nerve is damaged.
- It spreads back into infratemporal fossa, causing restriction of mouth opening due to pterygoid muscle damage and pain.
- Or spread down in the mouth, loosening of the teeth and malocclusion of the teeth.

SN-122 Pterygopalatine ganglion

Introduction: Ganglion is a collection of cell bodies. It is the largest peripheral parasympathetic ganglion.[NEET] It is present in the course of parasympathetic nerve. It is situated in the peripheral part of cranium.

A. Structurally, it belongs to trigeminal nerve since it is suspended from the maxillary nerve.

B. Functionally, it is related to greater petrosal nerve (facial nerve).

  Eponym – Meckel's ganglion.

1. **Gross**

  A. **Situation:** Pterygopalatine fossa.

  B. **Relations**

    a. Medially: Pharyngeal artery.

    b. Laterally: Artery of pterygoid canal.

    c. Superiorly: Maxillary nerve.

    d. Posteriorly: Pterygoid canal.

2. **Connections**

  A. **Parasympathetic (motor root)** (Fig. 15.22)

    a. Preganglionic fibres arise from lacrimatory nucleus (pons)—facial nerve (VII)—geniculate ganglion—greater petrosal nerve—deep petrosal nerve (plexus around internal carotid artery)—nerve of pterygoid canal—pterygopalatine ganglion— relay.

    b. Postganglionic fibers—maxillary nerve—zygomatic branch—zygomatic-otemporal branch—communicating branch to lacrimal nerve.

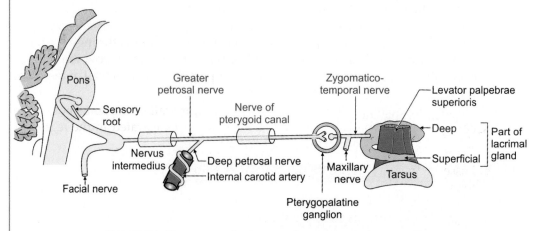

Fig. 15.22: Parasympathetic root of pterygopalatine ganglion

Head, Neck and Face

B. **Sensory:** From maxillary nerve passes through pterygopalatine ganglion without relay (Fig. 15.23).

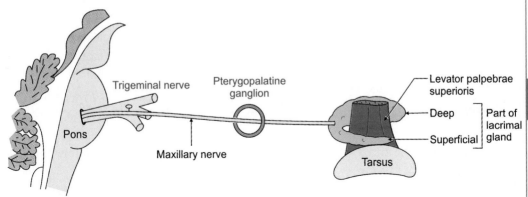

Fig. 15.23: Sensory root of the pterygopalatine ganglion carrying sensations of lacrimal, nasal and palatine glands

C. **Sympathetic** (Fig. 15.24)
   a. Preganglionic fibres—spinal nerve—superior cervical sympathetic ganglion.
   b. Postganglionic fibres—plexus around internal carotid artery (deep petrosal nerve) passes without interruption.

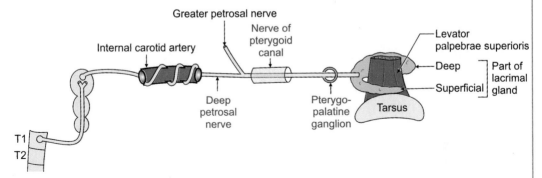

Fig. 15.24: Sympathetic fibres of pterygopalatine ganglion

3. **Branches:** They are virtually derived from maxillary nerve.
   A. **Orbital branch supplies**
      a. Orbitalis muscle,
      b. Mucous membrane of sphenoid, and
      c. Mucous membrane of posterior ethmoidal sinus.
   B. **Palatine**
      a. Greater palatine nerve—supplies mucous membrane of lateral wall of nose.
      b. Lesser petrosal nerve—supplies mucous membrane of soft palate and palatine tonsil.
   C. **Nasal branches**
      a. Posterior superior lateral nasal.
      b. Medial nasal.

4. **Applied anatomy**

> It is called ganglion of hay fever and produces running of nose and eyes.
> Injection of alcohol is occasionally employed in intractable cases of allergic rhinitis.

LAQ-38	Describe maxillary nerve under

1. Embryology,

2. Course, and

3. Branches and distribution of the branches

Introduction: It is the 2nd division of trigeminal nerve (5th cranial nerve). It is purely/completely sensory. It innervates meninges,

- Skin of
  - Temporal region,
  - Scalp,
  - Lower eyelid,
  - Side of nose,
  - Nasal septum,
  - Cheek, and
  - Upper lip
- Air sinus
  - Ethmoidal air sinus,
  - Maxillary air sinus,
- Teeth of upper jaw,
- Upper gingivae and adjoining part of cheek,
- Lateral wall of nose,
- Floor of nasal cavity,
- Adjoining part of nasal septum,
- Lacrimal gland, and
- Hard palate.

1. **Embryology:** It is said to be the pretrematic branch of trigeminal nerve. It supplies the derivative of the maxillary process.

2. **Course:** The nerve runs in the lateral wall of cavernous sinus, below the ophthalmic nerve. In the middle cranial fossa, it has a short course. It gives a meningeal branch.

   A. It leaves the skull via foramen rotundum and leads directly into posterior wall of pterygopalatine fossa. It gives two larger ganglionic branches containing fibres to nose, palate and pharynx.

   B. It inclines on the posterior surface of palatine bone and reaches on posterior surface of maxilla, runs through inferior orbital fissure. It lies outside orbital periosteum and gives zygomatic and posterior superior alveolar branch. In the midway of orbit, it enters infraorbital canal as infraorbital nerve. It gives terminal branches which supply the skin.

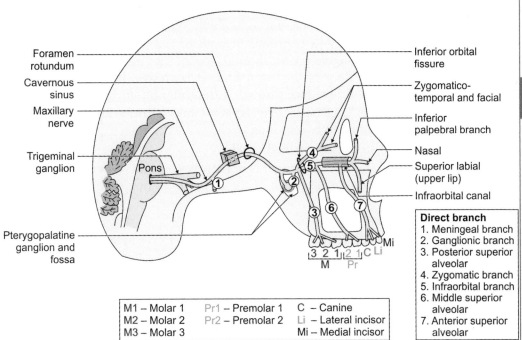

Foramen rotundum
Cavernous sinus
Maxillary nerve
Trigeminal ganglion
Pons
Pterygopalatine ganglion and fossa

Inferior orbital fissure
Zygomatico-temporal and facial
Inferior palpebral branch
Nasal
Superior labial (upper lip)
Infraorbital canal

Mi
3 2 1 2 1 C Li
M Pr

Direct branch
1. Meningeal branch
2. Ganglionic branch
3. Posterior superior alveolar
4. Zygomatic branch
5. Infraorbital branch
6. Middle superior alveolar
7. Anterior superior alveolar

M1 – Molar 1	Pr1 – Premolar 1	C – Canine
M2 – Molar 2	Pr2 – Premolar 2	Li – Lateral incisor
M3 – Molar 3		Mi – Medial incisor

Fig. 15.25: Sagittal section of skull showing origin, course, and branches of maxillary nerve

3. **Branches and distribution of the branches—My good pretty zoology instructor**

A. **Branches from the trunk of maxillary nerve** 🔑 **MG PZI**

a. *Meningeal:* It is 1st branch arising from the trunk of mandibular nerve. It is given in the middle cranial fossa. It supplies the dura mater of anterior part of middle cranial fossa.

b. *Ganglionic* branches: They are two in number. They suspend the ganglion.

c. *Posterior superior alveolar* nerves (posterior superior dental): They are usually three in number. The branches are given in the pterygopalatine fossa. They pass downwards and laterally through pterygomaxillary fissure to reach posterior surface of maxilla. Here, they divide into numerous small branches. They enter the maxilla through posterior superior alveolar foramina. They supply
   I. Maxillary sinus,
   II. Upper molar teeth, and
   III. Adjacent gum of the vestibule.

d. *Zygomatic:* It arises from the trunk of maxillary nerve just before maxillary nerve enters the inferior orbital fissure. It enters the inferior orbital fissure and divides into
   I. *Zygomaticotemporal:* It is one of the terminal branches of zygomatic nerve. It traverses through a canal in the zygomatic bone to emerge into anterior part of temporal fossa. It supplies

    i. Skin above zygomatic arch.

    ii. Communicating twig to lacrimal nerve.

   II. *Zygomaticofacial:* It is one of the terminal branches of zygomatic nerve. It passes through zygomaticofacial foramen. It supplies skin over the bone.

  e. *Infraorbital nerve*: It is a terminal branch of maxillary nerve. It leaves pterygopalatine fossa and passes through the inferior orbital fissure. It passes forward along the floor of the orbit, sinks into groove. It enters infraorbital canal and emerges on the face through infraorbital foramen.

B. **Branches on the face:** They lie between levator labii superioris and levator anguli oris. They are described in two groups.

 I. Branches given in the infraorbital canal

  i. *Middle superior alveolar nerve*: It is not always present. When present, most frequently arises as a branch of the infraorbital nerve. It supplies upper premolar

   • Variations:

    * It may directly arise from the maxillary nerve in the pterygopalatine fossa.

    * It may arise as a branch of the anterior superior alveolar nerve.

  ii. *Anterior superior alveolar nerve:* It arises at midpoint of infraorbital canal and enters the fine sinuous canal which passes downwards in the maxilla. It supplies

   • Incisor and

   • Canine teeth.

   • It gives a nasal branch which supplies

    * Anteroinferior quadrant of the lateral wall of nasal cavity.

    * Floor of the nasal cavity

    * Adjoining part of nasal septum.

 II. Branches outside the infraorbital canal. They are divided into three groups.

  i. Palpebral branches: They supply skin in the lower eyelid

  ii. Nasal branch: It supplies

   • Skin of the

    * Side of nose

    * Movable part of nasal septum.

  iii. Superior labial branches: They are large and numerous. They supply

   • Skin of the

    * Upper part of cheek

    * Upper lip.

C. *Branches from the pterygopalatine ganglion:* There are five branches that are distributed to nose, palate and nasopharynx. Every branch carries sensory, secretomotor and sympathetic fibres.

 a. **Orbital branches:** It enters the inferior orbital fissure and supply

  I. Orbital periosteum,

II. Sphenoidal air sinus,

III. Ethmoidal air sinus,

Orbital branches join branches of carotid plexus. The plexus supplies

   i. Orbitalis, and

   ii. Lacrimal gland.

b. **Nasal branches:** These enter the sphenopalatine foramen and divide into

  I. Posterior superior medial nasal nerves: They are 2 to 3 in number. One of the largest branches is called nasopalatine nerve. As the word suggests, they supply medial part of nose, i.e.

    • Nasal septum

    • Mucosa of posterior part of roof

  II. Nasopalatine (long sphenopalatine): It is the largest branch of posterior superior medial nasal branch. It enters the posterior part of septum and turns down through incisive fossa and reaches the anterior part of hard palate. As the name suggests, it supplies

    • Lower part of nasal septum

    • Anterior part of hard palate.

  II. Posterior superior lateral nasal nerve (short sphenopalatine): As the name suggests, it supplies

    i. Posterior superior quadrant of lateral wall of nose which includes

      • Superior concha and superior meatus,

      • Middle concha, middle meatus, and

      • Posterior ethmoidal sinus.

c. **Palatine branches:** They pass downwards. They are greater palatine and lesser palatine nerves.

  I. Greater palatine nerve (anterior palatine nerve) descends through greater palatine canal and emerges on hard palate and runs forwards up to the incisor teeth. It supplies

    i. Gingivae

    ii. Mucosa and glands of hard palate and communicate with the terminal filaments of the nasopalatine nerves.

    iii. In the greater palatine canal, it gives

      • Posterior superior nasal branch which pierces the perpendicular plate of palatine bone and supply

        * Mucous membrane of posterior superior quadrant of the lateral wall of nose.

    iv. Outside the greater palatine canal, it gives branches to both surfaces of adjacent part of soft palate.

  II. Lesser palatine nerves: They are much smaller than greater palatine. They are descending through greater palatine canal and emerge through lesser palatine foramen. They innervate.

    i. Uvula,

    ii. Tonsil, and

    iii. Soft palate.

d. **Pharyngeal branches:** It leaves the ganglion posteriorly. It passes through palatovaginal canal and supplies mucosa of nasopharynx behind pharyngotympanic tube.

e. **Lacrimal branches:** They carry secretomotor fibres to the lacrimal gland. They travel through zygomaticotemporal branch of zygomatic nerve.

Table 15.6: Maxillary teeth nerve blocks

Teeth	Nerves to be blocked	Blocks
• Incisor and canine	• Anterior superior alveolar • Incisive	• Incisor orbital + nasopalatine
• Premolar	• Middle superior alveolar and • Greater palatine nerve	• Infraorbital +greater palatine
• Motor	• Posterior superior alveolar • Middle superior alveolar • Greater palatine	• Posterior superior alveolar + 1st molar by local infiltration+ greater palatine nerve block

LAQ-39 Describe sphenoidal air sinus under the following heads:

1. Morphology,

2. Relations,

3. Communication,

4. Blood supply,

5. Lymphatic drainage,

6. Nerve supply,

7. Development, and

8. Applied anatomy

(*Sphenoid*—wedge-like)

Introduction: These are paired sinuses located within the body of sphenoid bone.

1. **Morphology**
   A. **Situation:** Above and behind the nasal cavity.
   B. **Dimensions**
      a. **Vertical:** 2 cm
      b. **Anteroposterior:** 2 cm
      c. **Transverse:** 1.5 cm
   C. **Extent**
      a. **Anteriorly:** Roof of the orbit.
      b. **Posteriorly:** Anterior margin of foramen magnum.
      c. **Laterally:** Pterygoid canal.
   D. **Types**
      a. **Sellar:** The commonest type, where the sinus extends for a variable distance beyond tuberculum sellae.
      b. **Presellar:** It doesn't extend beyond tuberculum sellae.
      c. **Concha:** It is rarest type. Here, a small sinus is separated from the sella turcica.

2. **Relations**
 A. **Above**
  a. Optic chiasma
  b. Hypophysis cerebri
 B. **Below:** Roof of nasopharynx.
 C. **On each side**
  a. Cavernous sinus, and
  b. Internal carotid artery.
 D. **Behind**
  a. Pons, and
  b. Medulla oblongata.
 E. **Front:** Sphenoethmoidal recess.
3. **Communication:** Sphenoidal air sinus opens into sphenoethmoidal recess, present above superior concha of nose.
4. **Blood supply:** Posterior ethmoidal vessels (branches/tributaries of ophthalmic vessels).
5. **Lymphatic drainage** : Retropharyngeal nodes
6. **Nerve supply**
 A. Posterior ethmoidal nerve (branch of ophthalmic division of trigeminal nerve).
 B. Orbital branch of pterygopalatine ganglion.
7. **Development:** At birth, the sinuses are minute and main development occurs after puberty.
8. **Applied anatomy**
 ➤ Pituitary tumours are commonly approached via sphenoidal air sinus (transnasal approach). The septal mucous membrane is elevated on both sides. A part of the septal bones and cartilages are removed. The nasal conchae are flattened against lateral nasal walls. The anterior wall and the roof of the sphenoidal sinus are removed to expose the floor of the sella turcica (Fig. 15.26).

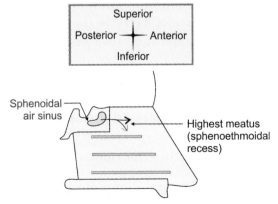

Fig. 15.26: Openings of sphenoidal air sinus

Head, Neck and Face

Larynx

SN-123 Recurrent laryngeal nerve

Introduction: It is the nerve of 6th pharyngeal arch supplying muscles of larynx, pharynx and soft palate and mucous membrane of most posterior part of tongue.

1. **Origin**
   A. Right recurrent laryngeal nerve arises from right vagus nerve in the neck.
   B. Left recurrent laryngeal nerve arises from the left vagus nerve in the thorax.
2. **Course and relations:** The relations are slightly different for the right and left recurrent laryngeal nerves (Fig. 16.1).
   A. **Right recurrent laryngeal nerve**
      a. Winds around the right subclavian artery.
      b. Runs upwards and medially behind the subclavian and common carotid arteries and reaches the tracheo-oesophageal groove.
      c. In the upper part of groove, it is related to the inferior thyroid artery.
      d. The nerve passes deep to lower border of inferior constrictor. It enters the larynx behind cricothyroid joint.
   B. **Left recurrent laryngeal nerve**
      a. It crosses the left side of arch of the aorta.
      b. It loops around the ligamentum arteriosum and reaches the tracheo-oesophageal groove.
      c. It is not have to pass behind the subclavian and carotid arteries.
   C. **Distribution**
      a. It supplies all the intrinsic muscles of larynx except cricothyroid.
      b. It carries the sensations of the larynx below the vocal cords.
      There are four cardiac branches from the right and left recurrent laryngeal nerves. These are
      I. Two superior, and
      II. Two inferior branches.

   i. Out of the four cardiac branches, the left inferior branch goes to superficial cardiac plexus.

   ii. The other three cardiac branches join the deep cardiac plexus.

c. Branches to trachea and oesophagus

d. Branch to the inferior constrictor.

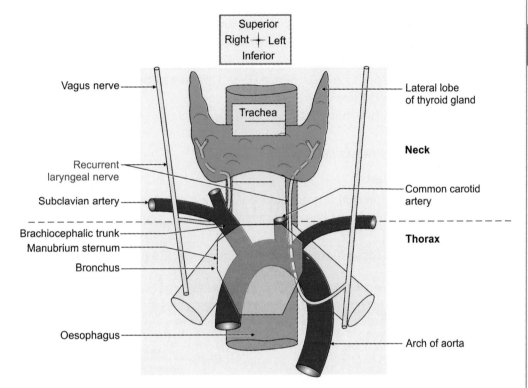

Fig. 16.1: Course of recurrent laryngeal nerve

3. **Applied anatomy**

➢ During thyroidectomy, the right recurrent laryngeal nerve is injured because of variable relation with inferior thyroid artery on right side.

➢ Left recurrent laryngeal nerve is damaged because of left atrial enlargement. The enlargement of left atrium compresses the left recurrent laryngeal nerve.

➢ Recurrent laryngeal nerves may be injured in thyroid surgery or compressed by a growing tumour, aortic aneurysm or from other causes.

➢ If only one recurrent laryngeal nerve is paralyzed, the affected vocal cord remains in the paramedian position and the vocal cord on the normal side compensates for phonation.

➢ If both recurrent laryngeal nerves are paralyzed, the vocal cords remain in the paramedian position (in between abduction and adduction). This results in

   • Loss of phonation,

   • Dyspnoea (difficulty in breathing) and respiratory stridor.

Head, Neck and Face

SN-124   Stylopharyngeus

Introduction: It is the longitudinal muscle of pharynx.

1. **Origin:** It arises from medial side of base of styloid process.
2. **Insertion:** Along with palatopharyngeus, it is inserted in the posterior border of lamina of thyroid cartilage.
3. **Action:** It lifts the larynx during swallowing and phonation.
4. **Development:** It is developed from 3rd pharyngeal arch.
5. **Features:**
   A. Along with glossopharyngeal nerve (IX), it passes between two branches of common carotid arteries.
   B. It passes between two constrictors.

OLA-71   Give sensory nerve supply of larynx.

It is divided into two parts

A. Above the glottis—internal laryngeal nerve, branch of external laryngeal nerve.
B. Below the glottis—recurrent laryngeal nerve, branch of vagus nerve.

OLA-72   Describe the movements of vocal cords. Name the muscles causing them.

Table 16.1: Movements and muscles of vocal cords

S. no.	Movements	Muscle producing
1.	• Elevation of larynx	• Thyrohyoid • Mylohyoid
2.	• Depression of larynx	• Sternothyroid • Sternohyoid
3.	• Abductor of vocal cords	• Posterior cricoarytenoid
4.	• Adduction of vocal cords	• Lateral cricoarytenoid • Transverse arytenoid
5	• Tensor of vocal cords and modulation of voice	• Cricothyroid
6	• Relaxer of vocal cords	• Thyroarytenoid and vocalis

SN-125   Vocal and vestibular folds

1. Inside the cavity of larynx, there are two folds of mucous membrane on each side.
   A. The upper fold is the vestibular fold. The space between the right and left vestibular folds is the rima vestibule.
   B. Lower fold is the vocal fold. The space between the vocal folds is the rima glottidis.
      a. **Attachments**
         I. Anteriorly to the posterior aspect of middle of the angle of the thyroid cartilage.
         II. Posteriorly to the vocal process of the arytenoid cartilage.

b. **Features**
    I. The rima glottidis is limited posteriorly by interarytenoid fold of mucous membrane.
    II. The rima has an anterior intermembranous part (3/5th) and a posterior intercartilaginous part (2/5th).
       i. The rima is the narrowest part of the larynx.
       ii. It is longer (23 mm) in males ♂ than in females ♀ (17 mm).
2. The vestibular and vocal folds divide the cavity of the larynx into three parts.
  A. **Supraglottic part:** Part above the glottis.
  B. **Sinus or ventricle of the larynx:** Part between the vestibular and vocal folds.
  C. **Infraglottic part:** Part below the glottis.

SN-126 Rima glottidis

Introduction: It is the narrowest anteroposterior cleft, or space of laryngeal cavity. It is lined by a stratified squamous non-keratinized epithelium. It is without submucous coat (Fig. 16.2).
1. **Attachments:**
  A. **Anteriorly:** The middle of angle of thyroid cartilage.
  B. **Posteriorly:** Vocal process of arytenoid cartilage.
    Limited: Posteriorly by an interarytenoid fold of mucous membrane.
    - Shape and size of rima glottidis is changed by movements of vocal cords.

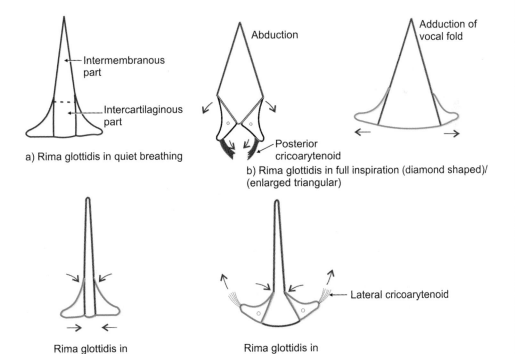

Fig. 16.2: Various positions of rima glottidis in different pitches of voice

Table 16.2: Difference between intermembranous and intercartilaginous part of rima glottidis

Particulars	Intermembranous	Intercartilaginous
• Contribution phase	• 3/5	• 2/5
• Quiet breathing	• Triangular	• Quadrangular
• Forced inspiration	• Triangular	• Triangular
• Phonation: Speech	• Chink	• Chink
• Whispering	• Closed	• Widely open

2. **Nerve supply**: All muscles of larynx are supplied by recurrent laryngeal nerve (vagus nerve) except cricothyroid, which is supplied by external laryngeal nerve (superior laryngeal, branch of vagus nerve).

LAQ-40 **Describe larynx under the following heads:**

1. Formation,

2. Cartilages of larynx,

3. Muscles of larynx,

4. Actions,

5. Nerve supply, and

6. Applied anatomy

1. **Formation:** Larynx is formed by paired and unpaired cartilages. They are
   A. **Unpaired:** Thyroid, cricoid and epiglottis.
   B. **Paired:** Arytenoid, corniculate and cuneiform cartilages.
2. **Cartilages of larynx:** They are 11 in number. Four are paired and three are unpaired.[NEET]
   A. Paired cartilages of larynx: They are 1 on each side.
   B. Unpaired
   A. **Paired** (Fig. 16.3): There are four paired cartilages
      a. **Arytenoid cartilage:** It is a 3-sided pyramid with anterolateral, medial and posterior surfaces.
         I. **Apex:** It is directed upwards and articulates with corniculate cartilage. It gives attachments to oblique arytenoid muscle.
         II. **Base:** It is directed downwards and forms cricoarytenoid joint.
         III. **Vocal process:** It is pointed and projects horizontally forwards from the base. It gives attachment to vocal ligament by its tip and vocalis ligament by its lateral aspect.
         IV. **Muscular process:** It gives attachment to
            i. Posterior cricoarytenoid by the posterior aspect, and
            ii. Lateral cricoarytenoid by its anterior aspect.
         V. **Medial surface:** It is flat and narrow and faces similar surface of the other arytenoid. It forms the lateral boundary of the intercartilaginous part of rima glottidis.

VI. **Posterior surface:** It is deep to oblique arytenoid muscle.

VII. Anterolateral surface is convex and rough. It gives attachment to

    i. Vestibular ligament,

    ii. Vocalis, and

    iii. Lateral cricoarytenoid muscles.

    iv. Thyroarytenoid muscle.

  b. **Corniculate cartilage** (of Santorini): It is conical nodule enclosed in the dorsal part of aryepiglottic fold.

  c. **Cuneiform cartilage:** It is present in the aryepiglottic fold and lies ventral and superior to the corniculate cartilage.

  d. **Cartilago triticea:** They are present at lateral part of thyrohyoid membrane.NEET

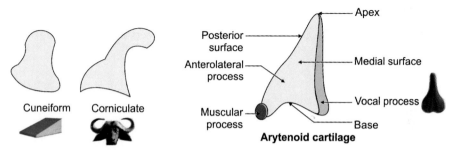

Fig. 16.3: Paired cartilages of larynx

B. **Unpaired cartilages**

  a. Cricoid cartilage: Refer SN-127

  b. Thyroid cartilage: Refer SN 128

  c. Epiglottis:

    I. It is slightly curved, resembles a leaf. It is prolonged below into a slender process, the stalk of the leaf. It is attached in the midline to the back of laryngeal prominence.

    II. The posterior surface above the apex is pitted by mucous glands.

3. **Muscles of larynx:** Muscles of larynx are divided into extrinsic and intrinsic groups.

  A. Intrinsic muscles take origin and get inserted in the same organ. They are described as given in Table 16.3.

Table 16.3: Origin and insertion of intrinsic muscles of larynx

Muscle	Origin	Insertion
• Posterior cricoarytenoid	• Posterior surface of cricoid cartilage	• Muscular process of arytenoid cartilage
• Lateral cricoarytenoid	• Upper border of lateral surface of cricoid cartilage	• Muscular process of arytenoid cartilage
• Cricothyroid	• Arch of cricoid cartilage	• Inferior horn of thyroid cartilage

Contd.

Head, Neck and Face

Table 16.3: Origin and insertion of intrinsic muscles of larynx (Contd.)

Muscle	Origin	Insertion
• Thyroarytenoid	• Deep surface of thyroid cartilage	• Lateral surface of arytenoid cartilage
• Thyroepiglotticus	• Thyroarytenoid cartilage	• Epiglottis
• Oblique arytenoids	• Muscular process of one arytenoid cartilage	• Apex of other arytenoid cartilage
• Vocalis	• Posterior surface of thyroid cartilage in midline	• Vocal process of arytenoid cartilage
• Transverse arytenoid	• Posterior surface of arytenoid cartilage of one side	• Posterior surface of other side
• Aryepiglotticus	• Muscular process of arytenoid cartilage	• Epiglottis

   B. Extrinsic muscles take origin outside and get inserted inside the organ. They are
      a. Sternothyroid,
      b. Thyrohyoid,
      c. Omohyoid and
      d. Digastric.

4. **Actions of intrinsic muscles**

Table 16.4: Muscles acting on vocal cords

Actions on vocal cords	Muscles
Abduction	Posterior cricoarytenoid
Adduction	Lateral cricoarytenoid
Tensor	Cricothyroid
Relaxation	Vocalis

Table 16.5: Muscles acting on larynx

Actions on larynx	Muscles
Opening of inlet of larynx	ThyrO-epiglottic
Closing of inlet of larynx	Aryepiglottic
Elevation	Thyrohyoid, mylohyoid
Depression	Sternohyoid, sternothyroid

5. **Nerve supply**

   A. **Sensory**
      a. Above vocal fold: Internal laryngeal nerve, a branch of superior laryngeal nerve, a branch of vagus nerve.
      b. Below the vocal fold: Recurrent laryngeal nerve (branch of vagus nerve).
   B. **Motor (muscle):** All muscles of larynx are supplied by recurrent laryngeal nerve, a branch of vagus except cricothyroid, which is supplied by external laryngeal nerve, a branch of superior laryngeal nerve, a branch of vagus nerve.

a. Embryological (developmental) correlation

I. Cricothyroid muscle develops from 4th pharyngeal arch. Nerve of the 4th pharyngeal arch is superior laryngeal nerve, which gives external laryngeal nerve. Hence, cricothyroid is supplied by external laryngeal branch.

II. Remaining all muscles of larynx are developed from 6th arch. The nerve of 6th pharyngeal arch is vagus nerve which gives a recurrent laryngeal nerve. Hence, remaining all muscles are supplied by a recurrent laryngeal nerve.

b. **Physiological (functional correlation):** The cricothyroid muscle acts as a tuning fork. First, it receives impulses and starts vibrating. The remaining muscles receive impulses few milli-second afterwards, which help in producing voice.

6. **Applied anatomy**

➤ Examination of larynx is called laryngoscopy.

➤ Laryngitis is inflammation of larynx. It occurs in common cold.

➤ The swelling of vocal cords is rare in acute laryngitis because of following reasons:

- The vocal cords are lined by stratified squamous epithelium (rest of the larynx is lined by pseudostratified ciliated columnar epithelium).

- The mucous membrane is firmly attached to the underlying vocal ligaments.

- **There is no submucous tissue and there are no glands over the vocal cords.** For the same reason, the vocal cords appear pearly white in colour.

➤ Damage to internal laryngeal nerve produces anaesthesia (loss of sensation in supraglottic part of larynx).

➤ Foreign bodies can readily enter the larynx, if internal laryngeal nerve is damaged.

➤ Damage to the external laryngeal nerve causes paralysis of cricothyroid muscle. It results in weakness of phonation.

➤ When both recurrent laryngeal nerves are injured, vocal cords lie in cadaveric position.

➤ During swallowing, the larynx moves up and down by extrinsic laryngeal muscles (viz. palatopharyngeus, salphingopharyngeus and stylopharyngeus).

➤ Compression of larynx due to thyroid swelling may produce hoarseness of voice called dysphonia.

➤ Removal of foreign bodies from the piriform fossa may damage internal laryngeal nerve, leading to anaesthesia of the supraglottic portion of the larynx.

➤ **Teacher's nodules** (or singer's nodules): These nodules are seen in the vocal cords of the teachers and singers. They are usually located at the junction of anterior and middle third of vocal cord.

SN-127 Cricoid cartilage

(Cricoid Gr. *Krikos*—a ring, *-oid*—resemblance)

Introduction: It is a midline unpaired cartilage of larynx. It forms the foundation of larynx (Fig. 16.4).

Head, Neck and Face

1. **Morphology**
    A. **Shape:** It is only complete ring ◯ in all the structres of respiratory tract.^{NEET}
    B. **Situation:** It encircles the larynx and is present at the level of 6th cervical vertebra.
    C. **Parts:** It has
        a. **Arch:** The narrow anterior part is called arch. It has upper and lower borders and outer and inner surfaces.
        b. **Lamina:** Cricoid cartilage has broad, quadrilateral posterior part called lamina. It has upper and lower borders, anterior and posterior surfaces.

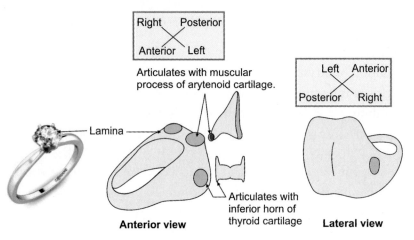

Fig. 16.4: Cricoid cartilage

2. **Attachments**

Table 16.6: Structures attached to various borders and surfaces of cricoid cartilage

Particulars	Area of cricoid cartilage	Structures attached
• Outer	• Surface	• Cricothyroid muscle
• Posterior surface	• Of lamina	• Posterior cricoarytenoid • Tendon of oesophagus
• Lateral surface		• Lateral cricoarytenoid
• Upper border	• Of anterior arch	• Cricoarytenoid
• Lower border		• Trachealis, • Cricotracheal ligament.
• Arch of cricoid		• Anterior cricothyroid ligament

3. **Joints:** It forms joint with thyroid and arytenoids. Both are synovial joints.

SN-128 Thyroid cartilage

(Gr. *thyreos*—a shield—*oid*—like)

Introduction: It is one of the unpaired cartilages of larynx.
1. **Parts**
    A. It has two conjoined laminae whose posterior borders are free. They are projected upwards and downwards as superior and inferior cornua.

B. The two laminae fuse in the midline and form the laryngeal prominence (Adam's apple).

C. Oblique line: It extends on the outer surface. It is bounded below and above by a tubercle.

2. **Joints:** Inferior horn articulates with the cricoid cartilage and forms cricothyroid joint.

3. **Relations:** The common carotid artery bifurcates at the tip of superior cornu into internal and external carotid arteries.

4. **Attachments**

A. Superior border gives attachment to thyrohyoid membrane.

B. Oblique line gives attachments to the following muscles ●━▼ SIT .

   Sternothyroid

   Inferior constrictor of pharynx

   Thyrohyoid

C. Inferior cornu and lower border of thyroid lamina give attachment to cricothyroid muscle.

D. Superior cornu gives attachment to thyroepiglottic ligaments.

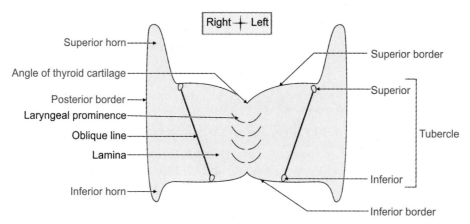

Fig. 16.5: External features of thyroid cartilage

5. **Applied anatomy** : The upward enlargement of the thyroid gland is prevented by the sternothyroid muscle attached to oblique line of thyroid cartilage.

SN-129 Inlet of larynx

Introduction: It is the continuation of laryngopharynx.

1. **Boundaries** (Figs 16.6 and 16.7)

A. **In front and above:** Upper free margin of epiglottis.

B. **Below and behind:** Interarytenoid fold of mucous membrane.

C. **Laterally:** Aryepiglottic fold.

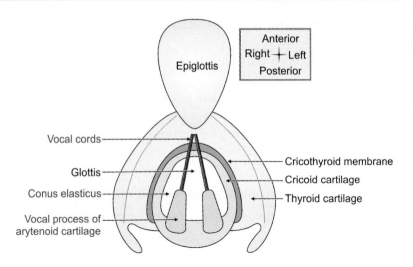

Fig. 16.6: Boundaries of inlet of larynx

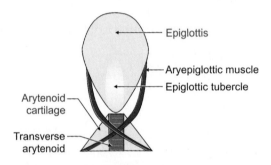

Fig. 16.7: Epiglottis and arytenoid cartilage

2. **Placement:** Obliquely. The anterior wall is much longer than the posterior wall.

3. **Communication**

   A. **Above:** Laryngopharynx

   B. **Below:** Trachea.

4. **Muscles acting on inlet of larynx**

   A. **Thyroepiglotticus:** It helps in active opening of laryngeal inlet.

   B. **Aryepiglotticus:** It closes the inlet of larynx (Fig. 16.8).

5. **Relations:** On either side of inlet of larynx, there is a small recess termed the piriform fossa.

6. Applied anatomy

   ➤ A malignancy tumour may grow in the piriform fossa without producing symptoms, until the patient presents with metastatic lymphadenopathy.

   ➤ The recesses are dangerous sites for perforation by an endoscope.

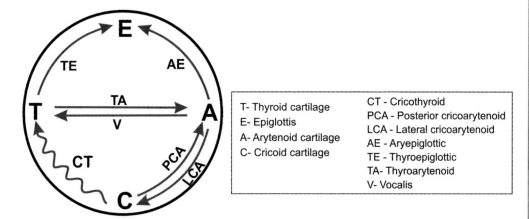

Fig. 16.8: Nomenclature and action of the muscles of larynx

| SN-130 | **Thyrohyoid membrane** |

Introduction: It is extrinsic membrane extending from
- Upper border of thyroid laminae, and
- Superior horns of thyroid cartilage to
  - Greater cornu of hyoid bone, and
  - Upper border of body of hyoid bone.

1. **Modifications**
   A. Median thyrohyoid ligament: It is midline thickened part of thyrohyoid membrane.
   B. Lateral thyrohyoid ligament: It is thickening on the posterior free border.

2. **Relations**
   A. It forms the lateral boundary of piriform fossa.
   B. A bursa lies between the membrane and back of hyoid bone.

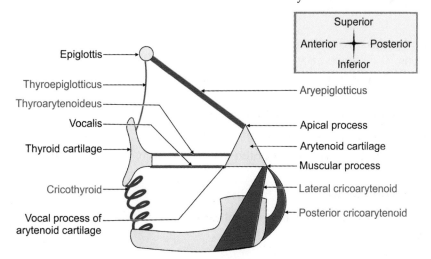

Fig. 16.9: Schematic diagram to recollect the attachments of muscles of larynx

Head, Neck and Face

3. **Structures piercing**
   A. Internal laryngeal nerve.
   B. Superior laryngeal vessels.

SN-131 Cricothyroid muscle

Introduction: It is the only intrinsic muscle present outside the larynx. It is ▲ lar.
1. **Proximal attachment:** It arises from the arch of cricoid cartilage.
2. **Distal attachment:** Inferior horn and lower border of thyroid cartilage.

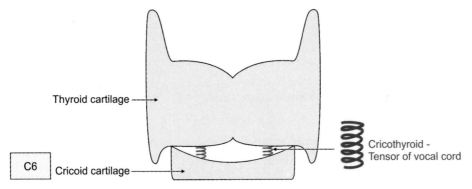

Thyroid cartilage

C6 | Cricoid cartilage

Cricothyroid - Tensor of vocal cord

Fig. 16.10: Cricothyroid muscle

3. **Action:** It brings the arch of cricoid cartilage near thyroid cartilage. Hence, tensor of the vocal cord.
4. **Development:** It develops from the skeletal element of 4th pharyngeal arch.
5. **Nerve supply**: External laryngeal nerve, branch of superior laryngeal nerve (branch of vagus nerve).

SN-132 Posterior cricoarytenoid

Introduction: It is the intrinsic and most important muscle of larynx and probably in the body.
1. **Origin:** It arises from the posterior surface of lamina of cricoid cartilage. It is also known as, *"safety muscle of larynx"*.[NEET]
2. **Insertion:** Posterior aspect of muscular process of arytenoid cartilage of the same side.
3. **Action:** It abducts the vocal folds and opens the glottis.
4. **Nerve supply**: Recurrent laryngeal nerve, branch of vagus nerve.
5. **Development:** It develops from 6th pharyngeal arch.

SN-133 Piriform fossa

Introduction: It is a space present on each side of inlet of larynx. It is broad above and narrow below.
1. **Boundaries**[NEET]
   A. **Medially:** By the quadrate membrane below the aryepiglottic fold.

B. **Laterally:** Mucosa covering the thyroid lamina and thyrohyoid membrane.

C. **Superiorly:** Lateral glossoepiglottic fold. It separates pyriform fossa from vallecula of oropharynx.

2. **Structures deep to piriformis**

A. Internal laryngeal nerve, and

B. Superior laryngeal vessels.

3. **Relations:** It is traversed by internal laryngeal nerve.

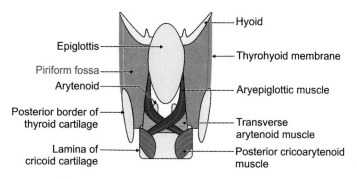

Fig. 16.11: Posterior view of larynx showing piriform fossa

4. Applied anatomy

➢ Foreign body in larynx: At times fish bones may get impacted in the vallecula or piriform fossa. These foreign bodies scratch the mucosa. The person feels discomfort and uneasiness due to a dull visceral pain.

➢ The fossa is artificially deepened by smugglers to carry smuggled goods. In old days, it was used to smuggle gold coins. After introduction of metal detectors, it is used to carry precious stones, diamonds, etc. Hence, it is called *smuggler's fossa*.

➢ Tumours in the piriform fossa cause dysphagia. These also cause referred pain in the ear. Pain of pharyngeal tumours may be referred to the ear, as vagus nerve supplies larynx, tympanic membrane and external acoustic meatus.

➢ By laryngoscope, one can visualize piriform fossa.

➢ A malignancy may grow in the space without producing symptoms unless the patient presents with metastatic cervical lymphadenopathy.

➢ The recess is dangerous site for perforation by an endoscope.

➢ It acts as a site for lodgment of foreign body.

Head, Neck and Face

Tongue

OLA-73 | Why genioglossus is called 'safety muscle'?

1. Genioglossus is protractor of tongue. It prevents falling back of tongue and prevents the choking of the air passage. Hence, it is called "safety muscle of tongue".[NEET]

OLA-74 | Name the muscles required for changing the shape of the tongue.

Intrinsic muscles of tongue change the shape of the tongue. They are

1. Longitudinal
   A. Superior
   B. Inferior
2. Transverse
3. Verticalis

OLA-75 | What is the effect of bilateral paralysis of genioglossus?

If both genioglossi are paralyzed, the tongue may fall backwards. It obstructs the airway (oropharynx) which may lead to death of an individual due to suffocation.

OLA-76 | Why jugulo-omohyoid node is called 'lymph node of tongue'?

The jugulo-omohyoid node is situated close to the omohyoid muscle. It is mainly associated with drainage of the tongue.

OLA-77 | Name different types of papillae present on dorsum of tongue and give their functions.

Table 17.1: Different types of papillae

Papillae	Site and number	Shape	Lining epithelium	Taste buds	Function
• Filiform	• Numerous and fills dorsum of tongue in anterior 2/3rd of tongue	• Conical projection of lamina propria	• Stratified squamous keratinised	• Absent	• Help to hold the food • Increase friction between tongue and food
• Fungi-form	• Dispersed in dorsum of tongue in anterior 2/3rd of tongue	• Mushroom shaped	• Stratified squamous non-kera-tinised	• Present on upper surface of expanded part	• Increase the area of con-tact between food and tongue
• Circu-mvallate	• Largest, 10–12 in number, arranged in V shaped in front of sulcus terminalis	• Circular surrounded by sulcus	• Stratified squamous non kera-tinised	• Present on the walls of sulcus	
• Foliate	• Poorly dev-eloped in humans. Present in rows on lateral aspect of dorsum of tongue infront of sulcus ter-minalis		• Stratified squamous non-keratinised		

Head, Neck and Face

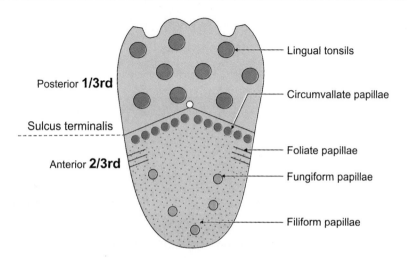

Posterior **1/3rd**

Sulcus terminalis

Anterior **2/3rd**

Lingual tonsils

Circumvallate papillae

Foliate papillae

Fungiform papillae

Filiform papillae

Fig. 17.1: Different types of papillae present on dorsum of tongue

SN-134 Define a lingual papilla. State its four types, salient features, differences and functions of each

Table 17.2: lingual papilla

Particulars	Filiform	Fungiform	Circumvallate	Foliate
• Epithelium	• Stratified squamous keratinised	• Stratified squamous non-keratinised	• Stratified squamous non-keratinised	• Stratified squamous non-keratinised
• Structure	• Conical projection of lamina propria	• Mushroom shaped and consists of a care of lamina propria which expands in the upper part	• Large, circular and surrounded by sulcus	
• Size	• Smallest	• Intermediate	• Largest	
• Quantity	• Numerous		• 10 to 12	
• Site	• Fills the dorsal surface of tongue. It is present on anterior 2/3rd of tongue	• Dispersed among filiform papillae in the anterior two-thirds of the tongue	• In front of sulcus terminalis	• Infront of sulcus terminalis on lateral border of tongue
• Taste buds	• Absent	• On the upper surface of the expanded part	• Walls of the sulcus	
• Features			• Ducts of numerous serous glands open into the sulcus. These glands are known as **von Ebner's** glands	• Poorly developed in humans.
• Functions	• Holds the food		• Make the food soluble by the secretion of **Von Ebner's** gland	

OLA-78 Which lingual papilla does not contain taste buds?

Filiform papilla.

OLA-79 What are Von Ebner's, and Nuhn's glands?

These are serous glands. The ducts of these glands open into sulcus present around each circumvallate papilla.

OLA-80 State the two types of epithelia found in lip and explain why these epithelia are found there.

1. Outer surface lined by stratified squamous keratinised epithelium. The outer surface of the lip is dry. The cells on the surface loose nuclei and become dead and the epithelium is called stratified squamous keratinised epithelium.
2. Inner surface is lined by stratified squamous non-keratinised epithelium. Inner surface of the lip remains moist. The most superficial cells are living and nuclei can be seen in them. This kind of epithelium is described as stratified squamous non-keratinised epithelium.

OLA-81 What is vermilion zone, border?

1. In between the outer and inner surfaces, there is a zone of transition called vermilion zone.
2. It is lined by modified skin which does not have glands and hairs.
3. It has highly vascular dermis and because of this, it appears pink.
4. It lacks glands, so it remains dry and cracks in the dry weather.
5. It is kept moist by saliva to prevent cracking.

SN-135 Vagus nerve (Alderman's nerve) in neck

Introduction: It is Xth cranial nerve supplying mainly the muscles of larynx and sensations to most posterior part of tongue.

1. **Functional components:**

Table 17.3: Functional components

S. no.	Functional components	Nucleus	Function	Distribution
1	• General somatic afferent	• Nucleus of spinal tract of trigeminal nerve	• General sensation	• Skin of the auricle, • External auditory meatus via the auricular branch of the vagus.
2	• Special visceral afferent (SVAd)	• Lower part of nucleus tractus solitarius	• Taste sensation	• From the epiglottis, most posterior part of the tongue near the valleculae, and valleculae via the internal laryngeal nerve

Contd.

Head, Neck and Face

Table 17.3: Functional components (Contd.)

S. no.	Functional components	Nucleus	Function	Distribution
3	• General visceral afferent		• General sensation	• Larynx, trachea • Pharynx, oesophagus • Foregut and midgut
4	• General visceral efferent (GiVE)	• Dorsal nucleus of vagus	• Movements	• Smooth muscles of the heart, trachea, bronchi, foregut and midgut
5	• Somatic Visceral efferent • SaVE- BRANCHial • ArchES	• Nucleus ambiguus	• Movements	• Skeletal muscles of pharynx except stylopharyngeus • Intrinsic muscles of larynx • Soft palate except tensor veli palatini through vagus

2. **Exit from**
   A. Brainstem: Post-olive sulcus.
   B. Cranium: Through the jugular foramen but separated from the glossopharyngeal nerve by a fibrous septum.

3. **Ganglions**
   A. *Superior (jugular):* It lies in jugular foramen. It is connected with
      a. Inferior ganglion of the **IXth** (glossopharyngeal nerve),
      b. Cranial root of the **XIth** (accessory nerve),
      c. Sympathetic trunk. It sends auricular branch which joins with the facial nerve by a twig. *This ganglion is concerned with general somatic sensations via its auricular branch.*
   B. *Inferior ganglion (ganglion nodosum):* It lies just below the jugular foramen. It is connected with
      a. Hypoglossal.
      b. Superior cervical ganglion of the sympathetic.
      c. Loop between **C1** and **C2** nerves. This ganglion is concerned with special sense (taste) from the epiglottis, valleculae and general visceral sensory from the larynx, pharynx, heart, lungs, oesophagus, stomach and intestine.

4. **Course**

A. *In the neck:* The nerve descends vertically lying within the carotid sheath.

   a. Up to the level of the upper border of the thyroid cartilage, the nerve lies in between and behind the internal jugular vein and internal carotid artery.

   b. Below the level of the upper border of the thyroid cartilage, the nerve lies in between and behind the internal jugular vein and common carotid artery.

B. *Entrance in the thorax:*

   a. *Right vagus crosses*

      I. Right subclavian, and

      II. Right common carotid arteries from front and enters the thorax.

   b. *Left vagus enters* the thorax and lies between left common carotid and left subclavian arteries. It lies behind the left brachiocephalic vein.

5. **Branches**

A. From superior cervical ganglion

   a. Auricular,

   b. Meningeal,

B. From inferior ganglion

   a. Pharyngeal,

   b. Superior laryngeal,

      I. Internal laryngeal

      II. External laryngeal

C. Sinus branch

   a. Carotid body

   b. Carotid sinus

D. Superior and inferior cardiac branch.

E. Right vagus gives right recurrent laryngeal nerve, only on the right side in the neck.

F. Left vagus gives left recurrent laryngeal nerve, in the thorax.

6. **Development:** It is the nerve of 6th branchial arch.

7. Applied anatomy

   ➤ Isolated lesions of the vagus nerve are uncommon but they may be involved in injuries or disease of related structures.

   ➤ Damage or compression of the vagus and/or recurrent laryngeal nerves during surgical dissection of the carotid triangle may produce an alteration in the voice.

   ➤ **Ramsay-Hunt syndrome:** It is due to herpes zoster infection of the geniculate ganglion of the facial nerve. It is associated with ipsilateral facial paralysis. It is usually transient. There are vesicles on the external ear or tympanic membrane. If the nerve is irritated, there is spasm and irritation of the muscles of the pharynx. It causes cough.

Head, Neck and Face

➢ Auricular branch of vagus nerve is stimulated by

- Impacted wax, or
- By syringing the external ear. It can give rise to reflex cough.

➢ If the nerves of both sides are cut, both the vocal folds are paralysed and take the paramedian position.

➢ If left nerve is cut, the left vocal fold will be paralysed and become motionless. The right vocal fold will cross the midline of the rima glottidis as a compensatory phenomenon. As a result, the voice is possible but very weak.

8. **Testing of the nerves**

A. The pharyngeal reflex may be tested by touching the lateral wall of the pharynx with a spatula.

B. The innervation or the soft palate can be tested by asking the patient to say "ah". Normally, the soft palate rises and the uvula moves backward in the midline.

C. Hoarseness or absence of the voice may occur. Laryngoscopic examination may reveal abductor paralysis.

D. The lesions of the vagus nerve will produce following effects:

a. Nasal regurgitation of the swallowed liquids.

b. Nasal twang of the voice.

c. Flattening of the palatal arch.

d. Hoarseness of the voice.

e. Cadaveric position of the vocal cords and dysphasia.

LAQ-41	Describe tongue under the following heads:
	1. Muscles of tongue,
	2. Blood supply,
	3. Lymphatic drainage,
	4. Applied anatomy of lymphatic drainage,
	5. Nerve supply,
	6. The 4 varieties of papillae,
	7. Development, and
	8. Applied anatomy

1. **Muscles of tongue:** These are grouped into intrinsic and extrinsic muscles.

A. **Intrinsic muscles:** The muscles having origin a nd insertions in the tongue. They alter the shape and size of tongue (Table 17.4 and Fig. 17.2).

B. **Extrinsic muscles of tongue** (Table 17.5 and Fig. 17.3)

Table 17.4: Origin insertion and action of intrinsic muscles of tongue

Muscle	Origin	Insertion	Action
• Superior longitudinal	• Posterior part of median fibrous septum	• Sides of tongue	• Shortens the tongue
• Inferior longitudinal	• Posterior part of side of tongue	• Anterior part of median fibrous septum	• Shortens the tongue
• Transversus	• Median fibrous septum	• Sides of tongue	• Reduces the width
• Vertical	• Lamina propria of dorsum of tongue	• Sides of tongue	• Reduces the thickness of tongue

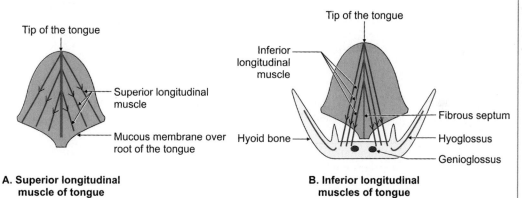

A. Superior longitudinal muscle of tongue

B. Inferior longitudinal muscles of tongue

C. Intrinsic muscles of tongue

Fig. 17.2: Dorsal surface of tongue showing superior longitudinal muscle

Head, Neck and Face

Head, Neck and Face

Table 17.5: Origin, insertion and action of extrinsic muscles of tongue

Muscle	Origin	Insertion	Action
• Genioglossus: Fan shaped (It is the safety muscle of tongue)	• Superior genial tubercle • Symphysis menti present on the inner surface of mandible	• Upper fibres: Root to apex of the tongue • Middle fibres: Mixes with constrictor of pharynx • Lower fibres: Body of hyoid bone	• Protrusion of tongue • Safety muscle of tongue • Saves the life by preventing the backward fall
• Hyoglossus: Quadrilateral	• Upper surface of greater cornu of hyoid bone • Body of hyoid bone	• Side of the tongue between styloglossus laterally and inferior longitudinal muscle medially	• Makes dorsum of the tongue convex • It retracts the protruded tongue
• Chondroglossus: Detached part of the hyoglossus	• Lesser cornu of hyoid bone • Part of body of hyoid bone	• Side of tongue	• Depression of tongue
• Styloglossus	• Tip of styloid process and stylomandibular ligament	• Side of tongue	• Retraction of tongue
• Palatoglossus	• Under surface of palatine aponeurosis	• Side of tongue	• Elevation of tongue

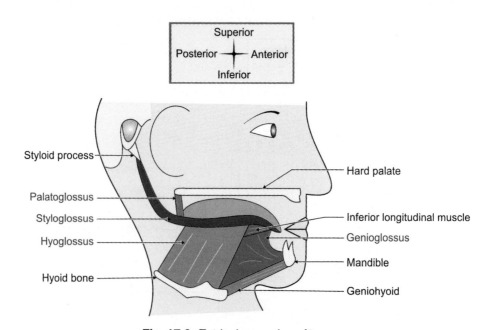

Superior
Posterior ——+—— Anterior
Inferior

Styloid process

Hard palate

Palatoglossus

Styloglossus

Inferior longitudinal muscle

Hyoglossus

Genioglossus

Mandible

Hyoid bone

Geniohyoid

Fig. 17.3: Extrinsic muscles of tongue

2. Blood supply

A. **Arterial supply**:

  a. Lingual artery (chief artery of tongue), branch of external carotid artery supplies tongue through

  I. Profunda lingual artery: It supplies oral part of tongue.

  II. Dorsal lingual artery: It supplies pharyngeal part of tongue.

  b. Facial artery through

  I. Ascending palatine.

  II. Tonsillar branch.

  c. Ascending pharyngeal branch of external carotid artery.

B. **Venous drainage**: Veins are arranged in two sets. Mainly drain into profunda lingual vein.

Table 17.6: Superficial and deep veins of tongue

Particulars	Superficial	Deep
• Location	• Superficial to hyoglossus	• Deep to hyoglossus
• Distribution	• Tip and under surface of tongue	• Dorsum of tongue
• Structures accompanied	• Hypoglossal nerve (XII)	• Lingual artery
• Drains into	• Internal jugular vein	• Internal jugular vein

3. Lymphatic drainage

A. **Peculiarities**

  a. Do not accompany the blood vessels.

  b. The tip of the tongue has richest lymphatic plexus.

  c. Lymphatics in the posterior one-third of tongue drain bilaterally.

  d. Lymphatics of the tongue ultimately drain into Jugulo-OmoHyoid Nodes. Hence, they are called *lymph nodes of tongue*. JOHN has TONGUE.[NEET]

Lymphatics drainage of tongue consists of following sets (Table 17.7).

Table 17.7: Lymphatic drainage of the tongue (Figs 17.4 and 17.5)

Lymph node	Afferent (receiving)	Efferent (draining)
• Apical	• Tip • Frenulum	• Submental (major lymph node) Bilateral
• Marginal	• Side of tongue in front of sulcus terminalis	• Submandibular node
• Central	• Anterior 2/3rd of tongue (in front of vallate papillae.)	• Jugulodigastric • Jugulo-omohyoid
• Dorsal	• Posterior 1/3rd	• Bilaterally into jugular and digastric (major part) • Jugulo-omohyoid lymph nodes.

4. Applied anatomy of lymphatic drainage

➢ Malignancy in the tip and posterior one-third of tongue is more dangerous since it drains bilaterally.

➤ Lymph vessels piercing mylohyoid are often closely related to the periosteum of mandible accounting early spread to the bone.

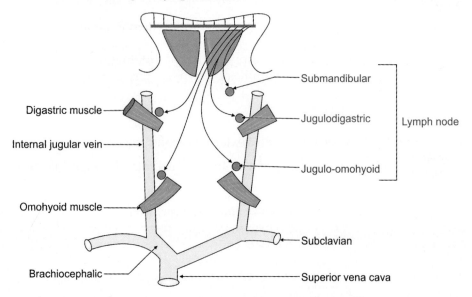

Fig. 17.4: Internal arrangement of lymph nodes

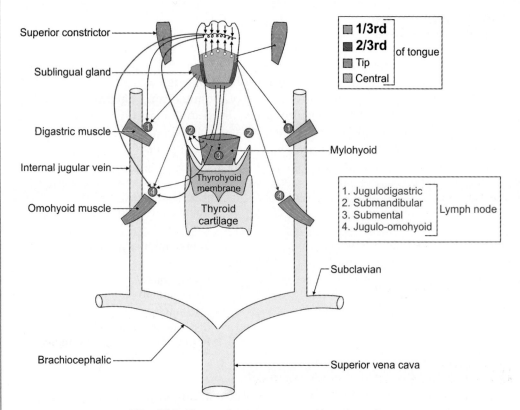

Fig. 17.5: External arrangement of lymph nodes

5. **Nerve supply of tongue** : It is divided into motor and sensory.

A. **Motor**

a. **Somatomotor:** All the extrinsic and intrinsic muscles of tongue are supplied by hypoglossal nerve (nerve of occipital myotome) except palatoglossus which is supplied by pharyngeal plexus.

b. **Secretomotor fibres** are derived from superior salivatory nucleus—facial nerve—chorda tympani—lingual nerve—submandibular ganglion—lingual glands.

c. **Vasomotor nerve** arises from spinal cord—superior sympathetic ganglion—plexus around external carotid artery (plexus around lingual artery).

B. **Sensory**

Table 17.8: Sensory nerve supply of tongue

Particulars	Anterior 2/3rd	Posterior 1/3rd	Most posterior part
• General sensation: Touch, pain and temperature	• Lingual branch of mandibular (trigeminal): Nerve of 1st pharyngeal arch	• Glossopharyngeal (IX) nerve, a nerve of 3rd pharyngeal arch	• Vagus (nerve of 4th and 6th arches)
• Special sensation: Taste	• Chorda tympani (facial) pretrematic nerve (of 2nd pharyngeal arch)	• Glossopharyngeal (IX) nerve, a nerve of 3rd pharyngeal arch	• Vagus (nerve of 4th and 6th arches)
• Circumvallate papillae	• Glossopharyngeal nerve, nerve of 3rd pharyngeal arch	—	—
• Fungiform, filiform and foliate	• Lingual nerve (branch of mandibular nerve)		

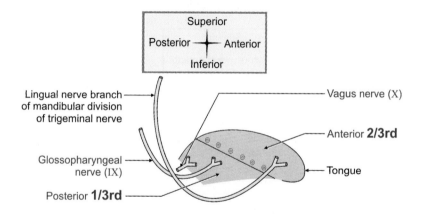

Fig. 17.6: Nerves carrying general sensations of tongue

Table 17.9: Filiform and fungiform papillae

Particulars	Filiform	Fungiform
• Number	• Numerous	• Few
• Arrangement	• Uniform	• Irregular
• Distribution	• All over tongue	• Tip and sides
• Shape	• Thread-like pointed ▪━━━━━	• Club ♣ shaped
• Taste buds	• Absent	• Few

6. **The papillae are of four varieties**
   A. Filiform
   B. Fungiform
   C. Vallate, and
   D. Foliate.

   They consist of a fibrous core derived from the tunica propria, covered with stratified squamous epithelium.
   A. The *filiform papillae* are tapering and thread-like. They are arranged in V-shaped rows present over the dorsum of the oral part of the tongue. They contain touch corpuscles. Their epithelium is scaly. In some animals (e.g. cat, cow), it is cornified and is used as a rasp (grating noise) to grasp food.
   B. The *fungiform papillae* have globular heads and are red. The core is more vascular and the epithelium is not scaly. They lie scattered singly among the filiform papillae. They are present at the tip and margin of the tongue. They do not rise above them.
   C. The *vallate papillae* are circular, about 2 mm in diameter. They are a dozen in number. They are also arranged in a V-shaped row just in front of the sulcus terminalis. Their fiat tops hardly rise above the general surface.
   D. The *foliate papillae*, rudimentary in man, are 3–4 vertical folds at the hinder part of the sides of the tongue.
   Taste buds occur on most fungiform papillae, on the opposed sides of the foliate and on both walls of the vallate. They also occur sparsely on the soft palate, epiglottis and posterior wall of the pharynx.

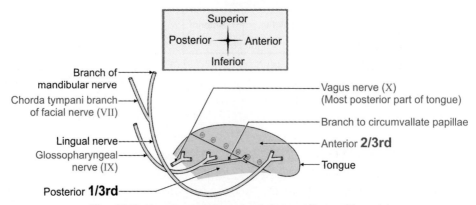

Fig. 17.7: Nerves carrying special sensations of tongue

7. Development of the tongue
   A. **Chronological age:** It develops in the 4th week of intrauterine life.
   B. **Germ layer**
      a. Tip of tongue—surface ectoderm
      b. Base of tongue—endoderm
      c. Muscles—mesoderm
   C. **Site:** Floor of the pharynx just cranial to median thyroid diverticulum.
   D. **Sources**
      a. *Muscles:*
         I. All the muscles of tongue are developed from occipital myotome except palatoglossus. The nerve of the occipital myotome is hypoglossal (12th cranial nerve). Hence, all the muscles are supplied by hypoglossal nerve.
         II. Palatoglossus developed from pharyngeal arches which develop from neural crest cells.[NEET]
      b. *Mucous membrane:* It is developed from endoderm of the floor of pharynx and is subdivided into
         I. Anterior 2/3rd is developed from:
            i. Fusion of a pair of *lingual swelling* arising from pouch of the 1st branchial arch, and
            ii. *Tuberculum impar* (*impar* unpaired) a midline swelling arises from 1st pouch and gives a very little contribution. The post-trematic nerve of 1st arch is lingual nerve and pre-trematic nerve of 2nd arch is chorda tympani nerve.
         II. Posterior 1/3rd is developed from cranial part of hypobranchial eminence, which is formed by fusion of 3rd and 4th branchial arches only. The eminence is divided by a transverse groove into cranial and caudal part. The nerve of 3rd arch is glossopharyngeal nerve, nerve of 4th arch is superior laryngeal nerve and the nerve of the 6th arch is recurrent laryngeal nerve.
      c. *Fibrous stroma:* Blood vessels and lymphatics are developed from mesoderm of the adjacent arches.
      d. *Papillae:*
         I. Formed by thickening of epithelium of dorsum of tongue.
         II. Fungiform and filiform papillae develop in anterior two-thirds of tongue.
         III. Circumvallate papillae develop in posterior one-third of tongue which is developed from 3rd pharyngeal arch. The nerve of posterior one-third of tongue is glossopharyngeal nerve. It gets submerged by the overgrowth of 3rd arch and these papillae occupy the anterior wall of sulcus terminalis. Hence, they are supplied by glossopharyngeal nerve (9th nerve).
   E. **Anomalies**
      a. **Ankyloglossia:** Restricted movements of tongue. It may be
         I. **Ankyloglossia superior:** Tongue is adherent to palate.
         II. **Ankyloglossia inferior or tongue-tie:** Tongue is adherent to floor of the mouth.

b. **Microglossia:** Too small tongue.

c. **Aglossia:** Absence of tongue. This is due to complete agenesis of the tongue.

d. **Hemiglossia:** Suppression of one of the lingual swellings.

e. **Macroglossia:** Too large tongue.

8. Applied anatomy

➤ Injury to the hypoglossal nerve produces paralysis of the muscles of the tongue on the side of the lesion. Infranuclear lesion shows ipsilateral hemiatrophy of the tongue. Supranuclear lesion produces paralysis without wasting.

➤ In unconscious patient, the tongue may fall back and obstruct the air passage. This can be prevented by keeping the tongue on one side or pulling the tongue anteriorly.

➤ Carcinoma of the tongue is quite common. It is better treated by radiotherapy than by surgery.

SN-136 Occipital myotome

Introduction: The muscles of tongue are developed from occipital myotomes.

1. **Formation:** They are formed by occipital or precervical somites.

2. **Number:** They are four in number. The 1st somite disappears.

3. **Innervation:** Pre-cervical nerves. These nerves unite and form the hypoglossal nerve.

4. **Course:** As the tongue develops in the floor of pharynx, the occipital myotome migrates and invades the substance of the tongue.

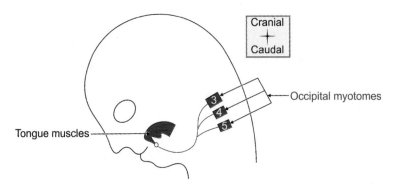

Fig. 17.8: Development of muscles of tongue

SN-137 Circumvallate papillae

1. **Papillae** surrounded by trench.

2. **Size:** 2 mm, pinhead size.

3. **Number:** About 10 to 12.

4. **Situation:** They are present in front of sulcus terminalis as a single row.

5. **Contains** taste buds, present on lateral wall of papillae.

6. **Taste buds:** They contain three types of cells.
   A. Gustatory cell or bipolar cells.
   B. Sustentacular or supporting cells.
   C. Basal cells.

7. **Nerve supply** : Glossopharyngeal nerve (**IXth cranial nerve**).

8. **Development:** It develops in posterior one-third of tongue, migrates and settles in anterior two-thirds of tongue in front of sulcus terminalis.

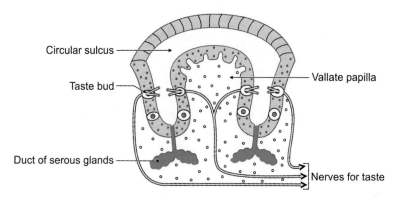

Fig. 17.9: Histology of circumvallate papillae

SN-138 Histological features of taste buds

1. These are end organs for taste sensations.

2. Each is barrel shaped and stands on the corium but extends through the whole thickness of the epithelium. It opens on the surface through a minute gustatory pore. They are formed of two types of cells.
   A. **The gustatory cells are**
     a. Slender, fusiform.
     b. Situated in the central part of the taste bud.
     c. The central part of each cell contains the nucleus.

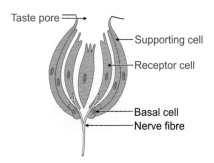

Fig. 17.10: Taste bud

Head, Neck and Face

d. The ends are tapering.

    I. At one end, it has a hair-like process which projects through the gustatory pore.

    II. The other end is branched and sensory nerve fibres end around these processes as well as between the cells.

B. **Sustentacular cells** form a lining for the taste buds and, therefore, surround the gustatory cells. They are also long and slender.

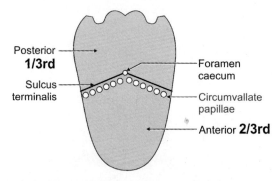

Fig. 17.11: Location of circumvallate papillae

SN-139   Foliate papillae of tongue

Introduction: They are vertical mucous folds occasionally noted on the side of tongue.

1. **Site:** They are present close to palatoglossal arch. Found in the anterior two-thirds of tongue in front of lateral end of sulcus terminalis.

2. **Number:** 3 to 4.

3. **Content:** Taste buds.

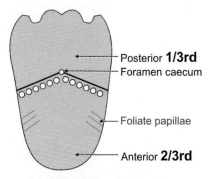

Fig. 17.12: Foliate papillae of tongue

> Word about foliate papillae—Tip

Box 17.1

Note: They are present in rabbit. They are not prominent in man.

AQ-42	Describe lingual nerve under following heads:
	1. Origin,
	2. Course,
	3. Branches,
	4. Distribution, and
	5. Applied anatomy

Introduction: It is sensory nerve of anterior two-thirds of tongue.

1. **Origin:** It is one of the two terminal branches of mandibular nerve.

2. **Course** (Fig. 17.13)

   A. It begins 1 cm below the base of skull.

   B. It runs between

      a. Tensor palatini and pterygoid, and then

      b. Lateral and medial pterygoids.

   C. It joins at an acute angle with chorda tympani nerve.

   D. At lower border of lateral pterygoid, it runs downwards between medial pterygoid and mandible.

   E. It lies anterior to inferior alveolar nerve.

   F. It lies in direct contact with mandible. It is medial to the third molar tooth. It is covered only by mucous membrane. Hence, it is palpated from within the mouth.

   G. It runs forwards across the floor of the mouth and supply the mucous membrane.

   H. It lies on hyoglossus muscle. Here, it has connections with submandibular ganglion.

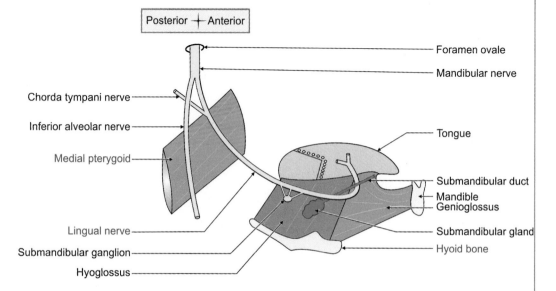

Fig. 17.13: Course of lingual nerve

Head, Neck and Face

I. It lies deep to submandibular duct. It runs forward and upwards between sublingual and genioglossus. It then divides into terminal branches.

3. **Branches**

A. Gingival branch that supplies all the lingual gum and mucous membrane.

B. Communicating branches to
   a. Submandibular ganglion, and
   b. Hypoglossal nerve

4. **Distribution**

A. It carries general sensations (of touch, pain and temperature) and special sensations (of taste through chorda tympani) from anterior two-thirds of tongue.

B. It carries pre- and post-ganglionic secretomotor fibres to salivary glands in the floor of the mouth.

C. It has sensory fibres to the
   a. Mucous membrane lining the floor of the mouth, and
   b. Lingual surface of the mandibular alveolar process.

5. **Applied anatomy**

➢ Lingual nerve is closely related to 3rd molar tooth. Care is taken while extracting misplaced wisdom tooth to avoid injury to lingual nerve.

➢ **Lingual nerve block:** It is approached from premolar teeth of the opposite side, a small injection is made 0.5 cm from the mucosal surface, when the needle is above the lingual nerve (Fig. 17.14).

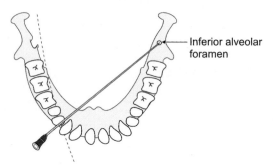

Inferior alveolar foramen

Fig. 17.14: Lingual nerve block

Ear

SN-140 Pinna (ear)

1. **Features**
   A. The greater part of it is made up of a single crumpled plate of elastic cartilage.
   B. It is lined on both sides by skin.
   C. The lowest part of the auricle is soft.
   D. It is made up of fibrofatty tissue covered by skin.
   E. This part is called the lobule used for wearing the ear rings.
   F. The rest of the auricle is divided into a number of parts.
      a. These are helix, antihelix, concha, tragus, scaphoid fossa.
      b. The large depression called the concha.
      c. It leads into the external acoustic meatus.
      d. The external ear has following muscles.
         I. Auricularis anterior,
        II. Auricularis superior, and
       III. Auricularis posterior.

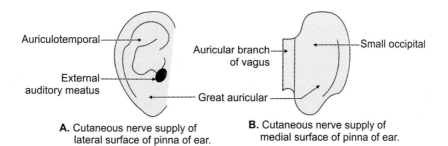

A. Cutaneous nerve supply of lateral surface of pinna of ear.

B. Cutaneous nerve supply of medial surface of pinna of ear.

Fig. 18.1: Pinna (ear)

2. Nerve supply

Table 18.1: Nerve supply of pinna of ear

Motor	Sensory		
	Region	Medial	Lateral
• All muscles of the external ear are supplied by auricular branch of facial nerve	• Upper 2/3rd	• Lesser occipital nerve (C2, C3)	• Auriculo-temporal nerve, branch of mandi-bular nerve
	• Lower 1/3rd	• Great auricular nerve (C2, C3)	

3. **Blood supply**
    a. Posterior auricular, 2nd dorsal branch of external carotid artery, and
    b. Superficial temporal arteries, one of the small terminal branches of external carotid artery given at the neck of mandible.

4. **Lymphatic drainage**
    a. Preauricular, and
    b. Postauricular lymph nodes.

SN-141 Chorda tympani nerve

1. **Origin:** It is a branch of facial nerve (VIIth cranial). It arises from the facial nerve about 6 mm above the stylomastoid foramen.
2. **Functions**
    A. It conveys the preganglionic secretomotor fibres to the
        a. Submandibular,
        b. Sublingual glands, and
    B. Taste fibres from the anterior two-thirds of the tongue except circumvallate papillae.
3. **Development:** It is pretrematic branch of 1st pharyngeal arch.
4. **Course**
    A. It passes through the tympanic membrane.
    B. It runs between mucous and fibrous layers of tympanic membrane.
    C. The course is at the junction of pars flaccida and pars tensa.
    D. It enters the infratemporal fossa through the medial end of the petrotympanic fissure. The anterior ligament of malleus and anterior tympanic artery accompany it.
    E. It passes downward and forward under cover of the lateral pterygoid.
    F. It crosses the medial side of the spine of sphenoid bone.
    G. It joins the posterior border of the lingual nerve at an acute angle.
5. **Relations**
    A. In the infratemporal fossa,
        a. Laterally with

    I. Middle meningeal artery,

    II. Auriculotemporal nerve, and

    III. Inferior alveolar nerve.

b. Medially with

    I. Tensor palati

    II. Auditory tube

c. Anteriorly with

    I. Trunk of mandibular nerve, and

    II. Otic ganglion.

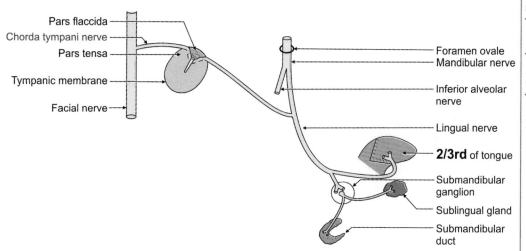

Fig. 18.2: Chorda tympani nerve

6. **Communication branches** to the otic ganglion, which probably forms an alternate root of taste sensations from the tongue.

7. Applied anatomy

> ➤ For the operation in the tympanic membrane, the incision is taken posteromedially to avoid the injury to chorda tympani.

> ➤ Damage to 7th nerve proximal to the origin of the chorda tympani results in
> - Loss of taste sensation of anterior two-thirds of tongue.
> - Decrease salivation.

> ➤ A lesion in the region of spine of sphenoid may involve chorda tympani and auriculotemporal nerves. It results in loss of secretion of submandibular, sublingual and parotid glands.

SN-142 **External auditory canal (external auditory meatus)**

1. It conducts sound waves from the concha to the tympanic membrane.

    A. **Shape:** S-shaped.

Head, Neck and Face

B. It has three parts
    a. Outer part is directed medially, forwards and upwards.
    b. Middle part is directed medially, backwards and upwards.
    c. Inner part is directed medially, forwards and downwards.
C. It can be straightened for examination by pulling the auricle *upwards, backwards and slightly laterally.*
D. **Dimensions**
    a. **Length:** 24 mm long.
        I. Medial two-thirds or 16 mm is bony. It is narrower than the cartilaginous part. It is formed by the tympanic plate of the temporal bone which is C-shaped in cross-section.
        II. Lateral one-third or 8 mm is cartilaginous. The *cartilaginous part is* also C-shaped in section, and the gap of the 'C' is filled with fibrous tissue. The lining skin is adherent to the perichondrium and contains hair, sebaceous glands and ceruminous or wax glands. *Ceruminous glands* are modified sweat glands.
          i. Due to the obliquity of the tympanic membrane, the anterior wall and floor are longer than the posterior wall and roof.
          ii. The canal is oval in section. The greatest diameter is vertical at the lateral end and anteroposterior at the medial end.
          iii. The narrowest point, the *isthmus lies* about 5 mm from the tympanic membrane.
          iv. The posterosuperior part of the palate is deficient. Here the wall of the meatus is formed by a part of the squamous temporal bone.
    b. **Epithelium lining:** The meatus is lined by thin skin, firmly adherent to the periosteum.
2. **Blood supply**
    A. Outer part:
        a. Superficial temporal and
        b. Posterior auricular arteries } Branches of external carotid artery
    B. Inner part: Deep auricular branch of the maxillary artery.
3. **Lymphatic drainage**
    A. Preauricular,
    B. Postauricular, and
    C. Superficial cervical lymph nodes.
4. **Nerve supply** (Fig. 18.3)
    A. The skin lining the anterior ½ is supplied by auriculotemporal nerve branch of mandibular nerve.
    B. Posterior ½ is supplied by auricular branch of the vagus.
5. **Applied anatomy**
    ➢ Backward dislocation of temporomandibular joint destroys the external acoustic meatus.
    ➢ Parotid gland disease often causes pain in the external acoustic meatus because of the same innervation by auriculotemporal nerve.

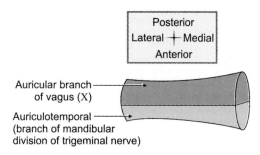

Fig. 18.3: Nerve supply of external auditory canal (meatus)

➤ Examination of the external acoustic meatus and tympanic membrane begins by straightening the meatus.

➤ In adults, the pinna is grasped and pulled posterosuperiorly (up, out and back). These movements reduce the curvature of the external acoustic meatus. It makes cartilaginous and bony canal in one line.

➤ The meatus is straightened in infants by pulling the auricle inferoposteriorly (down and back).

LAQ-43	Describe the external acoustic meatus under the following heads:

1. External features,

2. Relations,

3. Blood supply,

4. Lymphatic drainage,

5. Nerve supply, and

6. Applied anatomy

Introduction: It is a passage connecting the external ear to the tympanic membrane (Fig. 18.4A).

1. **External features**
   A. **Parts** (Fig. 18.4B)
      a. **Outer:** It forms one-third of external acoustic meatus. It is 8 mm long. It is formed by cartilage. The skin of the cartilaginous part shows many hair follicle and numerous ceruminous glands. It secretes wax.
      b. **Inner:** It forms two-thirds part and measures 16 mm in length. It is Bony. (B is the 2nd alphabet and is two-thirds of the external acoustic meatus.) Please associate with auditory tube. In auditory tube, bony part is one-third and cartilaginous part is two-thirds. The medial end of the bony part is smaller in diameter than its lateral part. It is not developed in newborn and hence, the meatus is much shorter.
   B. **Attachments**
      a. Medial end is fixed by the fibrous tissue to the circumference of lateral end of bony part.
      b. Lateral end is continuous with the auricular cartilage.

Head, Neck and Face

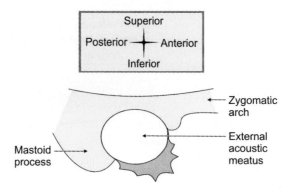

Fig. 18.4A: External acoustic meatus

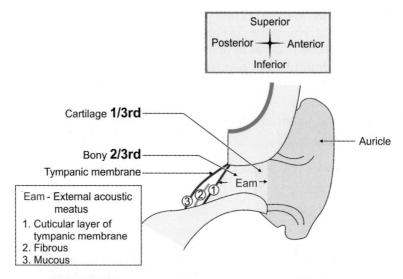

Fig. 18.4B: External acoustic meatus—coronal section

   C. Diameter is less in the middle. It forms the narrowest region of the meatus.

   D. **Surfaces:** The inner surface is lined by skin which is closely adherent to the perichondrium.

   E. **Constrictions:** There are two constrictions.

      a. One at the junction of bony and cartilaginous part (at 8 mm depth)

      b. One at the middle of meatus (at 12 mm depth).

2. **Relations**

   A. **Anterior:** Temporomandibular joint

   B. **Posterior:** Mastoid air cells.

   C. **Superior:** Middle cranial fossa.

3. **Blood supply**

   A. **Arterial supply**

      a. Anterior auricular artery, branch of superficial temporal artery.

b. Posterior auricular artery, branch of external carotid artery.

c. Deep auricular artery, branch of 1st part of maxillary artery.

B. **Venous drainage**

a. Anterior auricular vein drains into superficial temporal vein which drains into retromandibular vein—external jugular vein.

b. Posterior auricular vein drains into posterior division of retromandibular vein—external jugular vein.

c. Deep auricular vein drains into maxillary vein—pterygoid venous plexus.

4. **Lymphatic drainage**

A. Parotid group of lymph nodes.

B. Mastoid group of lymph nodes.

5. **Nerve supply**

A. Auriculotemporal branch of mandibular nerve supplies upper and anterior walls.

B. Auricular branch of vagus supplies posterior wall and floor.

6. **Applied anatomy**

➢ For visualizing tympanic membrane, one has to pull the pinna of ear upwards, backwards and laterally.

➢ Since external acoustic meatus is shorter in newborn, the tympanic membrane is likely to be damaged.

➢ Infection in the external acoustic meatus is extremely painful due to tightly adherent skin of the unyielding subcutaneous tissue.

➢ Removal of the foreign body behind cartilaginous part may be difficult due to hour glass constriction of the external acoustic meatus.

➢ Pain from the external acoustic meatus is referred to teeth because of same nerve supply.

➢ There may be cardiac arrest or vomiting while syringing during removal of foreign body because of vagal stimulation.

SN-143 Tympanic membrane

1. **Gross features:** It is a thin, translucent partition between the external and the middle ear. It is an ⬬ oval in shape, measuring 9 × 10 mm. It is placed obliquely at an angle of 55° with the floor of the meatus. It has outer and inner surfaces.

A. **Outer surface:** Covered by thin skin.

B. **Inner surface:** Provides attachment to the handle of malleus. The point of maximum convexity lies at the level of tip, called *umbo*.

The membrane is thick at its circumference, which is fixed to the tympanic sulcus. Superiorly, the sulcus is deficient. Here, the membrane is attached to the tympanic notch. Greater part of the tympanic membrane is tightly stretched and is called *pars tensa*. The part between the two malleolar folds is loose and is called *pars flaccida*. The pars flaccida is crossed by the chorda tympani, which passes between middle fibrous layer and inner mucous layer.

Head, Neck and Face

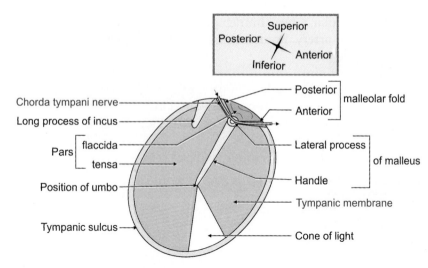

Fig. 18.5: Medial surface of tympanic membrane

2. **Structure:** Composed of three layers.
   A. Outer cuticular layer.
   B. Middle fibrous layer made up of superficial radiating fibres and deep circular fibres. The circular fibres are sparse at the centre and dense at the periphery.
   C. Inner mucous layer is lined by low ciliated columnar epithelium.

Table 18.2: Blood supply, lymphatic drainage and nerve supply of tympanic membrane

Particulars	Outer surface	Inner surface
• **Arterial supply**	• Deep auricular branch of maxillary artery	• Anterior tympanic branch of maxillary artery • Posterior tympanic branch of stylomastoid branch of posterior auricular artery
• **Venous drainage**	• External jugular vein.	• Transverse sinus • Venous plexus around auditory tube
• **Lymphatic drainage**	• Preauricular lymph nodes	• Retropharyngeal
• **Nerve supply**	• Auriculotemporal nerve	• Tympanic branch of glossopharyngeal nerve

3. **Applied anatomy**

   ➤ The otoscopic examination reveals the redness, bulging, perforation or retraction of the tympanic membrane.

   ➤ The membrane is incised to drain the pus present (acute otitis media) in the middle ear. The incision is called *myringotomy*. It is usually made in the *posteroinferior quadrant* of the membrane. In giving an incision, it has to be remembered that the chorda tympani nerve runs downwards and forwards across the inner surface of membrane. It is lateral to the long process of incus, but medial to the neck of mandible.

Table 18.3: Development of tympanic membrane

Particulars	Cuticular layer	Fibrous layer	Mucous layer
• Germ layer	• Ectoderm	• Mesoderm	• Endoderm
• Source	• Dorsal end of the 1st branchial cleft	• Mesoderm between two layers	• Dilated part of tubotympanic recess

OLA-82 **Name the bones in the middle ear**

Ear ossicles
1. Malleus
2. Incus, and
3. Stapes

LAQ-44 **Describe middle ear under the following heads:**

   1. Gross anatomy,

   2. Contents,

   3. Blood supply,

   4. Nerve supply, and

   5. Applied anatomy

Introduction: Narrow space situated between external and internal ear present in the petrous part of temporal bone.

1. **Gross anatomy**
   A. **Dimensions:** It is biconcave ⬤ in shape.
      a. **Vertical:** 15 mm.
      b. **Anteroposterior:** 15 mm.
      c. **Transverse**
         I. Roof: 6 mm.
         II. Centre: 2 mm.
         III. Floor: 4 mm.
   B. **Communication**
      a. **Anteriorly:** Nasopharynx through auditory tube.
      b. **Posteriorly:** Mastoid antrum and air cells through aditus to antrum.
   C. **Boundaries**
      a. **Roof or tegmental wall:** Separates ear from middle cranial fossa. It is formed by thin bone called tegmen tympani which also forms the roof of
         I. Canal for tensor tympani, and
         II. Mastoid antrum.
      b. **Floor or jugular wall**
         I. It is pierced by inferior canaliculus. It transmits tympanic branch of glosso-pharyngeal nerve.

II. Separates middle ear from superior bulb of internal jugular vein.

III. Formed by jugular fossa of temporal bone.

c. **Anterior wall or carotid wall**

I. It is constricted.

II. Consists of three parts:

i. Upper part forms canal for tensor tympani.

ii. Middle part forms opening of auditory tube.

iii. Lower part forms the posterior wall of carotid canal.

III. There is a septum between canal for tensor tympani and canal for auditory tube.

d. **Posterior wall or mastoid wall:** Represents following features from above downwards:

I. Superiorly: Aditus to mastoid antrum.

II. Fossa incudis: Depression for incus.

III. Pyramid (projection): Apex of pyramid presents an opening for tendon of stapedius.

IV. Lateral to pyramid: Posterior canaliculus for chorda tympani.

e. **Lateral or membranous wall.**

I. Separates middle ear from external ear.

II. Formed mainly by:

i. Tympanic membrane.

ii. Partly by squamous part of temporal bone.

III. Near the tympanic notch, there are two apertures

i. Petrotympanic fissure.

ii. Anterior canaliculus for chorda tympani.

f. **Medial or labyrinthine wall:** It separates middle ear from internal ear. It presents following features (Fig. 18.6):

I. Promontory produced by 1st turn of cochlea.

II. Fenestra vestibuli: Oval opening leads to vestibule of internal ear.

III. Prominence of facial canal.

IV. Fenestra cochlea ends in scala tympani and closed by secondary tympanic membrane.

V. Sinus tympani depression behind promontory.

2. **Contents**

A. Air is the main and important content.

B. **Bone:** Ear ossicles namely malleus, incus and stapes.

C. Vessels, which supply and drain middle ear.

D. **Muscles:** Tensor tympani and stapedius.

E. Ligaments of ear ossicle.

F. Tympanic cavity proper: Lies opposite to tympanic membrane.

G. Epitympanic recess above tympanic membrane.

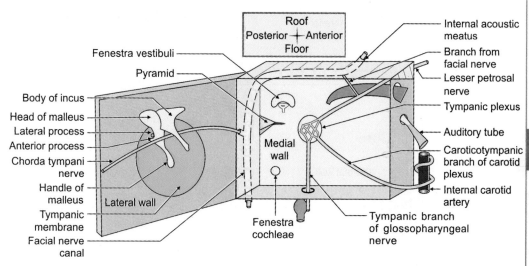

Fig. 18.6: Middle ear showing roof, anterior, posterior and medial walls

Note: Lateral wall is opened laterally

3. **Blood supply**

A. **Arterial supply**

   a. Main and large arteries

     I. Deep auricular

     II. Anterior tympanic } branch of 1st part of maxillary artery

     III. Posterior tympanic branch from stylomastoid, branch of posterior auricular artery.

   b. Small and less important arteries

     I. Superior tympanic (middle meningeal artery).

     II. Inferior tympanic (ascending pharyngeal).

     III. Tympanic branch (artery of pterygoid canal, branch of middle meningeal artery).

     IV. Caroticotympanic branch of internal carotid artery (ICA).

     V. Petrosal branch of middle meningeal artery.

B. **Venous drainage** : Veins from middle ear drain into:

   a. Superior petrosal sinus.

   b. Pterygoid plexus of vein.

4. **Nerve supply**: Tympanic plexus is formed by (Fig. 18.7)

A. Tympanic branch of glossopharyngeal nerve.

B. Caroticotympanic nerve (plexus around ICA).

5. **Applied anatomy** : Throat infections commonly spread to the middle ear through auditory tube, which are more common in children. In children, the tube is wide, small and horizontal. The pus may be discharged into one of the followings:

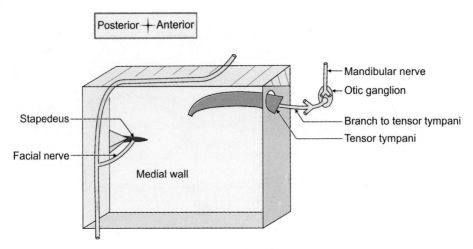

Fig. 18.7: Nerve supply of muscles of middle ear

➤ May be in the external ear following rupture of tympanic membrane.
➤ Posterior wall of middle ear is mastoid process. It contains mastoid air cells. They are not true air cells. They are air-filled pockets. It is related to posterior cranial fossa. The bone may be very thin and in some rare cases, it may be absent. The infection from middle ear can go posteriorly into mastoid air cells and may go to sigmoid air sinus present in posterior cranial fossa. It may end up in thrombophlebitis of sigmoid sinus and there may be severe and serious impairment of blood drainage of system. It can go back and produce infection of cerebellum.
➤ **Roof:** It is very thin and there is a petrosquamous suture. It may not be ossified and is weak in children and cause infection to spread to meninges or temporal lobe of brain. It results in
  • Extradural or subdural abscess.
  • Meningitis.
  • Temporal lobe abscess or infection (Fig. 18.8).
  • May erode the roof and results in meningitis.
  • May erode the floor and spread downward and causes thrombosis of internal jugular vein.
➤ Posterior wall
  • Mastoid air cells are connected to sigmoid sinus by emissary veins. The infection from posterior wall can go to sigmoid sinus and cause thrombosis.

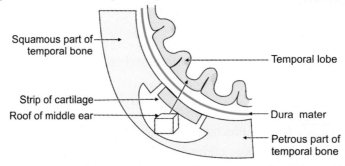

Fig. 18.8: Spread of infection from roof of middle ear to temporal lobe of cerebral cortex

Head, Neck and Face

• May cause mastoid abscess.
• Fracture of middle cranial fossa can cause bleeding through the ear.

SN-144 Muscles of tympanic cavity

1. **Tensor tympani**
   A. **Origin:** It lies in the bony canal and opens into anterior wall of middle ear. It arises from
      a. Bony canal
      b. Cartilaginous part of auditory tube.
      c. Inferior surface of greater wing of sphenoid bone.
   B. **Insertion:** Into upper end of handle of malleus.
   C. **Nerve supply**: The branch of the branch to medial pterygoid. Branch to medial pterygoid is a branch of mandibular nerve, arising from trunk.
   D. **Action:** It protects the ear from loud sound.

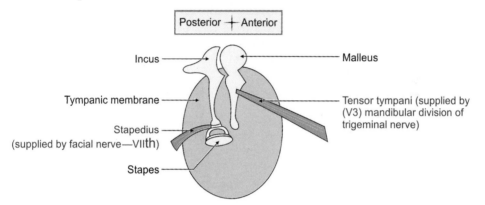

Fig. 18.9: Muscles of middle ear cavity

2. **Stapedius**
   A. **Origin:** It is a small muscle which lies in the bony canal. It arises from wall of bony canal.
   B. **Insertion:** Posterior surface of neck of stapes.
   C. **Nerve supply**: Branch of facial nerve.
   D. **Action:** It protects the ear from loud sound.
5. **Applied anatomy**: Paralysis of stapedius muscles gives rise to a condition called hyperacusis in which normal sound appears too loud.

SN-145 Spiral organ of Corti

Introduction: End organ for hearing.
1. **Gross:** It is located on basilar membrane of cochlear duct.
2. **Microscopic structure:** Consists of following parts (Fig. 18.10):
   A. **Basilar membrane:** Extends from osseous spiral lamina to the outer cochlear wall. It consists of collagen fibres.
   B. **Rods of Corti:** Enclose tunnel of Corti. The details of rods are as follows (Table 18.4).

Table 18.4: Details of inner and outer rods

Particulars	Inner rods (pillar)	Outer rods (pillar)
• Row	• Single	• Single
• Number	• 6000	• 4000

C. Hair cells are essential components of organ of Corti. It bears stereocilia.

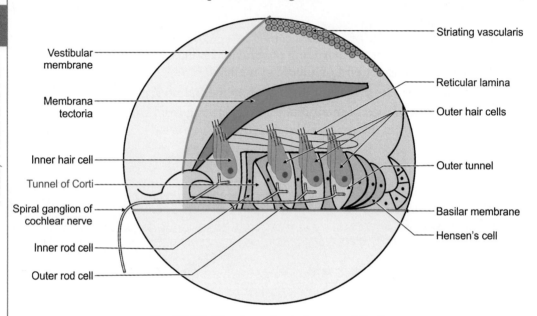

Fig. 18.10: Structure of spiral organ of Corti

3. **Functions**

   A. Detects the movements of endolymph.

   B. Detects the vibrations of basilar membrane.

   C. Transfers vibration into nerve impulse going to cochlear nerve.

4. The hair cells are divided into inner and outer hair cells.

Table 18.5: Details of inner and outer hair cells

Particular	Inner hair cells	Outer hair cells
• Situation	• Medial to inner rod of Corti	• Outer to outer rod of Corti
• Rows	• Single	• 3 to 4
• Number	• 3500	• 12000
• Shape	• Pear	• Cylindrical
• Type	• Predominantly afferent	• Afferent as well as efferent

Contd.

Table 18.5: Details of inner and outer hair cells (Contd.)

Particular	Inner hair cells	Outer hair cells
• Nerve supply	• Type I neuron • Frontal air sinus	• Type II, unmyelinated • Efferent from contralateral • Superior olivary nucleus
• Function	• Auditory sensation	• Auditory discrimination

SN-146 Cochlea

1. **Cochlea:** Shell of snail. Shape: conical ▲; 2 and 3/4 turns (Fig. 18.11).

2. **Location:** Anterior to the vestibule.
    A. Apex is towards anterosuperior part of the medial wall of middle ear.
    B. Base is at the floor of internal acoustic meatus, perforated by cochlear nerve.

3. **Dimension**
    A. From base to apex 5 mm.
    B. Width 9 mm (at base).

4. **Structure**
    A. **Central bony axis:** Modiolus (axis of wheel) with spiral bony canal around. The bony canal is divided into three channels which are spirally arranged.

    a. **Scala media (cochlear duct):** ▲ lar, bounded by
        I. Basilar membrane attached to osseous spiral lamina.
        II. Vestibular or Reissner's membrane.
        III. Outer wall of cochlea lies between basilar and vestibular membranes.

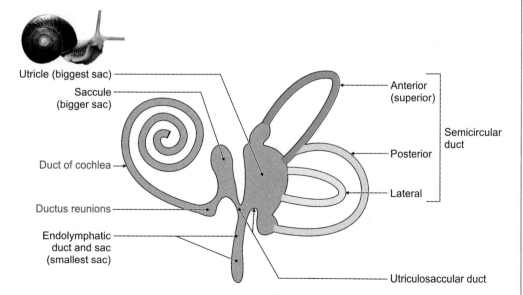

Fig. 18.11: Cochlea

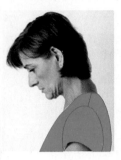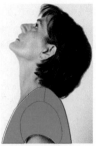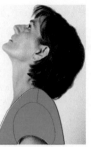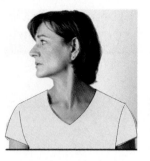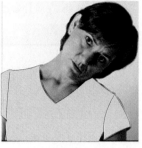

Deflection of fluid in superior semicircular canal detects when the head moves up and down

Deflection of fluid in lateral semicircular canal detects when the head turns to the left/right side

Deflection of fluid in posterior semicircular canal detects when the head tilts to the side

Fig. 18.12: Deflection of fluid in various semicircular canal

IV. The apex of the cochlea is blind. It contains endolymph.

V. Spiral organ of Corti lies on basilar membrane.

b. **Scala vestibuli**

  I. Canal above scala media.

  II. Communicates with

    i. Bony vestibule at base;

    ii. With scala tympani at apex of cochlea through *helicotrema* (spiral opening).

c. *Scala tympani:* Canal below scala media separated from the middle ear cavity by secondary tympanic membrane. Both scala vestibuli and scala tympani are filled with perilymph.

d. *Modiolus:* It is broad at the base, narrow at the apex, contains blood vessels and spiral ganglion. It gives out osseous spiral lamina which is attached to basilar membrane.

5. **Openings at basal turn of bony cochlea**

  A. **Oval window:** Occupied by foot plate of stapes.

  B. **Round window:** Closed by secondary tympanic membrane.

  C. **Cochlear canaliculus:** Communicates scala tympani with subarachnoid space.

Eyeball

OLA-83 What is glaucoma?

Raised intraocular pressure is called glaucoma. It may be due to
• Excessive production of aqueous humour, or
• Lack of its drainage, or
Combination of both raises the intraocular pressure.

OLA-84 What is lamina fusca of sclera?

It is thin layer of loose, pigmented cellular connective tissue. It is present in the perichoroidal space. It is delicate tissue. It is also called suprachoroidal lamina.

OLA-85 What is retinal detachment?

It is separation of single pigmented layer from remaining layers of retina. It is actually inter-retinal detachment.

OLA-86 What is fovea centralis?

(*Fovea* a pit or depression)
1. The centre of the macula is depressed to form the fovea centralis.
2. This is the thinnest part of the retina.
3. It contains cones only and is the site of maximum acuity (sharpness of vision).

Box 19.1
Fovea—FON—Fovea, Only cones

OLA-87 What is blind spot?

1. The depressed area of the optic disc is called the physiological cup.
2. It contains no rods and cones. It does not have sensory receptors, and is, therefore, insensitive to light.
3. It is the physiological blind spot.

OLA-88 **What is cataract?**

Increase in opacity of lens is called cataract. It occurs with increase in age.

OLA-89 **What is arcus senilis?**

It is a grey or white opaque ring in the corneal margin. It is present at birth or appears in later part of life. It is common after 50. It results from cholesterol deposit.

OLA-90 **Black eye (echymosis of the eye)**

1. **Definition:** It is small haemorrhagic spot, in the skin or mucous membrane. It is non-elevated, irregular blue or purplish patch.
2. **Cause:** It is the result of collection of blood in this space. It tends to gravitate in the eyelid. It is caused
   A. Due to local violence causing subcutaneous extravasation of blood into the eyelids. This is the most common cause. Haemorrhage occurs soon after the receipt of an injury and black discolouration of eyelids may occur within few hours of injury.
   B. Fracture of the anterior cranial fossa may cause bleeding.
   C. Bleeding in the loose areolar tissue of scalp causes generalized swelling of the scalp. The blood may extend anteriorly into the root of the nose and into the eyelids. This is because frontalis muscle has no bony origin.
   D. A blow to the superciliary arches (e.g. during boxing) may lacerate the skin and cause bleeding.

OLA-91 **Name the types of glands seen in eyelid. Classify them, state their mode of secretion and give their alternative names. Write the answers in a tabular form.**

Table 19.1: Glands in the eyelid and their details

Gland	Synonyms	Location	Classification	Mode of secretion
• Accessory lacrimal gland	• Glands of Wolfring or Krauses gland	• Above tarsal plate	• Serous	
• Tarsal gland	• Meibomian gland	• Tarsal plate	• Modified sebaceous gland	• Holocrine
• Sebaceous gland	• Glands of Zeiss	• Eyelash		• Holocrine
• Ciliary gland	• Glands of Moll	• Free margin of lid	• Modified sweat gland	• Apocrine

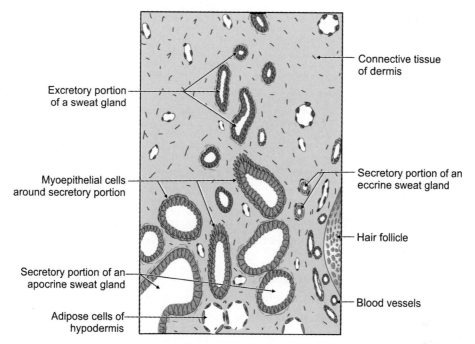

Fig. 19.1: Apocrine sweat gland: Secretory and excretory portions of the sweat gland. Stain: Hematoxylin and eosin. Medium magnification

OLA-92 **Enumerate the types of muscles seen in eyelid.**

Palpebral part of the orbicularis oculi muscle (skeletal muscle).

SN-147 **Orbicularis oculi**

(*Orbiculus*—orbit, *oculi*—eyeball)
Introduction: It is a muscle of face, the sphincter of orbital fissure.

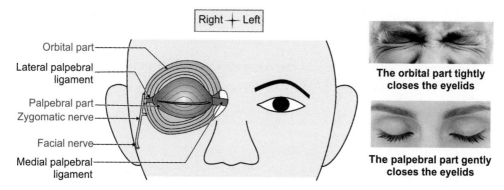

Fig. 19.2: Right orbicularis oculi

1. **Attachment:** It has three parts:
   A. **Palpebral part:** It is confined to the lids. It arises from medial palpebral ligament. It is inserted into lateral palpebral raphe.

B. **Orbital part:** It extends beyond orbit. It arises from
  a. Nasal part of frontal bone
  b. Anterior lacrimal crest
  c. Frontal process of maxilla
      I. It forms concentric rings and return to the point of origin.
C. **Lacrimal part** (deeper part): It is attached medially to the
  a. Posterior lacrimal crest
  b. Lacrimal sac
  They are inserted into upper and lower eyelids.

2. **Nerve supply**
  A. Mainly by zygomatic branch of facial nerve.
  B. It is also supplied by temporal branch of facial nerve.
3. **Actions**
  A. Palpebral part closes the eyelid gently.
  B. Orbital and palpebral part together closes the eyelid forcibly.
  C. Levator palpebrae superioris is the opponent of upper palpebral fibres of orbicularis oculi.
      Occipitofrontalis opposes the orbital part.
4. **Development:** They are developed from the mesoderm of the 2nd pharyngeal arch.

5. **Applied anatomy**: Infranuclear lesion to the facial nerve leads to paralysis of orbicularis oculi. Hence, the patient cannot close the eyelid tightly. Frequent closure of eyelids is required for the normal drainage of tears through the lacrimal ducts. Due to paralysis of orbicularis oculi, there is overflowing of tears through the eyelid.

SN-148 Fascial sheath of eyeball

Introduction: It is a thin fascial sheath surrounding the eyeball and separating it from the orbital fat.
Synonym: Tenon'scapsule, fascia bulbi.
1. **Attachments**
  A. **Anteriorly:** Sclera just behind the corneoscleral junction.
  B. **Posteriorly:** Fused with the dura mater.
2. **Structures piercing**
  A. Optic nerve.
  B. Ciliary vessels, and
  C. Tendons of
      a. Four recti and
      b. Two obliquii
3. **Supports of eyeball**
  A. **Medial and lateral check ligaments:** They are thickening of fascial covering of medial and lateral recti, respectively.

Head, Neck and Face

B. **Suspensory ligament of Lockwood:** It is thickening of inferior rectus with thickening of inferior oblique with the medial and lateral check ligaments. They act as a hammock like support to the eyeball.

4. Applied anatomy

> In case of the fracture of the orbit, the eyeball does not sag, if the suspensory ligament is intact.
> The fracture of the orbit associated with paralysis of inferior rectus manifests as double vision.

SAQ-2 What is the reason of papilloedema in raised intracranial tension?

1. Increased intracranial tension, papilloedema or choked disc is due to acutely obstructed venous return. The causes are
    A. Venous engorgement
    B. Retinal haemorrhages
2. Increased intracranial pressure is transmitted to the subarachnoid space around the optic nerve.
    A. There is excess of fluid in the subarachnoid space which extends as far as the lamina cribrosa sclerae.
    B. Venous return is through the central vein of the retina. It is blocked.
    C. There is leakage of fluid around the
        a. Optic disc, and
        b. Retina.
    D. Ophthalmoscopy examination shows
        a. Engorged veins,
        b. Swelling of the disc, and
        c. Obliteration of the physiological cup.
        This is known as *papilloedema.*

OLA-93 What is the applied importance of cornea?

Applied importance of cornea

1. Indications of corneal transplant
    A. Defective cornea interferes with the normal vision.
    B. Healthy cornea from a dead person (through eye donation).
2. The corneas are most common and successful organ transplants because of following reasons
    A. Cornea is avascular.
    B. There is no immunological reaction after corneal transplantation.
3. **Protection of cornea by ferritin:** Melanin pigment is absent in cornea. Melanin protects from ultraviolet light rays. Since eye is continuously exposed to UV light, it is likely to damage the DNA of nuclei.

Head, Neck and Face

4. Ferritin, an iron storage protein, is present in the eye. It prevents the damage of DNA present in nuclei. Therefore, the carcinoma of corneal epithelium is very rare.

SN-149 Cornea

1. It forms anterior 1/6th of the outer coat of eyeball. Cornea is transparent because of following reasons:

   A. Regular arrangement of fibres.

   B. Refractive index of ground substance and fibres is same.

   C. Thickness of each fibril is less than wavelength of light.

   D. Critical level of water is maintained by active absorption of water by endothelium.

   E. No blood vessels.

2. **Peculiarities:** Cornea has

   A. No blood vessels,

   B. No lymphatics, and

   C. Rich nerve supply. Nerves are non-myelinated.

3. **Layers:** There are **6** layers of the cornea.   A B C DD E

   A. **A**nterior epithelium (external epithelial layer):

      a. Stratified, squamous non-keratinised epithelium.

      b. Superficial cells are squamous and have flat nuclei.

      c. Deeper cells are columnar and have rod-shaped nuclei ▃▃▃▃.

      d. Cells rest on linear basement membrane.

      e. Cells never keratinise.

      f. Contain numerous *free nerve endings; hence, this layer is extremely sensitive.*

   B. **B**owman's membrane (anterior limiting membrane)

      a. Epithelium rests on this layer.

      b. Structure less, transparent and homogenous membrane.

      c. Contains collagen fibres which are produced by substantia propria.

   C. **C**onnective tissue proper (substantia propria)

      a. Main substance of cornea.

      b. Present deep to Bowman's membrane.

      c. Modified, transparent, flattened connective tissue.

      d. The connective tissue contains dens collagen fibres containing corneal spaces.

      e. It contains 200–250 lamellae and about 2000 fibres. It is embedded in ground substance containing sulphated glycosaminoglycans.

      f. The collagen fibres are of Type II (diameters 20 nm.)

      g. Arrangement of fibres is very regular.

      h. Fibres within lamellae are parallel to one another and are at obtuse angle to those of fibres adjacent to lamellae.

i. Contains fibroblast which is stellate or flat. They are also called keratocytes or corneal corpuscles or corneocytes.

D. <u>D</u>ua's layer (Dr Harminder Dua): It is strongest layer measuring 7 to 14 micron. It creates strongest barrier.

E. **<u>D</u>escemet's membrane**
   a. Formed by homogeneous material.
   b. Membrane breaks at the margin of the cornea into fibres which form inner wall of sinus venous sclera.
   c. Spaces between these trabeculae are called the *spaces of iridocorneal angle*.

F. **<u>E</u>ndothelium of anterior chamber**
   a. Bathed by aqueous humour. Hence, it is not a true endothelium.
   b. It is single layer.
   c. It is metabolically most active.[NEET]
   d. Lined by low cuboidal epithelium.
   e. Adapted for transport of ions.

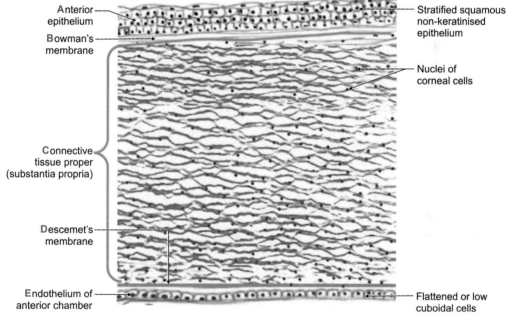

Fig. 19.3: Histology of cornea

OLA-94 **Layer of rods and cones consists of what?**

These are the photoreceptors; they pass through the external limiting membrane. Rods and cones are light receptors of the eye.

1. **The cones respond to** ⟨🔑 ABC⟩

   <u>A</u>cuity of vision.
   <u>B</u>rightness of vision.
   <u>C</u>olour vision.

2. Ro<u>d</u>s respond to <u>D</u>im light.

OLA-95 Draw pictures of rods and cones

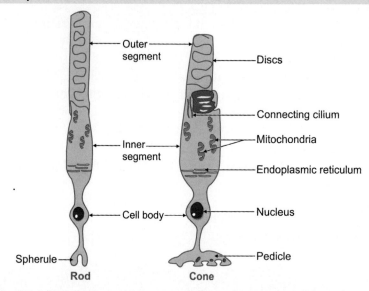

Fig. 19.4: The main parts of rods and cones (schematic representation)

OLA-96 What are the functions of pigment epithelium of retina?

1. It absorbs excessive light.
2. It prevents reflection of light.
3. It may play a role in regular spacing of rods and cones.
4. It provides mechanical support to rods and cones.
5. It has a phagocytic role. It "eats up" the ends of rods and cones.
6. It produces melanin.

OLA-97 Enumerate the neurons seen in retina.

1. Rods and cones
2. Bipolar neurons
3. Ganglion
4. Optic nerve

OLA-98 What are the cells in outer nuclear layer, inner nuclear layer and ganglion cell layer?

1. **Outer nuclear layer:** This layer consists of nuclei of photoreceptors.
2. **Inner nuclear layer:** It contains nuclei of
   A. Bipolar cells,
   B. Muller cells,
   C. Horizontal cells: They establish contact between different photoreceptors in the outer plexiform layer.

D. Amacrine cells (*A*—neg. + Gr. *makros*—long). Having no long processes. They connect ganglion cells and bipolar neurons to each other in the inner plexiform layer.

3. **Ganglionic cell layer:** This layer consists of large cell bodies of ganglion cells.

OLA-99 **Plexuses between processes of which cells are formed in outer and inner plexiform layers?**

1. **Outer plexiform layer:** The processes of adjoining gliocytes meet to form a thin external limiting membrane.
2. **Inner plexiform layer:** It is formed by synapse of axons of bipolar cells with the dendrites of ganglion cells.

OLA-100 **Layer of optic nerve fibres is formed by which processes of which cells?**

Axons of the ganglion cells travel in this layer towards the optic disc.

OLA-101 **What are outer and inner limiting membranes?**

1. **Outer limiting membrane** is a sieve-like membrane.
   A. It is present between 2nd and 3rd layer of retina.
   B. It looks like a pink linear marking lamina.
   C. It is a thin external limiting membrane.
   D. It is formed by
      a. Glial cells known as Muller cells with the
      b. Cell bodies of photoreceptor cells.
2. **Inner limiting membrane**
   A. It consists of the processes of Muller cells.
   B. Internally, the gliocytes extend to the internal surface of the retina and form an internal limiting membrane.
   C. This membrane separates the retina from the vitreous.
   D. The retinal gliocytes are neuroglial in nature.
   E. They support the neurons of the retina and may ensheath them.
   F. They probably have a nutritive function as well.

SN-150 **Retina**

It has 10 layers.
1. **Pigment cell layer:** It is single layer of cuboidal cells. The cells have rounded nuclei and the apical cytoplasm contains melanin granules.
2. **Layer of rods and cones**
   A. Rods and cones are light receptors of the eye.
   B. **The cones respond to** ⊶ ABC
      <u>A</u>cuity of vision.
      <u>B</u>rightness of vision.
      <u>C</u>olour vision.
   C. Ro<u>D</u>s respond to <u>d</u>im light.

Layers of retina

> **Box 19.2**
> **Outer L N P –Alternate letter after L, Inner N P**

3. **Outer limiting membrane:** Contains lateral process of radial fibres of nuclear cells.
4. **Outer nuclear layer:** Contains cell bodies of rods and cones which contain photosensitive process of neurons.
5. **Outer plexiform layer:** Contains axonal process of rods and cones, dendrites of bipolar.
6. **Inner nuclear layer:** It contains
   A. Cell bodies and nuclei of bipolar neurons (2nd order neurons of visual pathway).
   B. **Association neurons**
      a. Horizontal cells.
      b. Amacrine cells.
   C. Supporting cells (Muller's cells)

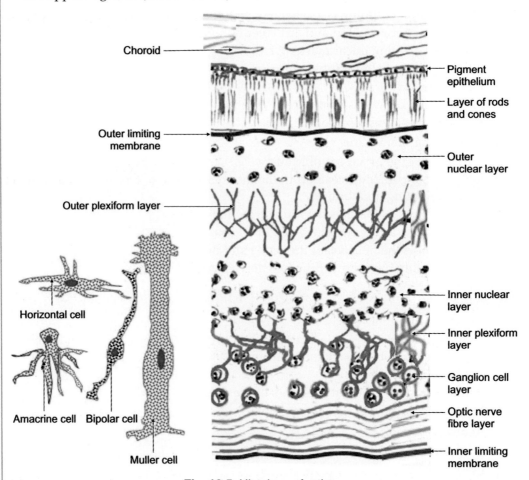

Fig. 19.5: Histology of retina

7. **Inner plexiform layer:** Contains synapse between axons of bipolar cells and also process of association cells or amacrine cells.

8. **Ganglion cell layer:** Contains cell bodies of ganglion cells. These are large multipolar cells with prominent Nissl's granules. The axons of ganglion layer form the optic nerve.

9. **Optic nerve layer:** Contains optic nerve fibres and Muller's fibres.

10. **Inner limiting membrane:** The surface facing next layer is thrown into processes which insinuate between rods and cones. It prevents diffusion of light. It is innermost layer of retina and represents a basal lamina formed by the expanded inner ends of Muller cells.

OLA-102 Name the different layers of eyelid.

1. **Skin**

   A. It forms the anterior surface.

   B. It is hairless except along margins of lid.

   C. Margins of lid have 3 to 4 rows of hair—eyelashes.

   D. It has modified sweat glands—the glands of Moll and sebaceous gland of Zeiss.

2. **Muscle layer**

   A. Orbicularis oculi, and

   B. Levator palpebrae superioris.

3. **Tarsal plate**

   A. It is dense connective tissue.

   B. It gives support to eyelids.

   C. It has sebaceous glands called tarsal glands or Meibomian glands. The ducts of these glands open into free margin of eyelid. The oily secretion forms a thin layer over tear and prevents evaporation of tears.

4. **Conjunctiva**

   A. It forms the posterior layer.

   B. It is lined by stratified columnar or cuboidal epithelium.

OLA-103 What is the nerve supply of eyelid?

1. The upper eyelid is supplied by the following nerves (from lateral to medial side).

   A. Lacrimal nerve, branch of ophthalmic division of trigeminal nerve.

   B. Supraorbital, branch of frontal nerve.

   C. Supratrochlear, branch of frontal nerve

   D. Infratrochlear nerves, smaller terminal branch of nasociliary nerve.

2. The lower eyelid is supplied by the

   A. Infraorbital nerve: It is the continuation of maxillary nerve, and

   B. Infratrochlear nerves: These are smaller terminal branches of nasociliary nerve.

Head, Neck and Face

OLA-104 Why the oedema in nephrotic syndrome appears first on face and eyelids?

1. Laxity of the greater part of skin of eyelid and face facilitates spread of oedema. Hence, oedema in nephrotic syndrome appears first in the face.
2. Superficial fascia of the eyelid is devoid of fat and composed of loose tissue. Hence, oedema of the eyelid is very common.

OLA-105 What is the advantage of blinking of eyelids?

Blinking of eyelids helps in uniform spread of tears over the eyeball and keeps the eyeball moist.

SN-151 Eyelid

Features

1. Both the surfaces of the eyelid are covered by epithelium.
   A. Skin of the eyelid is covered by stratified squamous keratinised epithelium.
   B. Mucous membrane of the eyelid is lined by stratified columnar epithelium.
2. Skeleton is formed by a mass of fibrous tissue called tarsus or tarsal plate.
3. Fat cells are absent in the subepithelial connective tissue.
4. Arrector pilorum muscle is absent in the hair follicle.
5. Glands: **A To Z**
   A. Accessory lacrimal glands are present. They are also called glands of Wolfring or Krause's gland. They are serous in nature.
   B. Tarsal glands (Meibomian gland): It is a modified sebaceous gland.
   C. **Glands of Zeiss:** These are sebaceous glands present along the eyelashes.
   D. **Moll's gland:** These are modified sweat glands.

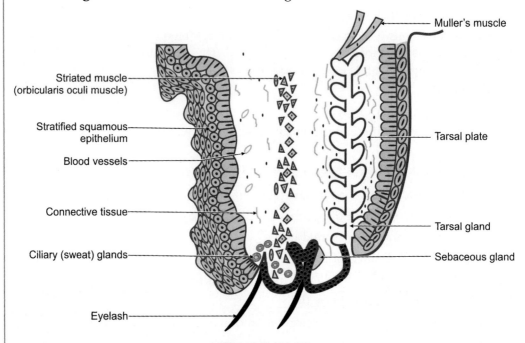

Fig. 19.6: Eyelid

OLA-106 What is the significance of colour of conjunctiva?

1. The *conjunctiva* is a moist, transparent membrane.
   A. The part lining the lids is called palpebral conjunctiva.
   B. The part lining the sclera is called the ocular or bulbar conjunctiva.
2. Significance of conjunctiva
   A. The conjunctiva is colourless, except when its vessels are dilated
      a. Eyes inflamed or tinged with blood is called "bloodshot eyes". It is congested conjunctiva.
      b. Hyperaemia of the conjunctiva is due to local irritation (e.g. from dust, chlorine, or smoke).
      c. Conjunctivitis ("pink eye") is contagious infection of the eye.
   B. Bulbar conjunctiva
      a. It is vascular.
      b. Inflammation of the conjunctiva leads to conjunctivitis.
      c. It is used to assess the depth of jaundice.
   C. Palpebral conjunctiva
      a. It is normally red and vascular.
      b. The look of palpebral conjunctiva is used to judge haemoglobin level.
      c. It is commonly examined in cases of suspected anaemia, a blood condition commonly manifested by pallor (paleness) of the mucous membranes.

SN-152 Sclerocorneal junction

1. It is junction of transparent cornea and opaque sclera (Fig. 19.7).
2. **At the junction**
   A. There is change of epithelium to that of conjunctiva.
      a. **The epithelium of the palpebral conjunctiva is typically two layered**
         I. Superficial columnar cells, and
         II. Deep flattened cells.
      b. **The epithelium of the sclera and fornix is three layered**
         I. Superficial columnar,
         II. Middle polygonal, and
         III. Deep flattened cells.
      c. At sclerocorneal junction: Stratified squamous epithelium.
      d. At cornea
         I. Anterior epithelium is stratified squamous non-keratinised.
         II. Posterior epithelium—cuboidal.
   B. Bowman's membrane changes into subepithelial layer of connective tissue.
   C. Collagenous bundles of the sclera continue as collagenous bundles of cornea. They become parallel with each other and appear homogenous and transparent.
   D. Posterior lip forms a projecting ridge in which the ciliary body is fastened.

Head, Neck and Face

E. Descemet's membrane terminates into trabecular meshwork. It encloses small spaces known as spaces of Fontana.
   a. They are lined by attenuated epithelium.
   b. They communicate with the anterior chamber of eye.
   c. There are several small cavities. They are lined by epithelium. They are anterior and lateral to trabecular meshwork. These cavities are the cross-sections of a circular canal. The canal is called *canal of Schlemm*. They are parallel to the cornea. The canal communicates with the venous spaces and is usually filled with clear aqueous humour.

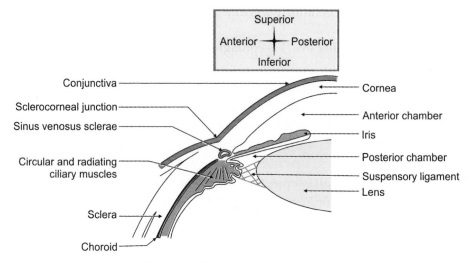

Fig. 19.7: Sclerocorneal junction

Table 19.2: Features of spaces of Fontana and canal of Schlemm

Particulars	Spaces of Fontana	Canal of Schlemm
• Shape	• Irregular	• Circular
• Position	• At the termination of Descemet's membrane at the sclerocorneal junction	• At anterior and lateral to the trabecular network
• Lining	• Attenuated epithelium	• Living epithelium
• Number	• Less	• More
• Size	• Small	• Small
• Communication with	• Anterior chamber	• Venous spaces.
• Content		• Clear aqueous humour

SN-153 **Give the nerve supply of iris**

1. Nerve supply of iris (Fig. 19.8)

   A. The long ciliary nerves convey the sensory fibres.
   B. Motor fibres to

a. Dilator pupillae are derived from sympathetic nerves.

b. Sphincter pupillae are derived from parasympathetic nerve.

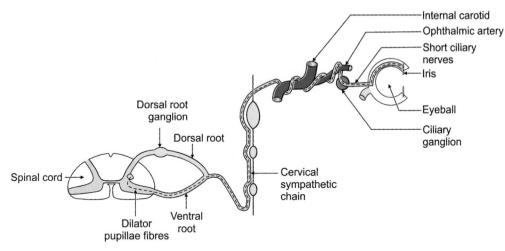

Fig. 19.8: Nerve supply of iris

2. Applied anatomy

> The injury to the cervical cord produces pupillary changes.

> Injury distal to the lowest trunk of brachial plexus does not produce pupillary changes.

> Constriction of pupil is one of the manifestations of Horner's syndrome. It results from paralysis of cervical sympathetic nerves (T1 fibres).

SN-154 Give the histology feature of olfactory epithelium.

1. The olfactory epithelium is pseudostratified. It is much **thicker** than the epithelium lining the respiratory system. There are three types of cells.

A. **Olfactory cells:** These are modified neurons. It has

a. Central part containing a rounded nucleus. The nuclei lie at various levels in basal two-thirds of the epithelium (Fig. 19.9).

b. Two processes

I. Proximal process represents the axon.

II. Distal process ends in a thickening called the rod or knob. Rods give rise to cilia.

c. Olfactory cells have short life. They are replaced by new cells produced by division of basal cells. **This is the only example of regeneration of neurons in mammals.**

B. **Sustentacular cells:** They support olfactory cells.

a. The nuclei are oval and lie on the free surface of the epithelium.

b. The cytoplasm contains yellow pigment. It gives yellow colour to olfactory mucosa.

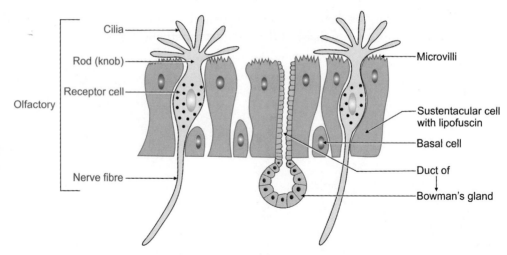

Fig. 19.9: Olfactory epithelium

C. **Basal cells**: They are placed deep. They do not reach the luminal surface. They divide to form new olfactory cells to replace dead.

SN-155 Development of eye

1. **Chronological age:** Fourth week of intrauterine life.
2. **Germ layers**
   A. **Surface ectoderm gives rise to L_3Ec_2**
      a. Lens
      b. Lacrimal apparatus
         I. Lacrimal gland
         II. Lacrimal sac
         III. Lacrimal duct
      c. Lid and its gland
      d. Epithelium of the
         I. Conjunctival sac
         II. Cornea.
   B. **Mesoderm**
      a. Choroid
      b. Hyaloid artery. It regresses it before birth. Remnant or hyaloid artery
         i. Muscae volitantes: Incomplete regression
         ii. Mittendorf's dot: Posterior pole at end.
         iii. Bergemeister's papilla: Attachments at optic disc
         iv. Persistent hyaline artery
         v. Tunica vasculosa lentis
         vi. Persistent pupillary membrane: Remnant of mesoderm.
         vii. Persistent hyperplastic primary vitreous

c. Temporal part of sclera

d. Fleshy belly of extraocular muscles.

C. **Neuroectoderm gives rise to**

a. RPE: Retinal pigment epithelium develops from outer lip of optic cup

b. Inner lip of optic cup: Neurosensory retina—all layers of retina

c. Ciliary epithelium

d. Iris epithelium

e. Sphincter pupillae

f. Dilator pupillae

g. Zonule: Tertiary vitreous

h. Vitreous gel: Secondary vitreous

i. Subretinal space

j. Optic stalk gives optic nerve.

D. Neural crest cells. They migrate to final destination.

a. Corneal endothelium

b. Trabecular meshwork

c. Descemet's membrane

d. Corneal stroma

e. Bowman's membrane

f. Iris stroma

g. Ciliary muscle

h. Ciliary storma

i. Sclera

j. Tendon of the extraocular muscle

k. Tenon's capsule

l. Oligodendrocytes

m. Meninges of optic nerve

n. Ciliary ganglion

o. Orbital bones

p. Melanocytes of iris.

E. Arrest or failure of neural cell migration

a. Congenital Horner's syndrome.

b. Neurocristopathy:

I. Congenital aniridia

II. Axenfeld-Rieger syndrome

3. **Source**

A. **Forebrain vesicle gives rise to**

a. Retina, and

b. Optic nerve,

4. Anomalies

A. **Coloboma (mutilation, defect):** Defective closure of optic fissure, site—ventromedial segment.

a. Coloboma of optic disc: It is congenital. Morning glory flower: Vessels come straight.

b. Chorioretinal coloboma: It favours retinal detachment.

c. Iris coloboma: Most commonly located.

  I. It is incomplete coloboma.

  II. Pear or tear shaped

  III. It is associated with lens coloboma.

B. **The causes of congenital cataract may be**

a. Hereditary

b. Infection by rubella virus.

C. **Astigmatism:** Faulty curvature of cornea or lens produces astigmatism.

D. **Rare anomalies are**

a. **Anophthalmos:** Absence of eye.

b. **Aphakia:** Absence of lens.

c. **Aniridia:** Absence of iris.

d. **Synophthalmia:** Fusion of eyes.

e. **Cyclopia:** Median eye.

f. **Microphthalmia:** Too small eye.

LAQ-45 Describe eyeball under the following heads:
1. Outer coat,
2. Middle coat, and
3. Inner coat

Coats: Eyeball has three coats (Fig. 19.10)

1. Outer coat

   A. Sclera

   B. Cornea

2. Middle coat

   A. Choroid

   B. Ciliary body

   C. Iris

3. Inner coat:

   A. Retina

   B. Lens

   C. Aqueous humour

1. **Outer coat**
   A. **Sclera (hard)**
      a. **External features**
         I. It is smooth and white in colour. It forms 5/6th of the fibrous layer.
         II. It receives insertion of
            i. Four recti muscles in front of the equator, and
            ii. Two obliques—behind the equator.
      b. **Ends**
         I. Anterior end continues with cornea at the sclerocorneal junction.
         II. Posterior end continues with dura mater of the optic nerve.
      c. **Surfaces**
         I. *Outer surface* is covered by a Tenon's fascia. The space between Tenon's fascia and sclera is called episcleral space or sub-Tenon's space. It is traversed by fibrous strands.
         II. *Inner surface* is covered by perichoroidal space. It is traversed by connective tissue that contains pigment cells. It is brown and has grooves for ciliary vessels and nerves.
      d. **Perforating structures**
         I. Optic nerve—3 mm medial to centre of the posterior aspect of sclera.
         II. Ciliary vessels and nerves—around the exit of the optic nerve.
         III. 2 or 5 venae vorticosae.
      e. **Lamina cribrosa** (*cribrum*—L. sieve): Posterior part of the sclera is perforated by structures. It gives the appearance of a sieve. The structures piercing are
            i. Optic nerve
            ii. Central artery, and
            iii. Vein of the retina.
               ✚ Applied anatomy: The lamina cribrosa is weak. In glaucoma, there is increased intraocular pressure. This results in bulging of the lamina outwards.
      f. **Sinus venosus sclerae:**
         I. There is an important venous structure at the sclerocorneal junction called *sinus venosus sclerae (canal of Schlemm)*.
         II. It is lined by endothelium.
         III. Between *canal of Schlemm* and the anterior chamber, there is only a meshwork. It is formed by trabeculated (partitioned) tissue.
         IV. The aqueous humour (*liquid*) > anterior chamber > trabeculated tissue > venous system.
         V. ✚ Applied anatomy: Any form of obstruction to this drainage may lead to a rise in intraocular pressure (*glaucoma*).
   B. **Cornea**
      a. **Features**
         I. It forms anterior 1/6th of the outer coat of eyeball. It is transparent because of the following reasons. Cornea ART

Head, Neck and Face

i. Critical level of water is maintained. It is done by active absorption of water by endothelium.

ii. Arrangement of fibres is regular.

iii. Refractive index of ground substance and fibres is same.

iv. Thickness of each fibril is less than wavelength of light.

II. **Peculiarities:** It has

i. No blood vessels. Nutrition is by aqueous humour.

ii. No lymphatics

iii. ✚ Therefore, cornea can be easily transplanted.

iv. Rich nerve supply. Nerves are non-myelinated.

III. **Layers:** There are **6** layers of the cornea. ⚷ A B C DD E

A̲nterior epithelium,

B̲owman's membrane (anterior limiting membrane),

C̲onnective tissue proper (substantia propria),

D̲escemet's membrane (true basement membrane)

D̲ua's layer

E̲ndothelium of anterior chamber

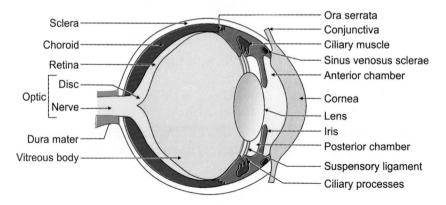

Fig. 19.10: Sagittal section showing coats of the eyeball

2. **Middle coat:** It is also called uveal tract (*uvea*—grape) or pigmented layer of eye. It consists of

A. **Choroid** (pigmented vascular layer of eyeball) (Fig. 19.11)

a. **Features**

I. It is present in the posterior 5/6th of the eyeball.

II. It is thin pigmented layer that lines the posterior part of sclera.

III. It is a vascular membrane of dark brown colour.

IV. It lines the inner surface of the sclera.

V. It can be readily stripped up.

VI. It is brown in man and black in many animals.

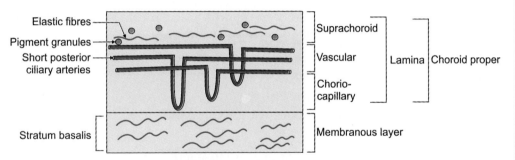

Fig. 19.11: Structure of choroid

b. **Surfaces:** It has two surfaces—outer and inner.

   I. The **outer surface** is loosely connected with the sclera by **suprachoroid membrane.** It is also called **lamina fusca** of the sclera.

   II. The **inner surface** is attached to the pigment layer of the retina.

c. **Histology of choroid:** It consists of masses of blood vessels sandwiched between two avascular membranes. From external to internal, they are:

   I. **Suprachoroid lamina**

     i. It is a non-vascular lamina of vascular coat.

     ii. It consists of elastic fibres having pigment granules.

       • Between the suprachoroid lamina and choroid proper, there is a thin layer of connective tissue called the **stratum intermedium**.

   II. **Choroid proper:** It consists of two layers

     i. The outer layer is called the **vascular lamina or stratum vasculosum.** It consists of larger arteries and veins, namely

       • Branches of short posterior ciliary arteries and

       • Veins which unite to form 4 to 5 large veins called venae vorticosae, and

       • Pigment cells.

     ii. The inner layer is called the **choriocapillary lamina**.

       • It is formed by capillary plexuses derived from branches of short posterior ciliary arteries.

   III. **Stratum basalis**

     i. It is a membranous layer of elastic fibres.

     ii. It lies on the outer surface of the pigmented layer of the retina.

     iii. It consists of cells or fibres deep to the choriocapillary lamina.

   IV. **Tapetum**

     i. In many animals, e.g. in bullock's eye, the back part of the choroid presents tapetum.

     ii. It reflects light and gives it a greenish appearance.

       ✚ **Uveitis:** It is inflammation of vascular layer of the eyeball. It may progress to severe visual impairment and blindness.

Head, Neck and Face

B. **Ciliary body:** The anterior end of the middle vascular coat is dilated and called ciliary body. It consists of the following structures.

  a. **Ciliary ring**

    I. It is a circular ring of 4 mm breadth.

    II. It is marked with ridges.

    III. Posteriorly, it is continuous with the choroid.

  b. **Ciliary processes**

    I. These are formed by infoldings of the layers of the choroid.

    II. They are 60 to 80 in number.

    III. **Types of fibre:** Short and long.

    IV. **Ends**

      i. Peripheral end of the process is attached to the ciliary ring.

      ii. Central ends of the processes are free. They are directed towards the posterior chamber of the eyeball and circumference of the lens.

    V. **Surfaces**

      i. Its anterior surface is continuous with the iris at its periphery.

      ii. Its posterior surface is connected with the suspensory ligament of the lens.

    VI. **Function:** The ciliary processes secrete the **aqueous humour,**

  c. **Ciliary muscles**

    I. Types of muscle. It consists of two sets:

      i. Radiating, and

      ii. Circular.

        i. Radiating fibres: They lie outside. They are attached

          • Anteriorly to scleral spur.

          • Posteriorly to ciliary ring and ciliary processes.

        ii. Circular fibres

          • These lie on the inner side of the radiating fibres.

          • They are arranged as a circular ring behind the iridocorneal angle.

          • It is close to the circumference of the iris.

           ✚ Circular fibres are well-developed in the hypermetropic and more or less absent in the myopic.

    II. **Action of ciliary muscles:** Accommodation of eye for near objects. This is done by changing the curvature of the lens. As the ciliary muscles contract, they draw the ciliary processes forwards. This causes the relaxation of the suspensory ligament of the lens. So, the anterior aspect of the lens will be more convex.

C. **Iris** (diaphragm)

  a. **Definition:** It is a **musculovascular contractile diaphragm** between the cornea and the lens (Fig. 19.12).

b. **Shape and situation:** It is a thin circular disc suspended in the aqueous humour between the cornea and lens.

c. **Pupil:** It is a circular aperture in the iris.

  I. **Surfaces**

    i. **Anterior surface:** It is convex and forms the posterior boundary of the anterior chamber of the eyeball.

    ii. **Posterior surface:** It is concave and forms the anterior boundary of the posterior chamber of the eyeball.

  II. **Colour:** It is produced by the reflection of light from the pigment cells and varies from individual to individual.

    i. White eyes: It is du e to absence of pigments.

    ii. Brown, black or grey eyes: Pigments lie in the stroma of the iris.

    iii. Blue eyes: Pigments lying on the posterior surface of the iris.

  III. **Muscles of iris:** They are involuntary and consist of circular and radiating fibres.

    i. **Circular fibres (sphincter pupillae)**
    * They form a circular band about 1 mm wide.
    * It is around the margin of the pupil towards the posterior surface of the iris.
    * Nerve supply: Parasympathetic via the oculomotor nerve.
    * Action: Constriction of the pupil.

    ii. **Radiating fibres (dilator pupillae):** These lie close to the posterior surface of the iris. These converge from the circumference to the margin of the iris.
    * Nerve supply: Sympathetic via the superior cervical sympathetic ganglion.
    * Action: Dilation of the pupil.

  IV. **Development of the muscles of iris**

    i. Germ layer: *Ectoderm*

    ii. Source: Outer cells of the optic cup.

      ✚ The lower division of oculomotor nerve supplies sphincter papillae. It may get compressed in the cavernous sinus. The 1st sign is ipsilateral slowness of the pupillary response to light.

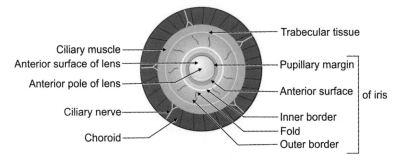

Fig. 19.12: Iris

3. **Inner coat**

A. **Retina**

a. **Definition:** It is the nervous coat, lying deep to the choroid. It is meant for the reception of the light stimuli.

b. **Fate**

 I. **Anteriorly:** It ends in a free serrated margin just behind the ciliary body.

 II. **Posteriorly:** It is continuous with the optic nerve.

c. **Parts of retina:**

 I. **Optic part:** It is the part from the optic disc up to the ora serrata. This part consists of all the functioning layers, i.e. nervous and pigmented layers.

 II. **Ciliary part** of the retina.

 III. **Iridial part** of the retina called **pars iridica retinae**.

 The last two layers are the prolongations of the pigmented layer. They are present only on the posterior surface of the ciliary processes and iris, respectively.

d. **Surfaces**

 I. **Outer surface:** It is in contact with the choroid.

 II. **Inner surface:** The following features are found:

   i. **Macula (spot) lutea (yellow):** It is an oval yellowish area near the centre of the posterior part of the retina. Here, the visual sense is *most perfect*. A depression at its centre is called **fovea centralis** where the retina is very thin.

   ii. **Optic disc**
   - It is the area which is pierced by the optic nerve.
   - The diameter is about 1–5 mm.
   - It is situated 3 mm medial to the macula lutea.
   - The central part of the disc is perforated by the central artery and vein of the retina.
   - This optic disc is insensitive to light and is called the **blind spot**.

   iii. On ophthalmoscopic examination,
   - Normally optic disc looks pink due to presence of the capillary vessels.
   - In optic atrophy, the disc looks white as the capillary vessels disappear.
   - In hypertension or thrombosis of central retinal veins, there is oedema of optic disc called papilloedema (chocked disc or oedema of disc).

   iv. **Arterial supply of retina** (Fig. 19.13)
   - **Up to the outer nuclear layer** from outside,
     * The retina has no direct arterial supply.
     * It gets its nutrition by diffusion from the choriocapillary layer of the choroid.
   - The remaining layers:

Head, Neck and Face

* By central artery of the retina, a branch of the ophthalmic artery. It is a classic example of an end artery.
  • Rupture of central artery of retina results in blindness of an individual.

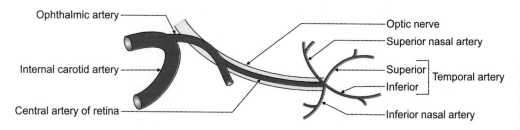

Fig. 19.13: Arterial supply of retina

v. **Venous drainage of retina**
  • The retinal veins end in the central vein of the retina.
  • The central vein ends in the cavernous sinus or superior ophthalmic vein.

SN-156 Contents of eyeball

1. Aqueous humour
2. Lens
3. Vitreous body.

1. **Aqueous humour**
   A. *Formation:* It is secreted from the capillaries of the ciliary processes into the posterior chamber of the eyeball.
   B. *Circulation:* From the posterior chamber pupil ⟶ anterior chamber ⟶
   C. It drains into space of the iridocorneal angle. (Here it is filtered by the lining membrane of the endothelial cells covering those spaces) ⟶ sinus venosus sclerae (canal of Schlemm) anterior ciliary veins ⟶ ophthalmic vein.
      a. Accessory route: A portion of the aqueous humour may be absorbed as follows:
         I. Via the blood vessels of the iris.
         II. Via the lymph spaces of the iris.
      b. Fluid from the posterior chamber ⟶ zonular space ⟶ hyaloid fossa
      c. Hyaloid canal ⟶ optic disc ⟶ perineural spaces around the nerve filaments of the optic nerve.
   D. Intraocular tension: Normal is 15–20 mm Hg. If there is interference in the absorption of the aqueous humour into the sinus venosus sclerae; there will be an increase in the tension which results in the formation of glaucoma.

2. **The lens**
   A. **Definition:** The lens is a transparent biconvex body, situated behind the iris and in front of the vitreous body (Fig. 19.14).
   B. **Capsule:** Lens is enclosed in a capsule which is a transparent elastic membrane.

C. **Features**

a. **Anterior surface** is less convex than the posterior surface.

    I. Its central part is in contact with the pupillary membrane till it disappears.

    II. After that, it forms the posterior boundary of the anterior chamber of the eyeball.

    III. Its periphery is separated from the iris by the aqueous humour of the posterior chamber.

    IV. Its curvature is regulated by the ciliary muscles for focusing the near or distant objects.

    V. These muscles are called *muscles of accommodation*.

b. **Posterior surface:** It is more convex and occupies the hyaloid fossa on the anterior aspect of the vitreous body.

c. **Poles:** The central points of the surfaces are called anterior and posterior poles.

d. **Axis:** It is the line joining the two poles.

e. **Equator:** The peripheral circumference of the lens is the equator.

f. **Dimensions:**

    I. Axis: 4 mm.

    II. Transverse diameter: 9 to 10 mm.

    III. Refractile index: 1.43.

    IV. Power of lens: 20 to 300

g. **Nutrition:** It is avascular. In foetal life, the posterior part of the lens capsule is supplied by hyaloid artery. It is a branch of the central artery of the retina.

h. **Structure**

    I. **Capsule:** The lens is composed of a series of more or less concentrically arranged fibres around a firm central part called the *lens nucleus*. So, the periphery is soft and the centre is hard.

        i. Deep to the anterior part of the capsule, *the lens is lined by epithelium.*

        ii. *It is formed by transparent, nucleated columnar cells.*

        iii. These cells grow and fill the cavity of the lens vesicle.

        iv. These elongated cells are called *lens fibres.*

        v. These fibres run from periphery to the centre but never from pole to pole.

    II. Applied: In foetus, lens is soft but in old age, it becomes harder and flattened, thereby reducing the focusing power. This condition is called **presbyopia**. In old age and also sometimes in early life, lens becomes opaque; this condition is called *cataract.*

3. **The vitreous body**

A. **Definition:** It is a colourless, transparent jelly-like substance, situated behind the lens and on the inner surface of the retina. It occupies the posterior 4/5th of the eyeball.

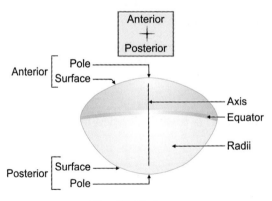

Fig. 19.14: Lens

B. **Composition:** It consists of
   a. 90% water,
   b. Salts,
   c. Mucoprotein, and
   d. Hyaluronic acid.
C. **Hyaloid canal:** It is traversed by a canal called hyaloid canal. In foetal life, it contains the hyaloid artery.
D. **Hyaloid fossa:** It is a fossa on the anterior surface of which lies the posterior surface of the lens.
E. **Hyaloid membrane:** Vitreous body is surrounded by its membrane. It is adherent to the retina in two places:
   a. **At optic disc:** Immediately in front of the ora serrata, it is thickened by radial fibres called **ciliary zonulae.**
   b. Ciliary processes.
F. **Nutrition:** No blood vessels pierce it. Nutrition is carried by vessels of the retina and ciliary processes.
G. **Suspensory ligament of the lens:** The ciliary zonule splits into two layers enclosing the lens:
   a. One layer is thin; it lines the hyaloid fossa.
   b. The other layer is thick and it is called the suspensory ligament.
      I. Its periphery is attached to the ciliary process and ora serrata.
      II. Centrally, it is attached to the lens slightly in front of its margin.
H. **Function:** In rest position, it keeps the anterior surface of the lens flattened under tension. When the ciliary muscles contract, this ligament is relaxed and causes the anterior surface to become convex thereby accommodating to focus near objects.
I. Applied anatomy : The zonular fibres constituting the suspensory ligament of lens are very tough structures. Hence, cataract extraction in immature state is not usually done because of the tough zonule. In immatue state, it is removed by zonulysis.

SN-157 Compartments of eyeball

1. **Chambers of the eyeball:** The eyeball is divided into two compartments by the lens and suspensory ligament
   A. Anterior compartment
   B. Posterior compartment

   A. **Anterior compartment:** It is further divided by the iris into
      a. Anterior chamber
      b. Posterior chamber

      a. **Anterior chamber:** It is 3 mm deep centrally.
         I. Boundary
            i. Anteriorly: Posterior surface of the cornea.
            ii. Posteriorly: Anterior surface of the iris and central part of the lens opposite the pupil.
               • At periphery: It is limited by the angle between the cornea and iris, called the **iridocorneal angle**. This angle is traversed by fibres called pectinate ligament. The spaces through this ligament drain into **canal of Schlemm**. Obliteration of this angle prevents the absorption of the aqueous humour, thereby increasing the interocular tension, i.e. glaucoma.
         II. **Contents:** Aqueous humour coming from posterior chamber through the pupil.

      b. **Posterior chambers**
         I. Boundary:
            i. Anteriorly: Posterior surface of the iris.
            ii. Posteriorly: Anterior surface of the lens and suspensory ligament.
               • ▲lar in cross-section, i.e. pupil and lens coming in contact form the apex, ciliary processes form the base.
         II. **Communication:** With the anterior chamber through the pupil.

   B. **Posterior compartment:** It contains the vitreous body.
      a. **Definition:** It is a colourless, transparent jelly-like substance, situated behind the lens and on the inner surface of the retina. It occupies the posterior 4/5th of the eyeball.
      b. **Composition:** It consists of
         I. 90% water,
         II. Salts,
         III. Mucoprotein, and
         IV. Hyaluronic acid.
      c. **Hyaloid canal:** It is traversed by a canal called hyaloid canal. In foetal life, it contains the hyaloid artery.
      d. **Hyaloid fossa:** It is a fossa on the anterior surface of the vitreous body. The lens is logged in the fossa. It is also called lenticular fossa or patellar fossa.

e. **Hyaloid membrane:** Vitreous body is surrounded by its membrane. It is adherent to the retina in two places:

    I. **At optic disc:** Immediately in front of the ora serrata, it is thickened by radial fibres called **ciliary zonulae,**

    II. Ciliary processes.

f. **Nutrition:** No blood vessels pierce it. Nutrition is carried by vessels of the retina and ciliary processes.

g. **Suspensory ligament of the lens:** The ciliary zonule splits into two layers enclosing the lens:

    I. One layer is thin; it lines the hyaloid fossa.

    II. The other layer is thick, and it is called the suspensory ligament.

        i. Its periphery is attached to the ciliary process and ora serrata.

        ii. Centrally, it is attached to the lens slightly in front of its margin.

h. **Function:** In resting position, it keeps the anterior surface of the lens flattened under tension. When the ciliary muscles contract, this ligament is relaxed and causes the anterior surface to become convex thereby accommodating to focus near objects.

2. Applied anatomy : The zonular fibres constituting the suspensory ligament of lens are very tough structures. Hence, cataract extraction in immature state is not usually done because of the tough zonule. In immature state, it is removed by zonulysis. Zonulysis causes melting of zonular fibres. The lens floats up and is removed.

Head, Neck and Face

Appendix

SN-158 Cervical sympathetic ganglion

They are three in number.

1. Superior cervical sympathetic ganglion.
2. Middle cervical sympathetic ganglion.
3. Inferior cervical sympathetic ganglion.

1. **Superior cervical sympathetic ganglion**
   A. **Features**
      a. It consists of 1 million cell bodies.
      b. Length: 3 cm.
      c. Situation: In front of transverse process of **C2** and **C3** vertebrae.
   B. **Branches**
      a. Gives grey rami to 1st four cervical nerves.
      b. Upper left ganglion gives branch to superficial cardiac plexus.
      c. It gives vascular branch to
         I. Internal carotid artery and forms plexus which runs along the
            i. Branches to the internal carotid artery,
            ii. Pterygopalatine ganglion, and
            iii. Dilator pupillae muscle of the eyeball.
         II. External carotid artery forms external carotid plexus and distributes along the
            i. Branches to external carotid artery.
            ii. Sympathetic fibres to pharyngeal plexus
            iii. Glandular branch to
               • Submandibular ganglion, and
               • Otic ganglion.

2. **Middle cervical sympathetic ganglion:** It is a small, inconstant ganglion.
   A. **Situation:** Medial to carotid tubercle.
   B. **Branches to**
      a. Grey rami of 5th and 6th cervical nerves.
      b. Branches to deep cardiac plexus.
   C. **Connection:** It is connected by two or more strands to the inferior cervical sympathetic ganglion, one of which passes in front of subclavian artery called ansa subclavia.

3. **Inferior cervical sympathetic ganglion**
   A. **Formation:** It is formed by fusion of 7th and 8th cervical ganglia at **C7** vertebra. It forms **stellate ganglion** with T1 ganglion (cervicothoracic ganglion).

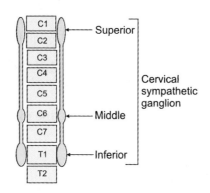

Fig. 20.1: Position of inferior cervical sympathetic ganglion

   B. **Relations**
      a. **Anterior:** 8th cervical spinal nerve.
      b. **Posterior:** 3rd part of vertebral artery.
   C. **Branches** (Fig. 20.2)
      a. Vascular branches:
         I. Vertebral artery, and
         II. Subclavian artery.
      b. Visceral branches: To the heart by deep cardiac plexus.
      c. Other branches: Grey rami communicantes to the ventral rami of **C7** and **C8** nerves.

5. 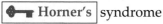 **Applied anatomy**

   Horner's syndrome

   ➤ **Horner's syndrome:** It is due to involvement of sympathetic nerve, which is contributed by **T1**. It is due to injury at the root of brachial plexus.
   ➤ **HORNER.** The letters of the word "Horner" give the information about clinical manifestations of Horner's syndrome.
   Hypohydrosis (*hypo*—less, *hydrosis*—sweating) is due to involvement of sympathetic nerves, which arise from first thoracic nerve. These are secretomotor fibres supplying the sweat glands of the skin of the face and forehead.

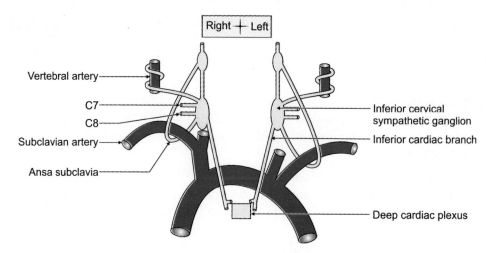

Fig. 20.2: Branches of inferior cervical sympathetic ganglion

Opening of eye is lost due to ptosis (drooping of the upper eyelid). It is caused by paralysis of Muller's muscle (smooth muscle of levator palpebrae superioris). In fact, it is pseudoptosis. [NEET]

Argyll-Robertson pupil [constricted pupil] is due to paralysis of dilator pupillae (unopposed action of sphincter pupillae).

Narrowing of palpebral fissure.

Elevation of lower eyelid.

Retraction of eyeball (sunken eyeball): Enophthalmos is due to involvement of orbitalis muscle.

➤ Absence of ciliospinal reflex.

SN-159 Killian's dehiscence

Killian's dehiscence: Part of posterior wall of pharynx between lower part of vocal folds and cricopharyngeus is weak and is not covered by the muscle. This weak area is called Killian's dehiscence (Fig. 20.3).

Pharyngeal diverticula are formed by out pouching of the dehiscence. The anatomical contributing factor for this condition is the neuromuscular incoordination of the two parts of inferior constrictor. The propulsive thyropharyngeus is supplied by pharyngeal plexus and sphincter of cricopharyngeus by recurrent laryngeal nerve.

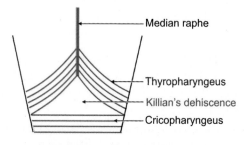

Fig. 20.3: Killian's dehiscence

Head, Neck and Face

Head, Neck and Face Embryology

Evolution of Pharyngeal Arches

In fishes, the region of the foregut is marked by slits. These are caudal to the stomodeum and the oral membrane. These slits are called gill slits and gill-bearing arches. With the evolution of lungs amongst land vertebrates, the region of the branchial (gill-bearing) arches underwent extensive modifications. This gives rise to the regions of the face, the pharynx and the associated structures. Hence, they are called **branchial arches**.

Their vascular supply is derived from a series of ventrodorsal aortic arches. Because of the peculiar nature of the blood supply, the mesoderm of the pharyngeal region shows localized thickenings. These are in the form of a series of dorsoventrally disposed bars. They are numbered from cranium to caudal as first to sixth. These bars appear temporarily as prominent "arches" on either side of the developing pharynx. Hence, they are called **"pharyngeal arches"**.

SN-160   First pharyngeal arch

First pharyngeal arch is also called mandibular arch.

Table 21.1: Derivatives of first pharyngeal arch

Muscles	Skeletal element	Ligament	Nerve and artery

• Temporalis
• Lateral pterygoid ⎫ Muscles of
• Medial pterygoid ⎬ mastication
• Masseter ⎭
• Mylohyoid
• Anterior belly of digastric
• Tensor tympani
	• Dorsal part forms
	  – Maxillary process
	  – Premaxilla
	  – Maxilla
	  – Zygomatic
	  – Temporal (partly)
	• Ventral part forms
	  – Meckel's cartilage
		• Anterior ligament of malleus
		• Spheno-mandibular ligament
			• Nerve of 1st pharyngeal arch is mandibular nerve, a branch of trigeminal nerve, (5th cranial nerve)

• Tensor palate	• Ventral part has ventral and dorsal end		• Artery of the 1st pharyngeal arch

Contd.

Table 21.1: Derivatives of first pharyngeal arch (Contd.)

Muscles	Skeletal element	Ligament	Nerve and artery
	– Ventral end forms mandible surrounding Meckel's cartilage – Dorsal end forms malleus and incus		mostly disappears • Part of this artery forms maxillary artery

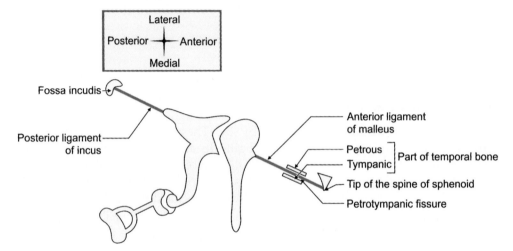

Fig. 21.1: Skeletal elements and ligaments developed from first pharyngeal arch

Anomalies of first pharyngeal arch

1. **Agnathia:** It is the most extreme form of 1st arch hypoplasia.

   A. There is failure of formation of lower jaw.

   B. In severe agnathia, the external ears remain in the ventral cervical region and may even join the ventral midline.

2. **Pierre Robin syndrome:** It consists of

   A. Extreme micrognathia (small jaw)

   B. Relatively large tongue

   C. Cleft palate

   D. Defects of the ear

   E. Leads to respiratory distress

3. **Treacher Collins syndrome** (mandibulofacial dysostosis—defective ossification of foetal cartilage)

   A. It is typically inherited as an **autosomal dominant** condition.

   B. Asymmetry of facial skeleton

   C. **Responsible gene:** *Treacle.*

D. **Manifestation**

   a. **C**oloboma-type defects of the lower eyelid

   b. High **c**left palate

   c. Faulty **d**entition

   d. Malformations of the **e**xternal and middle ears

   e. Hypoplasia of the mandible and **f**acial bones.

4. **Maxillary process defect** is recognized but with variable conditions with cleft lips and after facial fissures.

SN-161   Meckel's cartilage

1. **Definition:** Skeletal element of the 1st pharyngeal arch (mandibular arch) is called Meckel's cartilage.

2. **Extent:** It extends from the developing otic capsule to mandibular prominence.

3. **Derivatives:** Following are the structures given by different parts of Meckel's cartilage.

Table 21.2: Derivatives of Meckel's cartilage

Parts	Structures
• Dorsal	• Incus and malleus
• Intermediate	• Anterior ligament of malleus • Sphenomandibular ligament
• Ventral	• Body of mandible, and • Mental ossicle

SN-162   Give the persistent structures of fibrous envelop of Meckel's cartilage.

1. The cartilaginous bar of the mandibular part is known as Meckel's cartilage. It extends dorsally up to the cartilaginous ear capsule.

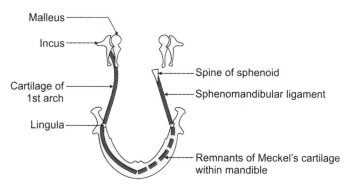

Fig. 21.2: Skeletal elements developed from first pharyngeal arch

2. The dorsal part of the cartilage is ossified to form the malleus and incus. The part of the cartilage extending from the region of the middle ear to mandible disappears. The sheath (perichondrium) forms
   A. Anterior ligament of the malleus
   B. Sphenomandibular ligament.
3. The fibrous membrane of ventral part of the Meckel's cartilage is ossified to form the body of the mandible. It extends from the inferior alveolar foramen to mental foramen. The cartilage cells disappear. The ossified remnants of the cartilage are mental ossicle of symphysis menti.

SN-163 Second pharyngeal arch

Reichert's cartilage and its pericondrium form the stapes, styloid process, stylohyoid ligament, lesser cornu and probably the upper part of the body of the hyoid bone.

The word "second" and the derivatives of the second pharyngeal arch begins with the letter "S"

Table 21.3: Derivatives of second pharyngeal arch

Muscles	Skeletal element	Ligament	Nerve and artery
• Stapedius • Stylohyoid • Posterior belly of digastric • Occipitofrontalis • Muscles of ear • Muscles of facial expression • Platysma	• Stapes • Styloid process of temporal bone • Smaller cornu of hyoid bone • Superior surface of body of hyoid bone	• Stylohyoid ligament	• Nerve of Second pharyngeal arch is facial nerve (Seventh cranial nerve) • Artery of Second pharyngeal arch mostly regresses except for dorsal part which forms Stapedial artery

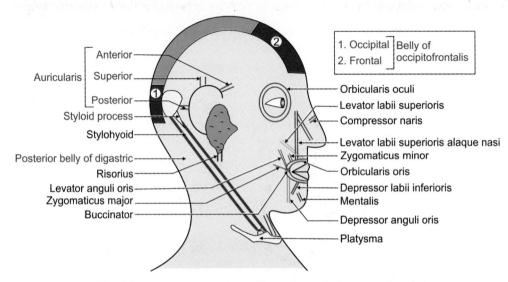

Fig. 21.3: Muscles developed from second pharyngeal arch

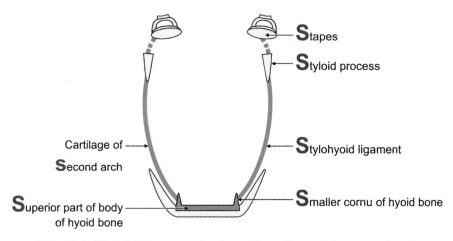

Fig. 21.4: Skeletal elements developed from Second pharyngeal arch

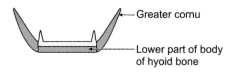

Fig. 21.5: Skeletal elements developed from third pharyngeal arch

---

SN-164   Pharyngeal pouches

The mesoderm between any two successive arches is very thin. This leads the ectoderm being drawn inwards to form clefts (grooves) and the ectoderm being pulled outwards to form pouches. Endodermal invaginations of each pharyngeal arch is called pharyngeal pouch. Following are the structures given by the respective pouches.

Table 21.4: Derivatives of pharyngeal pouches

Arch	Ventral end	Dorsal end
• 1st	• Tongue	• Dorsal ends of 1st and 2nd arches combine and form pharyngotympanic recess which gives rise to
• 2nd	• Tonsillar fossa • Tonsil develops from neural crest cell	– Proximal part: Pharyngotympanic tube, and – Distal part: Middle ear cavity.
• 3rd	• Thymus	• Inferior parathyroid gland
• 4th	• Ultimobranchial body which fuses with the thyroid	• Superior parathyroid gland

Note: Parafollicular cells of the thyroid which secrete calcitonin. They are derived from neural crest cells which are greater than ultimobranchial body.

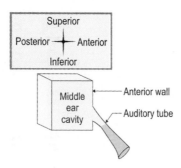

Fig. 21.6: Tubotympanic recess develops from dorsal end of 1st and 2nd pharyngeal pouches

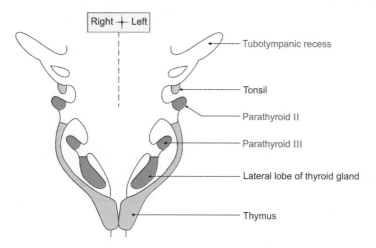

Fig. 21.7: Pharyngeal pouches

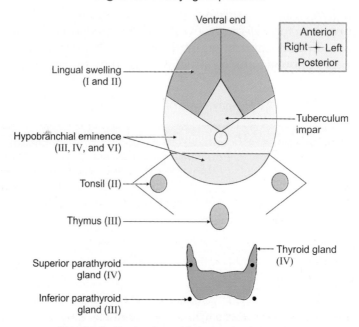

Fig. 21.8: Derivatives of pharyngeal pouches

SN-165 Abnormalities of pharyngeal pouches

1. Nezelof syndrome
   A. **Definition:** It is failure of development of only 3rd pharyngeal pouch.
   B. **Manifestations**
      a. Superior parathyroid glands are present.
      b. Inferior parathyroid gland and thymus are absent.
      c. There is normal function of parathyroid glands.
2. DiGeorge syndrome (3rd and 4th pharyngeal pouch syndrome) results from failure of development of 3rd and 4th pouches.
   A. **Manifestations**
      a. Thymic hypoplasia (resulting in selective T cell deficiency and greatly reduced cell-mediated immunity)
      b. Absence of parathyroid glands (resulting in hypocalcaemia and tetany).
      c. Immunodeficiency.
3. Catch 22 spectrum
   A. **Aetiology:** Deletion of long arm of chromosome 22 is the reason of the multiple anomalies.
   B. **Manifestations**
      a. Thymic hypoplasia (resulting in selective T cell deficiency and greatly reduced cell-mediated immunity)
      b. Absence of parathyroid glands (resulting in hypocalcemia and tetany).
      c. Cardiac defects
      d. Abnormalities of face and cleft palate.

SN-166 Pharyngeal cleft

Introduction: The depression between two arches on outer side is called pharyngeal cleft.

1. 1st pharyngeal cleft: Dorsal part of 1st pharyngeal cleft forms
   A. External acoustic meatus.
   B. Outer layer of tympanic membrane.
   C. Pinna of ear: Swellings on 1st and 2nd arches are called hillocks.
      These hillocks combine and form pinna of ear.
2. 2nd pharyngeal arch: It grows caudally over the 2nd and 3rd pharyngeal clefts. It encloses space lined by ectoderm called cervical sinus. The overhanging 2nd arch joins the epicardial ridge. Cervical sinus disappears (Fig. 21.9).
3. Anomalies: **Branchial cyst** is the persistence of cervical space. It is located below and behind the angle of mandible. Cholesterol crystal in the aspirate is diagnostic feature of branchial cyst.

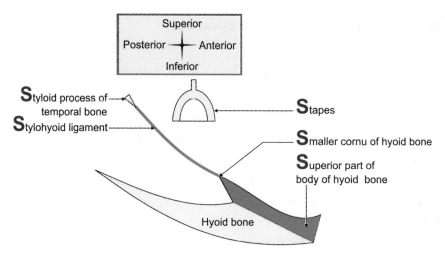

Fig. 21.9: Skeletal elements and ligaments of second pharyngeal arch

SN-167 Derivatives of 4th and 6th pharyngeal arches

1. **Muscles**
   A. Muscles of larynx
      a. Extrinsic—cricothyroid.
      b. Intrinsic muscles of larynx
   B. Constrictor of pharynx.
   C. Striated muscle of oesophagus.

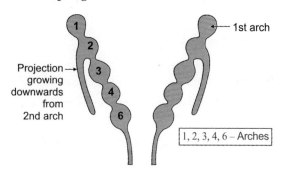

Fig. 21.10: Pharyngeal arches

2. **Skeletal element:** The 4th and 6th pharyngeal arches fuse together and form following cartilages (Fig. 21.11):
   A. Thyroid,
   B. Cricoid,
   C. Arytenoid,
   D. Corniculate, and
   E. Cuneiform.

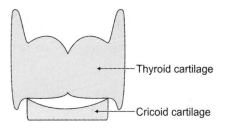

Fig. 21.11: Skeletal elements developed from 4th and 6th pharyngeal arches

3. **Nerves**
   A. Nerve of the 4th pharyngeal arch is superior laryngeal nerve, a branch of vagus nerve.
   B. Nerve of the 6th pharyngeal arch is recurrent laryngeal nerve, a branch of vagus nerve.
4. **Artery**
   A. **4th arch**
      a. Right side: Forms the proximal part of right subclavian artery.
      b. Left side: Arch of the aorta.
   B. **6th arch**
      a. Ventral part forms pulmonary artery.
      b. Dorsal part on right side forms ductus arteriosus which degenerates and forms ligamentum arteriosum.

SN-168 Ultimobranchial body (post-branchial or telobranchial body)

Introduction: It is the last structure derived from the pharyngeal pouches. Hence, it is called ultimobranchial body.

1. **Origin:** There are different views
   A. They arise purely from pharyngeal endoderm.
   B. Recent data suggests that neural cells migrate into post-branchial bodies and ultimately becomes secretory component of these structures.
2. **Comparative anatomy**
   A. This is a constant feature in all vertebrates.
   B. In sub-mammalian vertebrates, they remain as discrete bodies in the neck or mediastinum throughout adult life.
3. **Fate:** It fuses with the thyroid gland and its cells disseminate within it, giving rise to parafollicular cells of the thyroid gland. They are also called C cells to indicate that they produce calcitonin, a hormone that is involved in the regulation of the normal calcium level in the body fluid.
4. **Applied anatomy**: C cell hyperplasia is associated with medullary carcinoma and has been reported within the neck. These are presumed to be remnants of ultimobranchial body.

OLA-107 What are the various developmental anomalies of face?

1. **Anomalies:** Most of the anomalies of the face are due to failure of union of different processes, which form face.

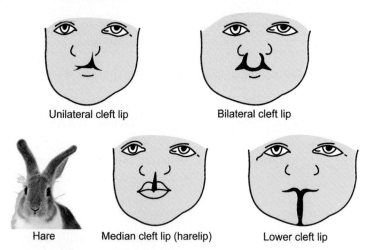

Fig. 21.12: Developmental anomalies of face

2. **Facial cleft or nasolabial furrow:** It is due to failure of fusion between lateral nasal process and the maxillary process. It may be unilateral or bilateral. Nasolacrimal duct is absent in this anomaly.

3. **Harelip** (usually upper harelip): It may be median or lateral. Lateral harelip may be unilateral or bilateral.
   A. Median harelip is due to failure of fusion of right and left median nasal processes of front nasal process.
   B. Lateral harelip: It is very common and due to failure of fusion of median nasal process and maxillary process.
   C. Very rarely there may be failure of fusion of mandibular arches and results into split lower lip.

4. **Macrostomia or wide opening of the mouth:** It is due to failure or lesser degree of fusion between mandibular and maxillary processes.

5. **Microstomia** (small oral fissure): It occurs due to excessive fusion of maxillary and mandibular processes.

6. Another rare anomalies area of nose may be absent.
   A. Proboscis: A cylindrical projection of nose below the forehead.
   B. Cyclops: Fusion of two eyeballs.

SN-169 Development of face

1. **Chronological age:** 5th month of intrauterine life.
2. **Germ layer**
   A. **Upper lip:** Ectoderm and mesoderm.
   B. **Lower lip:** Ectoderm and mesoderm.
   C. **Cheek and vestibule of mouth:** Ectoderm

3. **Sources:** It develops from 5 processes
   A. Unpaired frontonasal process which divides into medial and lateral nasal processes.
   B. Paired maxillary processes.
   C. Paired mandibular processes.

4. **Upper lip:** Frontonasal prominence appears cranial to stomodeum. Local thickenings of nasal placode appear on either side of frontonasal process. Nasal placodes dip to form nasal pit. Lateral to the nasal pit is lateral nasal prominence and medial to it is medial nasal prominence. Maxillary prominence moves medially and meets the medial nasal prominence, thus forming the upper lip. It is formed by
   A. Left and right medial nasal prominences
   B. Left and right maxillary prominences.

> **Box 21.1**
>
> **Note:** There is no role of lateral nasal prominence in the formation of upper lip.

Nasolacrimal groove: It is junction of lateral nasal process and maxillary process. Solid cords of ectodermal cells grow from the floor of the groove and get buried.

Nasolacrimal duct: The nasolacrimal groove gets canalized and forms the nasolacrimal duct.

Nasolacrimal sac: Upper part of nasolacrimal duct forms the nasolacrimal sac while the lower part forms the nasolacrimal duct.

5. **Lower lip** is formed by fusion of right and left mandibular processes.

6. **Anomalies:** Most of the anomalies of the face are due to failure of union of different processes, which form face.
   A. **Facial cleft or nasolabial furrow:** It is due to failure of fusion between lateral nasal process and the maxillary process. It may be unilateral or bilateral. Nasolacrimal duct is absent in this anomaly.
   B. Harelip (usually upper harelip): It may be median or lateral. Lateral harelip may be unilateral or bilateral.
      a. Median harelip is due to failure of fusion of right and left median nasal processes of front nasal process.
      b. Lateral harelip: It is very common and due to failure of fusion of median nasal process and maxillary process.
      c. Very rarely there may be failure of fusion of mandibular arches and results into split lower lip.
   C. **Macrostomia or wide opening of the mouth:** It is due to failure or lesser degree of fusion between mandibular and maxillary process.
   D. **Microstomia** (small oral fissure): It occurs due to excessive fusion of maxillary and mandibular processes.
   E. Another rare anomalies area of nose may be absent.

a. Proboscis: A cylindrical 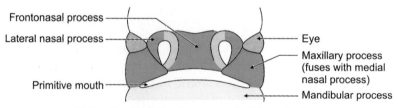 projection of nose below the forehead.

b. Cyclops: Fusion of two eyeballs.

Frontonasal process — Lateral nasal process — Primitive mouth — Eye — Maxillary process (fuses with medial nasal process) — Mandibular process

Nasal pits of both the sides come close to each other.
A naso-optic furrow separates lateral nasal process and maxillary process

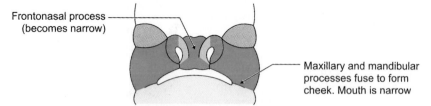

Frontonasal process (becomes narrow) — Maxillary and mandibular processes fuse to form cheek. Mouth is narrow

The naso-optic furrow obliterates as a result of fusion of
a. Maxillary process and
b. Lateral nasal process

Fig. 21.13: Development of face

SN-170   Frontonasal process of embryo

1. **Chronological age:** Fifth week of intrauterine life.
2. **Germ layer:** Core of mesoderm and is covered by ectoderm.
3. **Site:** Around stomodeum.
4. **Process:** The ectoderm which covers the caudal surface of the forebrain vesicle proliferates and together with the overlying surface ectoderm form the frontonasal process.
   A. It is divided into a
      a. Median nasal process. It extends more caudally and forms bilateral elevations known as the globular processes. It gives rise to the
         I. Nasal septum,
         II. Philtrum of the upper lip, and
         III. Primitive palate
      b. Two lateral nasal processes form the alae of the nose.
5. **Anomalies**
   A. **Central harelip:** It is produced by the failure of the fusion of the right and left globular swellings with each other.
   B. **Lateral harelip:** It is caused by failure of fusion between the maxillary process and globular swelling.
   C. **Facial cleft:** It is produced by failure of fusion of lateral nasal process with the maxillary process.

Index